Panic Disorder and Its Treatment

Compliments of

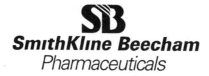

Medical Psychiatry

Series Editor

William A. Frosch, M.D.

Cornell University Medical College
New York, New York

1. Handbook of Depression and Anxiety: A Biological Approach, *edited by Johan A. den Boer and J. M. Ad Sitsen*
2. Anticonvulsants in Mood Disorders, *edited by Russell T. Joffe and Joseph R. Calabrese*
3. Serotonin in Antipsychotic Treatment: Mechanisms and Clinical Practice, *edited by John M. Kane, H.-J. Möller, and Frans Awouters*
4. Handbook of Functional Gastrointestinal Disorders, *edited by Kevin W. Olden*
5. Clinical Management of Anxiety, *edited by Johan A. den Boer*
6. Obsessive-Compulsive Disorders: Diagnosis • Etiology • Treatment, *edited by Eric Hollander and Dan J. Stein*
7. Bipolar Disorder: Biological Models and Their Clinical Application, *edited by L. Trevor Young and Russell T. Joffe*
8. Dual Diagnosis and Treatment: Substance Abuse and Comorbid Medical and Psychiatric Disorders, *edited by Henry R. Kranzler and Bruce J. Rounsaville*
9. Geriatric Psychopharmacology, *edited by J. Craig Nelson*
10. Panic Disorder and Its Treatment, *edited by Jerrold F. Rosenbaum and Mark H. Pollack*

ADDITIONAL VOLUMES IN PREPARATION

Panic Disorder and Its Treatment

edited by

Jerrold F. Rosenbaum

Mark H. Pollack

*Massachusetts General Hospital
and Harvard Medical School
Boston, Massachusetts*

MARCEL DEKKER, INC.   NEW YORK · BASEL · HONG KONG

ISBN: 0-8247-0216-6

This book is printed on acid-free paper.

Headquarters
Marcel Dekker, Inc.
270 Madison Avenue, New York, NY 10016
tel: 212-696-9000; fax: 212-685-4540

Eastern Hemisphere Distribution
Marcel Dekker AG
Hutgasse 4, Postfach 812, CH-4001 Basel, Switzerland
tel: 44-61-261-8482; fax: 44-61-261-8896

World Wide Web
http://www.dekker.com

The publisher offers discounts on this book when ordered in bulk quantities. For more information, write to Special Sales/Professional Marketing at the headquarters address above.

Current printing (last digit):
10 9 8 7 6 5 4 3 2 1

PRINTED IN THE UNITED STATES OF AMERICA

To the Massachusetts General Hospital
and Its Department of Psychiatry

Series Introduction

At the turn of the last century, the alienists (psychiatrists) were struggling to define the boundaries of the major psychoses and alcohol-related behavioral disorders. Emil Kraepelin is now safely ensconced, perhaps enshrined, in DSM-III, -IIIR, and -IV, where his manic depressive disease has become bipolar disorder illness, and dementia praecox has been transformed into schizophrenia. Most of us now know that we are "neo-Kraepelineans" when we use the current classification system.

We are less aware of the diagnostic mantle that we inherit from Freud. During that same period, the neurologists, among them Charcot and Freud, were attempting to separate the "neuroses" from "organic" illnesses, and from each other. For example, in 1893, Freud published "Some Points for a Comparative Study of Organic and Hysterical Motor Paralysis," in which he lays out the methods that we still use in making this important clinical distinction. Similarly, in 1895, he published the paper "On the Grounds for Detaching a Particular Syndrome from Neurasthenia Under the Description 'Anxiety Neurosis'." His description of the clinical picture encompasses both anxious expectation, and a variety of "physical" symptoms: palpitations, difficulty breathing, sweating, tremor and shivering, hunger, vertigo, paresthesias. He also describes the possible spread of the syndrome to include such phenomena as agoraphobia, obsessions, and compulsions. Across the century(ies), good clinicians see what the patient presents, although we may then organize our observations in different frameworks. Spitzer and Frances saw what Freud had seen. Plus ça change!

Freud also anticipated our current interest in the biological underpinnings and correlates of the anxiety disorders. He referred to them as the "real" neuroses, by which he meant that they had their origin in the individual's biology and biological sensitivities.

Drs. Rosenbaum and Pollack bring our view of the anxiety states up to date. They have gathered an unusually talented group of chapter authors from multiple medical centers across the country who provide us with a clear, comprehensive, and clinically relevant summary of current knowledge. We learn about symptoms, and course, care, and cost, comorbidities, and quality of life. May all the books we buy and read be as helpful to us in our care of those in need.

William A. Frosch

Preface

We are pleased to present this volume on panic disorder and its treatment, which offers comprehensive overviews by leading authorities on critical issues for clinicians who diagnose and manage this distressing and disabling disorder. Despite the considerable recent advances in understanding risk for panic disorder, and its prevalence, symptoms, course, outcome, and therapeutics, this disorder remains a challenge for diagnosis and treatment.

Although patients today may benefit from an array of available clinical options, far too many remain either unrecognized, untreated, or inadequately treated. The consequences of persistent suffering in terms of distress, impairment, and disability equal or exceed those of most major chronic medical conditions.

Testimonials from patients about the impact of panic disorder on their lives are poignant and compelling. A 60-year-old man who had endured panic disorder during an earlier period of his life awoke with crushing substernal chest pain radiating down his arm and up to his jaw. Observing him diaphoretic, nauseated, and in pain, his wife called an ambulance. On his arrival at the Massachusetts General Hospital emergency ward, he suffered cardiac arrest. Resuscitated and admitted to the coronary care unit, he was informed by the house officer that he had survived a myocardial infarction. He sighed with relief, and his first words were, "Thank goodness—I thought my panic attacks were coming back."

There is something so terrifying and painful about panic spells that patients would do almost anything to avoid having another, whether the costs are remaining homebound or self-medicating with alcohol. Why these spells are so seemingly aversive is unknown. The degree of autonomic arousal does not exceed that seen with intense excitement and the increases in heart rate and blood pressure are rarely more than those seen with vigorous exercise, yet the experience is one of memorable terror as if some primitive alarm intended for life-threatening events has been activated. One research group has compared the panic experience to the sensation of impending death from suffocation (1).

The first panic attack experienced by a patient is typically remembered for life as a major trauma. We have previously labeled the first such attack for panic disorder patients as the "herald attack," signaling as it does a watershed for the patient after which life may never be the same. The successful treatment of this disorder, however, is one of the most gratifying interventions in clinical medicine: patients get their lives back.

Untreated, many patients experience progressive restriction in their work, social, physical, and family lives. One of us (JR) recalls his experience 25 years ago as an intern in a busy urban emergency room, known as "the knife and gun club," where patients experiencing herald attacks were treated with bemusement and ignorance, at times given placebo (injections of normal saline), and observed with smugness as they reported the dissipation of distress. Unaware of the characteristic time-limited duration of panic, the intern would inform these otherwise healthy patients that they would be fine, and then discharge them home. Our own follow-up studies in a major academic center emergency room reveal that many patients who arrive with chest pain, and who in fact have had a panic attack, are still sent home as being free of "cardiac" pathology. Their health status and outcomes, however, are poor—often worse at follow-up than many who actually have coronary artery disease. May this volume prevent any future similar lost opportunities for early diagnosis and treatment.

Thus, a primary mission of this volume is to enhance recognition of panic disorder in medical settings. The first chapter, by James Ballenger, reviews the topic of panic disorder in primary care and general medicine. The pleomorphic physical manifestations of panic attacks account for the missed or delayed diagnosis of this condition, resulting in unnecessary or avoidable work-ups and testing, ineffective treatment, excessive cost, and, ultimately, patient suffering and demoralization.

Although from 10 to 30% of individuals in some populations experience occasional panic attacks, a smaller number (1 to 3%) actually develop panic disorder (2). The criteria required for a diagnosis of panic disorder, according to DSM-IV (*Diagnostic and Statistical Manual of Mental Disorders,* 4th ed., 1994) include 1) recurrent unexpected panic attacks and 2) at least one of the attacks followed by at least 1 month of one (or more) of the following:

1. Persistent concern about having additional attacks
2. Worry about the implications of the attack or its consequences
3. A significant change in behavior related to the attack

DSM-IV defines panic attacks as a discrete period of intense fear or discomfort, in which four (or more) of the following symptoms developed abruptly and reached a peak within 10 minutes:

1. Palpitations, pounding heart, or accelerated heart rate
2. Sweating
3. Trembling or shaking
4. Sensations of shortness of breath or smothering
5. Feelings of choking
6. Chest pain or discomfort
7. Nausea or abdominal distress
8. Feeling dizzy, unsteady, light-headed, or faint
9. Derealization or depersonalization
10. Fear of losing control or going crazy
11. Fear of dying
12. Paresthesias
13. Chills or hot flushes

For purposes of diagnosis, the panic attacks are not caused by the direct physiological effects of a substance or a general medical condition and are not better explained by another mental disorder such as phobia (social or specific), obsessive-compulsive disorder, or posttraumatic stress disorder. Panic disorder can occur with or without agoraphobia, which involves anxiety about places or situations from which escape might be difficult or embarrassing or where help would be unavailable in the event of a panic attack. These situations are either avoided or endured with great distress. Examples of agoraphobic setting are bridges, tunnels, elevators, restricted-access highways, movie theaters, dentist's chairs, supermarket lines, airplanes, and subways.

Although the diagnostic criteria provide a reliable definition of the disorder, they do not convey the complexity of the interplay between symptoms and behavior, as well as treatment and outcome. Most patients who seek treatment have other comorbid psychiatric disorders and multiple etiological or contributing factors. Among the most frequent, complicating comorbid conditions are agoraphobia, social phobia, obsessive-compulsive disorder, major depression, and personality disorders. In Chapter 2, Mark Pollack reviews the longitudinal course of panic disorder, emphasizing the potential for a chronic or recurrent course and the clinical features predictive of a poor prognosis.

As we advance in our knowledge of the neurobiology of panic disorder, we move closer to more precise and definitive interventions. Goddard and colleagues comprehensively detail in their chapter the body of knowledge of the disorder's biological substrate. Panic disorder likely represents the ultimate expression of the confluence of a variety of etiological factors from genetics to developmental experience and life events. In their chapter, "Early Antecedents of Panic Disorder: Genes, Childhood, and the Environment," Hirshfeld, Smoller, and coworkers review these contributions to vulnerability for the illness.

Rosenbaum and colleagues summarize available pharmacotherapies of panic disorder, in particular, the important contributions of the SSRIs as first established with the FDA approval of paroxetine for this condition. Otto and Deckersbach review the cognitive-behavioral therapies that have been developed specifically to target panic disorder and the cognitive responses to physical sensations that drive the impairment and distress of the condition. While most patients are benefited by pharmacotherapies, cognitive-behavioral therapies, or both, few are cured, and the therapeutic focus shifts to the residually ill and the nonresponder. Roy-Byrne and Cowley address the clinical strategies for assuring optimal diagnostic and therapeutic effort for these patients in their chapter, "Clinical Approach to Treatment-Resistant Panic Disorder."

As a disorder that predominantly afflicts women of childbearing potential, the course and treatment of panic disorder during pregnancy and the postpartum, as elaborated in the chapter by Nonacs and colleagues, is an unavoidable clinical challenge. Further, with up to a third of panic patients having a history of attempts at self-medication with substances of abuse, Jefferson and Greist address alcohol and substance abuse.

Despite the evident imperative to recognize and treat panic disorder and its comorbid conditions, the current health economic environment requires that we address issues relevant to health care utilization and allocation of resources. Connors and Davidson accomplish this goal in their chapter, "Panic Disorder, Quality of Life, and Managed Care: Cost-Effectiveness and Treatment Choices."

For clinicians seeking guidance to available measures and scales for use in assessing patients in documenting impairment, course, and outcome, Otto and colleagues provide an Appendix that reviews the most widely used or recommended instruments for evaluating panic disorder patients, either for clinical care or for research studies.

For psychiatrists, primary care doctors, or other clinicians working to treat panic disorder patients, this volume aims to provide preparation for the therapeutic challenges from recognition to treatment, while providing an up-to-date understanding of the disorder's etiology and outcome. We deeply hope this effort will enhance the reader's ability to improve the lives of his or her patients.

Jerrold F. Rosenbaum
Mark H. Pollack

REFERENCES

1. Klein DF. False suffocation alarms, spontaneous panics, and related con-

ditions: an integrative hypothesis. Arch Gen Psychiatry 1993; 50(4):306–317.

2. Eaton WW, Kessler RC, Wittchen Hu, Magee WJ. Panic and panic disorder in the United States. Am J Psychiatry 1994; 151(3):413–420.

Contents

Series Introduction   *William A. Frosch*   v

Preface   vii

Contributors   xv

1. Panic Disorder in Primary Care and General Medicine   1
   James C. Ballenger

2. The Longitudinal Course of Panic Disorder   37
   Mark H. Pollack

3. Neurobiology of Panic Disorder   57
   Andrew W. Goddard, Jack M. Gorman,
   and Dennis S. Charney

4. Early Antecedents of Panic Disorder: Genes,
   Childhood, and the Environment   93
   Dina R. Hirshfeld, Jordan W. Smoller,
   Steffany J. Fredman, Maria T. Bulzacchelli,
   and Jerrold F. Rosenbaum

5. The Pharmacotherapy of Panic Disorder   153
   Jerrold F. Rosenbaum, Steffany J. Fredman,
   and Mark H. Pollack

6. Cognitive-Behavioral Therapy for Panic Disorder:
   Theory, Strategies, and Outcome   181
   Michael W. Otto and Thilo Deckersbach

7. Clinical Approach to Treatment-Resistant Panic
   Disorder   205
   Peter Roy-Bryne and Deborah S. Cowley

8. Course and Treatment of Panic Disorder During
   Pregnancy and the Postpartum Period   229
   Ruta Nonacs, Lee S. Cohen, and Lori L. Altshuler

9. Panic Disorder: Alcohol and Substance Abuse   247
   James W. Jefferson and John H. Greist

10. Panic Disorder, Quality of Life, and Managed Care:
    Cost-Effectiveness and Treatment Choices   269
    Katherine M. Connor and Jonathan R. T. Davidson

    Appendix: Assessment and Measures of Panic
    Disorder and Treatment Outcome   323
    Michael W. Otto, Susan J. Penava,
    and Mark H. Pollack

    Index   341

Contributors

Lori L. Altshuler, M.D.   Associate Professor of Psychiatry and Behavioral Sciences, and Director, UCLA Mood Disorders Research Program, UCLA Neuropsychiatric Institute, UCLA Brain Research Institute and VA Medical Center, West Los Angeles, Los Angeles, California

James C. Ballenger, M.D.   Chairman and Professor, Department of Psychiatry and Behavioral Sciences, and Director, Institute of Psychiatry, Medical University of South Carolina, Charleston, South Carolina

Maria T. Bulzacchelli, B.A.   Senior Research Data Analyst, Clinical Psychopharmacology Unit, Massachusetts General Hospital, Boston, Massachusetts

Dennis S. Charney, M.D.   Deputy Chair for Academic and Scientific Affairs and Professor, Department of Psychiatry, Yale University School of Medicine, and Principal Investigator, Yale Mental Health Clinical Research Center, New Haven, Connecticut

Lee S. Cohen, M.D.   Director, Perinatal and Reproductive Psychiatry

Clinical Research Program, Clinical Psychopharmacology Unit, Massachusetts General Hospital, Boston, Massachusetts

Kathryn M. Connor, M.D. Clinical Associate, Department of Psychiatry and Behavioral Sciences, Duke University, Durham, North Carolina

Deborah S. Cowley, M.D. Professor, Department of Psychiatry and Behavioral Sciences, University of Washington School of Medicine, and Director, Psychiatry Resident Training Program, University of Washington Medical Center, Seattle, Washington

Jonathan R. T. Davidson, M.D. Director, Anxiety and Traumatic Stress Program, and Professor, Department of Psychiatry and Behavioral Sciences, Duke University, Durham, North Carolina

Thilo Deckersbach, Dipl. Psych. Research Fellow, Department of Psychiatry, Massachusetts General Hospital, and Department of Psychiatry, Harvard Medical School, Boston, Massachusetts

Steffany J. Fredman, B.A. Senior Research Data Analyst, Clinical Psychopharmacology Unit, Massachusetts General Hospital, Boston, Massachusetts

Andrew W. Goddard, M.D. Associate Professor, Department of Psychiatry, Yale University School of Medicine, New Haven, Connecticut

Jack M. Gorman, M.D. Department of Psychiatry, Columbia University, and New York State Psychiatric Institute, New York, New York

John H. Greist, M.D. Distinguished Senior Scientist, Dean Foundation for Health, Research and Education, Middleton, and Clinical Professor of Psychiatry, University of Wisconsin Medical School, Madison, Wisconsin

Dina R. Hirshfeld, Ph.D.   Staff Psychologist, Department of Psychiatry, Massachusetts General Hospital, and Instructor of Psychology, Department of Psychiatry, Harvard Medical School, Boston, Massachusetts

James W. Jefferson, M.D.   Distinguished Senior Scientist, Dean Foundation for Health, Research and Education, Middleton, and Clinical Professor of Psychiatry, University of Wisconsin Medical School, Madison, Wisconsin

Ruta Nonacs, M.D., Ph.D.   Perinatal and Reproductive Psychiatry Clinical Research Program, Clinical Psychopharmacology Unit, Massachusetts General Hospital, Boston, Massachusetts

Michael W. Otto, Ph.D.   Director, Cognitive-Behavior Therapy Program, Massachusetts General Hospital, and Department of Psychiatry, Harvard Medical School, Boston, Massachusetts

Susan J. Penava, Ph.D.   Cognitive-Behavior Therapy Program, Department of Psychiatry, Massachusetts General Hospital, and Instructor of Psychology, Harvard Medical School, Boston, Massachusetts

Mark H. Pollack, M.D.   Director, Anxiety Disorders Program, Department of Psychiatry, Massachusetts General Hospital, and Associate Professor of Psychiatry, Harvard Medical School, Boston, Massachusetts

Jerrold F. Rosenbaum, M.D.   Director, Outpatient Psychiatry Division, and Chief, Clinical Psychopharmacology Unit, Massachusetts General Hospital, and Associate Professor of Psychiatry, Harvard Medical School, Boston, Massachusetts

Peter Roy-Byrne, M.D.   Professor and Vice-Chairman, Department of Psychiatry and Behavioral Sciences, University of Washington

School of Medicine, and Chief of Psychiatry, Harborview Medical Center, Seattle, Wasington

Jordan W. Smoller, M.D., S.M.   Director, Psychiatric Genetics Program in Mood and Anxiety Disorders, Outpatient Division of Psychiatry, Massachusetts General Hospital, Boston, Masasachusetts

Panic Disorder in Primary Care and General Medicine

James C. Ballenger

Medical University of South Carolina
Charleston, South Carolina

INTRODUCTION

As we learn more about panic disorder (PD) and its frequent presentation in nonpsychiatric settings, and as recent trends make the primary care physician (PCP) more responsible for the recognition and care of PD and other psychiatric patients, greater knowledge of PD has become increasingly important for PCPs and generalists. Fully 60% of all the care delivered to patients with psychiatric conditions is in the primary care setting (1). Approximately 25% of primary care patients have a primary psychiatric rather than organic problem (2–6); others have suggested that the percentage may be as high as 79% (7).

Panic and anxiety are particularly prominent in primary care settings. In a survey of 250 PCPs, anxiety was rated the most prominent psychiatric problem seen in their practices (8). Zung (9,10) has documented that 20–32% of primary care patients have clinically significant anxiety symptoms. In one study, over 11% of visits to PCPs were shown to be for anxiety symptoms (11). In a study examining 1500 primary care visits, Wells and colleagues (12) documented that 18%

of patients received a minor tranquilizer, presumably in most cases for anxiety symptomatology.

PD patients often present in primary care, with over half being initially treated in that setting (13). They are seen first by a general internist or family practice physician in 35% of the cases, and usually continue to be treated by these practioners. Forty-three percent of patients are initially seen in the emergency room, 15% of them brought by ambulance.

PD has a 1-year prevalence of 2.3% in the general population and a lifetime prevalence of 3.5% (14). Katon and colleagues (15) have demonstrated that 13% of primary care populations have PD (6.5% with PD alone, and an additional 6.5% with PD and depression). More recent studies estimate that the prevalence of PD in primary care is between 8% (16) and 11% (17).

PROBLEM OF UNDERRECOGNITION

Goldberg and Blackwell (19) have referred to the problem of underrecognition of psychiatric problems in primary care as "hidden psychiatric morbidity" in pointing out how frequently psychiatric problems go unrecognized. As we review below, because PD patients often present in medical settings in a manner that leads to underrecognition, our knowledge about this condition in primary care is still limited (20).

Probably 50% or more of the psychiatric disorders in primary care are not properly diagnosed or treated (21–25). In recent studies by Fifer and colleagues (18) in an HMO setting, patients with anxiety disorders were not recognized over half of the time, although appropriate benefits were available in their insurance plan. The recent 14-country World Health Organization (WHO) Primary Care Study also found that 50% of patients with PD were not recognized (26,2,3,27).

It is not surprising that PCPs fail to recognize PD patients because an overwhelming percentage (>90%) present with somatic rather than psychological symptoms (28,29). Studies have shown that psychiatric conditions in primary care patients are correctly diagnosed 95% of the time if anxiety and depressive complaints are their principal presenting symptoms. This rate falls to 48% if the patients present with somatic symptoms (30). As discussed below, PD patients usually present with multiple, distressing physical symptoms in a variety of medical settings.

COST ISSUES

The underrecognition of PD in primary care is particularly critical because of its cost implications. A classic study by Clancy and Noyes (31) documented the high utilization of medical services in undiagnosed panic patients; 71 PD patients received 358 tests and procedures in 30 categories (range 0–11, mean 7.5) and 135 specialty consultations. The average panic patient sees 10 or more physicians before a correct diagnosis is made (28). It routinely takes more than 10 years to make a correct diagnosis, and Simpson and colleagues (32) have demonstrated that, during that time, PD patients utilize a continuously escalating number of health care procedures and services (more visits, medications, tests, admissions, and visits to the ER and mental health professionals).

PD patients are among the patient groups most likely to visit physicians. Males with PD are 8.5 times, and females 5.2 times, more likely to be high users of general health care services, defined as more than six outpatient visits over a 6-month period (33). PD increases utilization of primary care services threefold (34). In one study, PD patients saw the physician approximately three times as often as the average patient who goes three or four times per year (35). They frequently fall into the "high utilizer group" (top 10% of patients visiting health care facilities), i.e., more than 15 visits to a physician and 15 phone calls per year. In one large HMO, 22% of high utilizers had lifetime PD histories (36). Fully 85.9% of patients with PD (and 67.4% with panic attacks) sought care from a health care professional in the preceding year (vs. 31.3% with other psychiatric disorders) (37,33).

HOW CAN WE INCREASE RECOGNITION OF PANIC DISORDER IN GENERAL MEDICINE?

Recent attempts to increase recognition of psychiatric conditions in primary care have utilized brief paper-and-pencil screening questionnaires (e.g., the Prime-MD and SDDS-PC) to alert PCPs of the likelihood of psychiatric diagnosis (38–41). Although these tools are capable of reliably suggesting an anxiety or other psychiatric diagnosis, they have generally not been accepted for widespread use (42), in part because the time involved is often unacceptable in busy primary care practices (7). Efforts are now underway in many centers to improve the situation, including development of computerized diagnosis and management systems (43,44). Perhaps a more direct, and somewhat less apologetic, approach is currently indicated. As mentioned above and discussed in depth later in this chapter, PD is one of the more prevalent and important conditions seen in the primary care setting. Perhaps this is the time to give it greater emphasis. With a prevalence of 8–13% in primary care, it is among the most common conditions, joining hypertension and depression. It is also associated with significant functional difficulties (37) and is an extremely costly condition. (31,33,35). No one would question whether a screening blood pressure measurement is appropriate for every primary care patient. The situation is analogous for the screening of PD, which can be effectively accomplished by the utilization of a simple screening question with all primary care patients, and certainly any patients suggested by the symptom presentations discussed below. A question capable of identifying the overwhelming majority of PD patients can be asked simply and rapidly: "Have you ever experienced brief periods, lasting seconds or minutes, of intense, overwhelming panic or terror, usually accompanied by racing heart, shortness of breath, dizziness, or trembling?" Almost all PD patients would immediately identify themselves with a simple "yes," and proceed to vividly describe their panic attacks.

DIAGNOSING PANIC DISORDER PATIENTS IN THE PRIMARY CARE SETTING

Many unrecognized PD patients can be found in the most puzzling group of patients in medicine (i.e., those with multiple nonspecific and poorly understood symptoms). The work of Kroenke and colleagues (45) documents that over half of all primary care patients come to see the physician for one or more of the 11 most common symptoms, including fatigue, back pain, headache, dizziness, chest pain, dyspnea, and anxiety. These symptoms account for one of every seven primary care encounters and 23% of visits to internists (46). However, less than 10% of these patients have an organic diagnosis established after a full year of diagnostic evaluation (47,46). In other studies, 25–40% of patients have no medical diagnosis and 30–60% of primary care visits are for symptoms for which there is no known physical disorder (47).

Psychiatric disorders are much more common when the medical diagnosis is uncertain. In one study, 38–45% of patients with uncertain diagnoses (vs. 15% for whom the diagnoses were clear) had a psychiatric diagnosis (6); 12% had PD diagnoses. Simon and Von Korff (33) have demonstrated that patients with multiple unexplained symptoms are over 200 times more likely to have PD, an increased risk 10 times that of any other syndrome. Panic attacks are reported in over one-quarter of patients who experience five or more problems or symptoms, 18% meet full criteria for PD (33).

In an early classic study, Katon (29) described PD patients from primary care who were seen in consultation by a psychiatrist. They were referred by different types of specialists to whom the patients had gone because they were most concerned about a particular symptom in that specialist's area of expertise. Forty-four percent had been to see a neurologist, 39% had seen a cardiologist, and 33% a gastroenterologist. If PCPs raise their index of suspicion and address the screening question to the patients described below, a much higher percentage of PD patients could be effectively recognized and easily diagnosed, even within the constraints of a busy PCP setting.

Emergency Rooms

PD patients most commonly present initially to the ER. They may complain of chest pain, fearing that they are having a myocardial infarction. As many as 16–25% of patients who present to an ER with chest pain have PD (48,49), although this is undiagnosed 94% of the time (48–50). In one study, the prevalence of PD was essentially the same in patients with and without acute myocardial ischemia (19.4% vs. 16.6%), although the PD patients were significantly more likely to have visited the ER in the previous year (57.5% vs. 36%) (50). The best estimate is that approximately one of every three patients who visit the ER with acute chest pain has a psychiatric problem, most commonly PD.

Cardiovascular Symptoms

Cardiovascular symptoms, particularly tachycardia, palpitations, and chest pain, are the most common symptoms PD patients experience. In the Epidemiologic Catchment Area (ECA) study, individuals with chest pain symptoms were four times more likely to have PD (51,52). Chest pain is one of the most common complaints seen in primary care settings, but a specific medical diagnosis is not found in 80–90% of these individuals (36), often after a costly work-up (53). Chest pain patients seen in cardiology frequently undergo extensive testing, including coronary arteriography. Over half of such patients are found to have chest pain of noncardiac origin (53–55). In the 20–30% who have normal coronary arteries on arteriography (56), approximately 50% continue to experience significant symptoms, as well as occupational and social dysfunction, years after their normal angiograms (57–59). Fully 80% of patients with chest pain and negative coronary arteriograms have PD, depression, or both (60). Specifically, 43–61% have PD (60–62). Cormier and colleagues (63) reported that 11 of 20 (55%) patients who had normal studies on treadmill testing had PD. These patients can prospectively be identified in many cases by the facts that they tend to be younger and female, and have atypical chest pain, usually sharp and not related to exercise, and have positive symptoms of PD (64).

Even though it is more common to see PD in cardiology patients who have normal coronary arteries, it is also prevalent, as mentioned above, in patients with documented coronary artery disease (35). In a study of 1414 patients in a cardiology practice, Goldberg and colleagues (65) found that 9.2% had PD, but that 40–60% of these PD patients also had ischemic heart disease. PD has been diagnosed in 5–

23% of patients with angiographically proven significant coronary artery disease, and in 62% of patients with ECG abnormalities (60,66). Ischemic heart disease is present in 40–60% of patients followed in cardiology who have PD (67). It is, in fact, patients with documented coronary artery disease who are most likely to have their PD overlooked (30,68).

A particularly problematic issue is that panic, and particularly phobic symptoms, appear to be associated with increases in cardiac mortality. Several recent studies of males have demonstrated that increases in panic and phobic anxiety ascertained by questionnaire is associated with two to three times greater increases in sudden cardiac death years later (69,70). Variables leading to this small but significant increase are as yet undetermined but may have to do with decreased heart variability associated with phobic anxiety (71,72). The other hypothesis attempting to explain the association between PD and cardiovascular illness and mortality is the increased association between microvascular angina and PD. Roy-Byrne and colleagues (73) found that 40% of patients with microvascular angina also had PD and experienced chest pain during sodium lactate infusion. This suggests that PD and microvascular angina may be overlapping illnesses or that there may be two types of microvascular angina.

In summary, one-fourth of patients seen in cardiology practices have a current diagnosis of PD (74). Coupled with the fact that 33–40% of patients with chest pain will ultimately be shown to have PD (75,64), PD should be a prime differential in many cardiology patients. This is particularly true in acute chest pain clinics, in which, as shown in one study, 98% of patients not found to have coronary disease were found to have PD (76). In addition, findings of high rates of PD among patients admitted to inpatient cardiac units have important implications from a cost perspective. Carter and colleagues (77) reported that 30% of patients admitted to their University Hospital Coronary Care Unit had PD and no evidence of coronary artery disease. Of those admitted patients in which the coronary artery disease work up proved to be negative, 55% had PD (77). As with other symptom complexes in PD patients, the cardiovascular symptoms tend to resolve with treatment of the panic (78,79).

Palpitations

Palpitations are a common symptom in outpatient medical practice—
in one study, reported by 16% of all patients (45). Palpitations are also
common symptoms of PD; Weber and Kapoor (80) demonstrated that
almost one-third of patients complaining of palpitations in various medical settings have PD, panic attacks, or anxiety. Other studies suggest
that 27% of ER patients with palpitations, and 45% of those in medical
clinics, have PD (68).

Holter monitoring is often employed in the evaluation of patients
complaining of palpitations. Barsky and colleagues (81) demonstrated
that a high percentage of the patients undergoing Holter monitoring
evaluation have PD, 18.6% currently and 27.6% lifetime. A significant
percentage of the $250 million spent each year in the United States on
Holter monitoring evaluation of palpitations (81) may be unnecessary
because palpitations are frequently indicative of PD, which can be diagnosed with less extensive, and less expensive, strategies.

Mitral Valve Prolapse

The relationship between mitral valve prolapse (MVP) and PD is complex (82,85). While MVP itself occurs in 5–20% of the general population, 15–45% of patients with PD are affected (82,84). It appears that
the majority of PD patients with an echocardiographic diagnosis of
MVP actually have little valve redundancy and no regurgitation and
are at low risk of complications (82,85).

In addressing the relationship of PD and MVP, it is important to
neither underemphasize the PD nor overemphasize the MVP. Patients
with PD and MVP may or may not have a significant cardiac disorder.
Given the somatic preoccupations and pathological fears many PD patients have about their heart, what is told to them regarding MVP is
of critical importance. Since they fear dying suddenly of cardiac arrest,
it behooves the cardiologist or internist to exercise care in not overly
alarming these patients. It is also important that the PD be treated. Although few studies have been done in this area, it would appear that
PD patients with MVP respond as well to treatment as PD patients
without MVP (85,82,86,87). There is some evidence that the MVP in
these patients may be caused by the PD itself, and echocardiographic

evidence of MVP may resolve with appropriate treatment of the PD symptoms (82,85).

Hypertension

PD patients have higher rates of hypertension (88,29), which may be secondary to the hyperventilation associated with PD (89) or to increases in peripheral catecholamines (90). Katon and colleagues (29,15) observed that 13.6% of PD patients were hypertensive vs. 4.4% of a control population. PD is also associated with labile hypertension, particularly during a panic attack (91,92,88). Labile hypertension disappears with effective treatment of PD.

Perhaps one of the most striking examples of the need to consider PD in the differential diagnoses of medical symptoms occurs in the evaluation of hypertension. Pheochromocytoma accounts for less than 0.1% of cases of hypertension (93), but urinary studies are routinely performed in the work-up of hypertension to rule out a potential pheochromocytoma. These tests are costly and find a pheochromocytoma only one or two times out of 1000. However, almost two-thirds of the patients screened for pheochromocytomas have PD. Thus, when pheochromocytoma is considered in the differential of a patient displaying episodic symptoms of labile hypertension, PD should be the principal condition considered. Certainly screening questions and history would be far more cost-effective than extensive urinary testing to make the appropriate diagnosis in most cases.

Arrhythmias

A special mention should be made of the differential between paroxysmal supraventricular tachycardia (PSVT) and the sinus tachycardia seen routinely in PD patients. Lessmeier and colleagues (94) recently reported that almost two-thirds of patients with PSVT have panic symptoms. This has caused anxiety in PD patients and raised many questions as to whether they should have event monitoring or surgery. Although this area needs further research, most experts feel that it is unlikely that the average PD patient has PSVT or that event monitoring is indicated in routine cases. Most PD patients do not have the sudden "within one beat" onset and offset of their tachycardia and can accurately describe that difference. It is probably only in patients with symptoms suggestive of a sudden onset/offset that event monitoring is indicated.

Cardiovascular Risk Factors

It is important that PD patients be screened for cardiovascular risk factors. They have higher rates of smoking (95) and increased cholesterol (96), and are more likely to be socially isolated (97) and less likely to have a regular exercise program (99) than individuals without panic. Tricyclic antidepressants (TCAs), which are frequently utilized in the treatment of PD, have cardiotoxic side effects including cardiac conduction delay, orthostatic hypotension, and increased heart rate, as well as having interactions with antihypertensives (99), so patients receiving these agents should be carefully followed.

Neurological Symptoms

Headache

Headache is the third most common reason for primary care visits in the United States (100). Approximately 15% of males and 28% of females have consulted their physician complaining of headaches (101). A surprisingly high percentage of these patients have PD. Fully 15% of women and 12.8% of men (ages 24–29) who consult a physician for headache symptoms have PD (102). This is especially true with migraine headaches (103). Patients with PD are seven times more likely to report the occurrence of a migraine in the previous week than those without PD (104). Individuals with migraine headaches see physicians more frequently and make up twice the proportion of clinic patients as the remainder of headache patients. In one study, of those PD patients who consulted a physician for headache symptoms in the previous 2 weeks, 36% had a migraine headache (102). Migraine is more than three times more likely in females with PD and seven times more likely in PD males, compared to those without a history of PD (104).

Headaches in PD patients are also more severe than in non-panic patients. The proportion of PD patients who have frequent attacks is higher, with approximately half of females with PD or panic attacks having five or more headaches in a 4-week period. In males, 35–45% have frequent panic attacks (102). Disability is also more common in headache patients with PD. One-fourth to one-half of female patients with PD have significant disability attributable to headaches, a percentage that is three to five times higher than that of female headache patients without a history of PD (102).

Given that a high proportion of patients who go to physicians with a complaint of headache have PD, and the likelihood that the headaches they experience are more severe and frequent, it seems clear that PD should be commonly considered in the differential diagnosis of headache.

Cerebrovascular Disease

Utilizing data from the ECA study, Weissman and colleagues (105) observed a twofold increase in stroke in PD patients compared to other psychiatric disorders or normals. Although there is no clear explanation for this observation, the increases in hypertension and cholesterol and decreased exercise associated with panic may be pertinent risk factors.

Dizziness

Dizziness is a very common complaint of PD patients and, for some, is the most severe and disabling symptom (106). Jacob and colleagues (107) demonstrated abnormalities on otoneurological test batteries in patients with PD. They found that 75% of the patients with PD, and 60% with panic attacks and agoraphobia, had abnormal vestibular functioning. In PD patients selected for dizziness and imbalance symptoms, Jacob and colleagues (107) reported that 87.5% had abnormal vestibular results on at least one test. This observation has been replicated in some studies (108) but not others (109). Sklare and colleagues (108) identified vestibular abnormalities in 71% of their sample. In addition, abnormalities in these tests have been correlated with the amount of self-reported agoraphobic avoidance (110,111). Jacob and colleagues (112) have recently performed the largest and best controlled trial to date examining this issue. They continue to find a high rate of vestibular abnormalities in PD patients, especially those with agoraphobia.

However, it is important to note that the vestibular abnormalities in these studies do not fit any consistent or well-recognized pattern of dysfunction (e.g., Meniere's syndrome, vestibular neuritis), leaving this a controversial area with an uncertain connection between vestibular dysfunction and the frequent dizziness complaints in PD patients. However, PD patients are frequently seen in dizziness clinics, probably because dizziness is the second most common symptom of PD (113). Drachman and Hart (114) reported that 20% of patients in their dizziness clinic had "hyperventilation syndrome," usually thought to represent PD. Drachman and Hart (114) and Simpson and colleagues (115) reported that three-fourths of patients with so-called "psychogenic dizziness" met criteria for PD with or without agoraphobia. Clark and colleagues (116) studied 227 individuals in a balance disorder self-help group and found that 24% of these individuals met criteria for PD and 27% had a history of panic attacks. In a subsequent study with 50 patients visiting otolaryngologists with the primary complaint of dizziness, 20% met criteria for PD and another 24% had infrequent limited-symptom panic attacks; in contrast, none of a control hearing-loss patient group had PD and only 8% had infrequent panic attacks. These results are consistent with the findings of Frommberger and colleagues (117) in a study of patients referred to a neurological clinic for complaints of dizziness; 61% of that sample had a current or lifetime diagnosis of PD.

These findings suggest that one of the principal conditions in the differential diagnosis of the patient with dizziness, particularly in the younger patient, is PD. Whether ENT referral and work-up of dizziness in the primary care patient are necessary depends on the severity of symptoms and their response to traditional treatment of PD.

Syncope

In a study examining patients with medically unexplained syncope, the syncope was attributable to a psychiatric condition in 31% of patients (118); 63% had PD with or without agoraphobia (19% of all patients referred to the syncope clinic). Ten months after treatment, 76% of the PD patients were improved or very much improved, underscoring the importance of timely recognition and treatment.

Gastrointestinal Symptoms

The prevalence of unexplained gastrointestinal (GI) symptoms is surprisingly high in the general population (6–25%) (119). In the ECA study, subjects who reported at least one GI symptom were significantly more likely to have PD than those who did not report GI symptoms (2.5% vs. 0.7%). This also extended to agoraphobia (10.0% vs. 3.6%). Panic (5.2%) and agoraphobia (17.8%) were even more common in subjects reporting two GI symptoms. Lydiard and colleagues (120), also utilizing the ECA data, reported that individuals with PD have a higher incidence of nausea and irritable bowel syndrome (IBS) symptoms than those without panic.

There is significant concurrence between PD and IBS. It is estimated that IBS affects 8–17% of the general population (121,122). This syndrome accounts for 13–52% of new referrals to GI clinics and is a frequent problem in primary care settings (123,124). Even prior to inclusion of any GI symptoms in the diagnostic symptom picture for PD in DSM-III-R (125), it was apparent that PD could appear as IBS (126). Lydiard and colleagues (127) observed that 31% of patients in a GI clinic met lifetime criteria for PD and 26% met current criteria. This was higher than the 7% current PD observed by Walker and colleagues (128); however, that group also observed a 29% lifetime rate of PD and a 25% prevalence of agoraphobia lifetime. Subsequently, Walker and colleagues (129) compared 75 patients with IBS and 40 with inflammatory bowel disease (IBD). The IBS patients had a higher prevalence of current (28% vs. 3%) and lifetime (41% vs. 25%) PD. Consistent with findings with other somatic symptoms of PD, IBS patients treated with traditional treatments for PD (antidepressants or anxiolytics) experience decreased symptoms of IBS (125,128).

Respiratory Symptoms

Probably because of the choking, smothering symptoms, and dyspnea, 32% of asthmatic patients have panic attacks during an asthma attack and there is a greater prevalence (6.5–24%) of PD among patients with asthma (130–132). Shavitt et al. (132) examined 107 asthmatic outpatients and found that agoraphobia and PD were prevalent (13.1% and

6.5%, respectively). Interestingly, none of these patients had ever received a diagnosis of PD until questioned directly about the presence of panic anxiety symptoms and typical agoraphobic avoidances (132). In a subsequent study, Yellowlees and colleagues (133) found a high rate (24%) of PD in asthmatics. Carr et al. (131) reported that 22.6% of 93 individuals with asthma had panic attacks, with 9.7% meeting DSM-III-R criteria for PD.

Perna and colleagues (134) recently reported a prevalence of 19.6% for PD in asthma patients. In addition, 25% more had positive histories for unexpected sporadic attacks not meeting DSM-IV criteria for PD. Therefore, 45% of the asthmatics had at least one unexpected panic attack and 96% of them described their asthmatic attacks and panic attacks as being completely different. The onset of asthma preceded the onset of panic in 90% of the patients. The investigators also reported that the risk for PD was higher in first-degree relatives of the asthmatics with PD than in the first-degree relatives of asthmatics who had never experienced PD. They suggest that perhaps asthma tends to elicit panic attacks and PD in subjects with a familial predisposition to panic.

PD certainly complicates the course of asthma, including increased use of steroids and more frequent and longer hospitalizations (135). It is easy to imagine a vicious circle of airway obstruction causing anxiety, which exacerbates the obstruction. Although this area is understudied, treatment of panic attacks in asthmatic children with alprazolam and cognitive-behavioral therapy (CBT) did lead to improvement in both the asthma and the PD symptoms (136).

Similar findings have been reported in patients with chronic obstructive pulmonary disease (COPD). Karajgi and colleagues (137) and Smoller and colleagues (138) have both noted a high incidence of PD in patients with COPD. Yellowlees and colleagues (133) reported that 24% of their COPD patients had PD.

The prevalence of respiratory diseases is three times higher in PD patients than in patients without psychiatric illness or with other psychiatric disorders, and includes increases in asthma, bronchitis, emphysema, and allergic symptoms (139,140). Therefore, it is not surprising that a recent study found high rates of PD among patients referred for pulmonary functioning tests (PFTs). In that unselected sample, 17%

had panic attacks and 11% PD (141). These findings suggest that PD should also be considered in the differential when evaluating patients with significant complaints of dyspnea.

Alcohol and Substance Abuse

Certainly among the largest and most problematic groups of patients seen in primary care settings are those with alcohol or other substance abuse disorders. A number of studies have documented that the incidence of PD is higher among alcoholics (142–144). Inpatient alcohol treatment programs report rates of PD ranging from 2 to 21% (145–148). Johannesen and colleagues (147) report an 8% lifetime PD rate in alcoholics, with 14% having a history of frequent, isolated panic attacks. The association may be particularly pronounced in early-onset alcoholics, in whom the rate of PD was 15% if abusive drinking began before the age of 20 but 6% in those with onset after the age of 20 (149).

In anxiety disorder clinic samples, the prevalence of alcohol dependence or abuse is in the range of 7 to 28% (150,151); PD patients have elevated rates of alcohol abuse (152,153). PD complicated by substance abuse is less well studied; however, the ECA study does not report a higher risk of PD in cocaine abusers (154).

Lydiard and colleagues (155) reported that PD predated alcohol abuse in 15% of a sample of VA alcohol inpatients. In a study of imipramine treatment of PD in alcoholics, symptoms of PD and alcoholism improved in a significant number of patients who were compliant with treatment (156).

Premenstrual Syndrome and Late Luteal Phase Dysphoric Disorder

Anecdotal reports suggest that PD in some female patients worsens during certain phases of their menstrual cycle and that patients with late luteal phase dysphoric disorder (LLPDD) have a high (25%) incidence of PD (157). Deci and colleagues (158) reported a case of PD apparently stimulated by oral contraceptives, and Wagner and Berenson (159) a case with Norplant. It is well known that PD can either worsen or improve with pregnancy (160).

It is of interest that both premenstrual syndrome (PMS) and PD patients develop panic attacks in response to lactate infusion (161), suggesting that there is some shared pathophysiology between PMS and PD. This is supported by the findings of Harrison and colleagues (162) that patients with LLPDD responded to 35% CO_2 inhalation with panic symptoms quite similar to those of PD patients. Low-dose alprazolam is effective in reducing anxiety and mood swings in women with PMS (163) and is an effective treatment of PD (164).

Differential Diagnosis

The principal difficulty with the differential diagnosis of PD patients in primary care settings is the multiple physical symptoms reported by PD patients (165). They have symptoms across multiple organ systems and average more than 14 physical symptoms in a full review of systems (15). Therefore, it can be a complex differential between PD, hypochondriasis, and somatization disorder; in fact, 49–71% of panic patients actually meet the criteria for somatization disorder (166,167) and many meet criteria for hypochondriasis (168,169). Patients with somatization disorder may have a more tumultuous history, including multiple relationships and marriages—often abusive in nature—and alcohol and substance abuse, and they may have a history of physical or sexual abuse that may aid in the differential from PD.

The principal psychiatric differential to consider in panic patients is depression—60% of PD patients have clinical depression in their lifetime (30% of PD patients have current depression) (170–172). Posttraumatic stress disorder (PTSD) patients can have considerable symptomatic resemblance to PD patients but are differentiated by a history of trauma such as rape or a car accident that precipitated distress. Social phobics can also resemble PD patients, but their panic attacks occur only in social situations in which the patient might feel embarrassed (173).

The differential diagnosis of PD in the medical setting also includes consideration of a number of medical conditions and drugs. Boulenger and colleagues (174) reported that caffeine will worsen PD and may cause panic symptoms in sufficiently high doses. Withdrawal from alcohol or sedatives can also result in panic symptoms (175), as can

Table 1   Medical Conditions That Can Resemble Panic Disorder

Anemia
Angina
Arrhythmias (particularly paroxysmal supraventricular tachycardia)
Asthma
Congestive heart failure
COPD
Epilepsy
Hyperthyroidism
Mitral valve prolapse
Orthostatic hypotension
Paratyroid disorders
Pulmonary embolus
Transient ischemic attacks

the use of marijuana, amphetamines, and especially cocaine (176–178). The medical conditions listed in Table 1 can resemble PD. Lindemann and colleagues (179) found that 11% of patients with panic attacks had a history of thyroid disease, and PD patients were shown to have an increased rate in a recent large survey (180). Although PD patients often feel they have hypoglycemia, it is almost never the case (181,182). Hypoglycemia should be considered only in cases in which the symptoms are almost exclusively postprandial or associated with hunger. In those rare cases, endocrine abnormalities should be explored.

SUGGESTED MEDICAL WORK-UP

The proper diagnosis of PD can usually be made with an appropriate medical and psychiatric history, family history, and medication and drug history, and without the use of extensive laboratory testing. Physical and neurological examinations investigating the reported symptoms are important. An ECG may be indicated for patients with significant cardiovascular symptoms, especially if the patient is over age 40. This may be particularly important in patients who need reassurance that they do not have serious cardiac disorders. Other laboratory tests that are routinely helpful include routine blood count, chemistry panel, and thyroid function test (T_3, T_4, and perhaps TSH).

THE IMPORTANCE OF ISOLATED PANIC ATTACKS VS. PANIC DISORDER

The prevalence of single panic attacks isolated in time has been reported to be 3.6 to 10% in the community (183) and 0.4–8% in primary care (15). In the recent WHO 14-country primary care study, 2.4% of patients had experienced a panic attack in the past month. However, in sites in the United States and Europe where the diagnosis of PD is more familiar, the rates were as high as 16.5% in the previous month, which may be a more accurate figure (172).

In that same study, it was clear that a single panic attack carries much of the same importance as the full disorder (172). After even a single panic attack, over two-thirds of the patients developed PD over the next year and 51% of the patients developed major depression (a fourfold increase). Panic attacks are accompanied by increases in alcoholism, social phobia, and obsessive-compulsive disorder (OCD), and increases in morbidity and suicide risk. As we have reviewed, the presence of panic attacks is almost certainly associated with a higher incidence of headaches, IBS, multiple unexplained symptoms, and high utilization of health care resources.

An even more striking finding in the large WHO primary care study was that 99% of the patients who had had a panic attack in the previous month also had a depressive or anxiety disorder at a full syndromal or subthreshold level (26). In other words, if a panic attack occurred, it was almost always part of a complex anxiety and depressive picture, and almost all patients who had one panic attack had this important symptom cluster.

This study suggests that a panic attack is the "tip of the iceberg" and underscores the potential importance of recognizing even a single panic attack (172). Panic attacks are generally easy for patients to recognize and describe if they are asked even a brief screening question as described earlier. Thus, we should reorient our attention to recognizing panic attacks in primary care settings without requiring patients to meet full DSM-IV criteria for PD before initiating treatment.

TREATMENT

At this point, there are few studies focusing directly on the treatment of PD in primary care. There are no accepted models for the treatment of psychiatric problems in primary care (184) in general, and there are multiple obstacles to effective treatment of PD in the primary care setting. These obstacles include the briefness of the usual visit in primary care settings, high resistance on the part of the patient and most clinicians to open discussion of psychiatric problems (185), and very poor reimbursement for psychiatric problems treated by PCPs (186).

Despite these difficulties, we need to suggest models for treatment in primary care derived from psychiatric settings because of the pressing clinical need and the importance of appropriate research evaluation of this issue. At this point, no models have gained widespread acceptance. For a model to be accepted, it must fit the patient, the practice setting, and the PCP.

A useful treatment model needs to be appropriate to the type of difficulties raised by PD patients. PD patients visit physicians more than any other type of patient, hoping to find reassurance because of their tremendous anxiety about their complex and distressing symptoms. Therefore, care provided for PD patients in the primary care setting must provide patients with appropriate, but not excessive, medical work-up to allow the practitioner to effectively reassure the patient about what they do, and do not, have. Patients also benefit from reading materials about PD to augment what the PCP or physician's staff tell them. This is a critical issue in the recovery of PD patients, as well as in securing their compliance with recommendations. It is also helpful for spouses and other family members to read these materials in order to understand this puzzling condition.

Appropriate management of PD in primary care involves a series of steps: 1) early recognition and accurate diagnosis, 2) ruling out comorbid conditions, 3) education and support, 4) development of appropriate staff capabilities, and 5) development of a ''best practice model'' of treatment for the average patient.

The PCP should screen for even isolated panic attacks in most, if not all patients. Although consultations to psychiatrists from PCPs and their patients may be experienced negatively by the patient because of stigma, cost, or inconvenience (187,188), they may be quite useful. Since many of these patients have comorbid conditions such as depression, substance abuse, OCD, and social phobia, consultation with a psychiatrist with experience in the anxiety disorders may be helpful in working through diagnostic dilemmas. Consultation would also increase patient compliance through confirmation that the correct diagnosis has been made and the treatment plan initiated. If feasible, patients with PD can often be well treated in primary care after an initial consultation with an anxiety disorder expert, with a follow-up in 3 to 6 months later, especially if initial response to treatment is not optimal.

Successful treatment of PD patients in primary care generally requires development of new expertise within the practice. This could certainly be accomplished in a multispecialty practice in which a working relationship exists between the PCP and a psychiatrist with expertise in the anxiety disorders. However, these large multispecialty practices are still generally uncommon and the primary care practice may need to develop this expertise with a nonmedical physician extender— e.g., a social worker, physician-assistant, or nurse—who works full-time in the practice. Since 8–10% of primary care patients have PD and are already consuming considerable resources in the primary care practice, development of this expertise is important. In general, sufficient expertise can be developed through reading and perhaps a short clerkship (i.e., 1 week) in an anxiety disorders clinic. This physican extender could then work with the PCP to support, educate, and manage patients with anxiety disorders. A module for the treatment of PD in primary care has been developed by the American Psychiatric Association (44).

As is the case with most psychiatric patients, the principal difficulty in treatment is ensuring that they receive enough treatment for an adequate period of time. PD patients are almost phobic about taking medications and may develop multiple side effects that require attention, education, and reassurance. Most patients benefit from recommendations for consistent exposure to their phobic situations, as well as a modified form of CBT. CBT, in at least some form, is essential in helping patients learn to manage their panic symptoms, to understand and develop an appropriate cognitive model of the meaning of their symptoms, and to be desensitized to both external and internal stimuli that are frightening to them. There are numerous reading materials (189,190) that are helpful to the patients.

The psychopharmacological treatment of PD has been the subject of intense study over the past 25 years (191) and is reviewed elsewhere in this volume. Most of the tricyclic antidepressants are effective if given in appropriate doses. The monoamine oxidase inhibitors (MAOIs) are also effective but are usually not employed unless safer and easier interventions have been unsuccessful. High-potency benzodiazepines such as clonazepam and alprazolam are also effective for the treatment of PD. However, the current treatment of choice for PD has become the selective serotonin-reuptake inhibitors (SSRIs), because of their antidepressive properties and their popularity with patients and physicians due to a favorable side-effect profile. They are also likely to become widely utilized in primary care settings because of their ease of use with complicated medical conditions.

Most studies show that 50–60% of PD patients will have an excellent response to treatment and another 20–25% at least a moderate response (197). Approximately 10–25% of patients respond poorly to the first treatment offered; it is at least this group of patients who should be referred to an anxiety disorders program or psychiatric consultation. The NIH Consensus Conference recommended that patients who do not respond well after 6 weeks should be referred for consultation (198).

The physical symptoms associated with PD generally do resolve with effective treatment (199). Studies suggesting that cardiovascular symptoms (78,199), IBS and more nonspecific GI symptoms (125), and even hypochondriasis (168) all tend to improve with appropriate treatment for the panic disorder underscore the need for timely diagnosis and treatment to reduce patient distress, morbidity, and overutilization of medical resources.

REFERENCES

1. Regier DA, Goldberg ID, Taube CA. The de facto U.S. mental health services system: a public perspective. Arch Gen Psychiatry 1978; 35: 685–693.
2. Sartorius N. Ustun TB, Costa e Silva JA, Goldberg D, Lecrubier Y,

Ormel J, Von Korff M, Wittchen HU. An international study of psychological problems in primary care: preliminary report from the World Health Organization Collaborative Project on "Psychological Problems in General Health Care." Arch Gen Psychiatry 1993; 50: 819–824.

3. Sartorius N. Ustun TB, Lecrubier Y, Wittchen HU. Depression comorbid with anxiety: results from the WHO study on psychological disorders in primary health care. Br J Psychiatry 1996; 168(suppl 30):38–43.

4. Schulberg HC, Burns BJ. Mental disorders in primary care: epidemiologic, diagnostic, and treatment research directions [review]. Gen Hosp Psychiatry 1988; 10(2):79–87.

5. Barrett JE, Barrett JA, Oxman TE, Gerber PD. The prevalence of psychiatric disorders in a primary care practice. Arch Gen Psychiatry 1988; 45:1100–1106.

6. van Hemert AM, Hengeveld MW, Bolk JH, Rooijmans HG, Vandenbroucke JP. Psychiatric disorders in relation to medical illness among patients of a general medical out-patient clinic. Psycholog Med 1993; 23:167–73.

7. Higgins ES. A review of unrecognized mental illness in primary care: prevalence, a natural history, and efforts to change the course. Arch Fam Med 1994; 3(10):862–864.

8. Orleans CT, George LK, Houpt JL. How primary physicians treat psychiatric disorders: a national survey of family practitioners. Arch Gen Psychiatry 1985; 42:52–57.

9. Zung WWK. Assessment of anxiety disorder: qualitative and quantitative approaches. In: Fann WE, ed. Phenomenology and Treatment of Anxiety. New York: Spectrum, 1979:1–17.

10. Zung WWK. Prevalence of clinically significant anxiety in a family practice setting. Am J Psychiatry 1986; 143:1471–1472.

11. Shurman RA, Kramer PD, Mitchell JB. The hidden mental health network: treatment of mental illness by nonpsychiatrist physicians. Arch Gen Psychiatry 1985; 42:89–94.

12. Wells KB, Goldberg G, Brook RH, Leake B. Quality of care for psychotropic drug use in internal medicine group practices. West J Med 1986; 145:710–714.

13. Katerndahl DA, Realini JP. Where do panic attack sufferers seek care? J Fam Pract 1995; 40(3):237–243.

14. Kessler RC, McGonagle KA, Zhao S, Nelson CB, Hughes M, Eshleman S, Wittchen HU, Kendler KS. Lifetime and 12 month prevalence of

DSMIII-R psychiatric disorders in the US: results of the National Cormorbidity Study. Arch Gen Psychiatry 1994; 51:8–19.

15. Katon W, Vitaliano PP, Russo J, Jones M, Anderson K. Panic disorder: epidemiology in primary care. J Fam Pract 1986; 23:233–239.

16. Taylor CB, Russiter EM, Agras WS. Utilization of health care services by patients with anxiety and anxiety disorders. In press.

17. Shear MK, Pilkonis PA, Cloitre M, Leon AC. Cognitive behavioral treatment compared with nonprescriptive treatment of panic disorder. Arch Gen Psychiatry 1994; 51:395–401.

18. Fifer SK, Mathias SD, Patrick DL, Mazonson PD, Lubeck DP. Untreated anxiety among adult primary care patients in a health maintenance organization. Arch Gen Psychiatry 1994; 51(9):740–750.

19. Goldberg DP, Blackwell B. Psychiatric illness in general practice: a detailed study using a new method of case identification. Br Med J 1970; 1:439–443.

20. Shear MK, Schulberg HC. Anxiety disorders in primary care. Bull Menninger Clinic 1995; 59(2, suppl a):A73-A85.

21. Pierce C. Failure to spot mental illness in primary care is a global problem. Clin Psychiatry News 1993; 5.

22. Ormel J, Koeter MWJ, van den Brink W, van de Willige G. Recognition, management, and course of anxiety and depression in general practice. Arch Gen Psychiatry 1991; 48:700–706.

23. Jones LR, Badger LW, Ficken RP, Leeper JD, Anderson RL. Inside the hidden mental health network: examining mental health care delivery of primary care physicians. Gen Hosp Psychiatry 1987; 9:287–293.

24. Borus JF, Howes MJ, Devins NP, Rosenberg R, Livingston WW. Primary health care providers' recognition and diagnosis of mental disorders in their patients. Gen Hosp Psychiatry 1988; 10:317–321.

25. Kessler LG, Cleary PD, Burke JJ. Psychiatric disorders in primary care: results of a follow-up study. Arch Gen Psychiatry 1985; 42:583–587.

26. Lecrubier Y, Usten TB. Panic and depression: a worldwide primary care perspective. Int Clin Psychopharmacol 1997. In press.

27. Ormel J, vonKorff M, Ustun TB, Pini S, Korten A, Oldehinkel T. Common mental disorders and disability across cultures. JAMA 1994; 272: 1741–1748.

28. Sheehan DV, Ballenger JC, Jacobsen G. Treatment of endogenous anxiety with phobic, hysterical, and hypochondriacal symptoms. Arch Gen Psychiatry 1980; 37:51–59.

29. Katon W. Panic disorder and somatization: a review of 55 cases. Am J Med 1984; 77:101–106.

30. Bridges KW, Goldberg BP. Somatic presentation of DSM-III psychiatric disorders in primary care. J Psychsom Res 1985; 29:563–569.

31. Clancy J, Noyes R. Anxiety neurosis: a disease for the medical model. Psychomatics 1976; 17:90–93.

32. Simpson RJ, Kazmierczak T, Power KG, Sharp DM. Controlled comparison of patients with panic disorder. Br J Gen Pract 1994; 44:352–356.

33. Simon GE, Von Korff M. Somatization and psychiatric disorder in the Epidemiologic Catchment Area study. Am J Psychiatry 1991; 148:1494–1500.

34. U.S. Department of Health and Human Services. Public Health Service National Center for Health Statistics, National Medical Care Utilization and Expenditure Survey (NMCUES). Washington, DC: US Government Printing Office, 1985.

35. Katon W. Panic disorder: relationship to high medical utilization, unexplained physical symptoms and medical costs. J Clin Psychiatry 1996; 57(suppl 10):11–18.

36. Katon W. Chest pain, cardiac disease, and panic disorder. J Clin Psychiatry 1990; 51:27–30.

37. Klerman GL, Weissman MM, Ouellette R, Johnson J, Greenwald S. Panic attacks in the community: social morbidity and health care utilization. JAMA 1991; 265:742–746.

38. Bech P, Malt UF, Dencker SJ, Ahlfors. Scales for assessment of diagnosis and severity of mental disorders. Acta Psychiatr Scand 1993; S87:1–87.

39. Spitzer RL, Williams JB, Kroenke K, Linzer M, deGruy FV III, Hahn SR, Brody D, Johnson JG. Utility of a new procedure for diagnosing mental disorders in primary care: the Prime-MD 1000 study. JAMA 1994; 272:1749–1756.

40. Broadhead WE, Leon AC, Weissman M, Barrett JE, Gilbert TT, Keller MB, Olfson M, Higgins ES. Development and validation of the SDDS-PC screen for multiple mental disorders in primary care. Arch Fam Med 1995; 4:211–219.

41. Weissman MM, Olfson M, Leon AC, Broadhead WE, Gilbert TT, Higgins ES, Barrett JE, Blacklow RS, Keller MB, Hoven C. Brief diagnostic interviews (SDDS-PC) for multiple mental disorders in primary care: a pilot study. Arch Fam Med 1995; 4:220–227.

42. Mathias SD, Fifer SK, Mazonson PD, Lubeck DP, Buesching DP, Patrick DL. Necessary but not sufficient: the effect of screening and feed-

back on outcomes of primary care patients with untreated anxiety. J Gen Intern Med 1994; 9:606–615.

43. Higgins ES. Computerized Mental Health Lab Test. Submitted 1997.
44. Katon W, Gonzales J. A review of randomized trials of psychiatric consultation-liaison studies in primary care. Psychosomatics 1994; 35: 266–278.
45. Kroenke K, Arrington ME, Mangelsdorff AD. The prevalence of symptoms in medical outpatients and the adequacy of therapy. Arch Intern Med 1990; 150:1685–1689.
46. Kroenke K. Symptoms in medical patients: an untended field. Am J Med 1992; 92(suppl 1A):3S-6S.
47. Kroenke K, Mangelsdorff AD. Common symptoms in ambulatory care: incidence, evaluation, therapy and outcome. Am J Med 1989; 86:262–266.
48. Fleet RP, Dupuis G, Marchand A, Burelle D, Arsenault A, Beitman BD. Panic disorder in emergency department chest pain patients: prevalence, comorbidity, suicidal ideation, and physician recognition. Am J Med 1996; 101:371–380.
49. Wulsin L, Hillard JR, Geier P, Hissa D, Rouan GW. Screening emergency room patients with atypical chest pain for depression and panic disorder. Int J Psychiatry Med 1988; 18:315–323.
50. Yingling KW, Wulson LR, Arnold LM, Rouan GW. Estimated prevalence of panic disorder and depression among consecutive patients seen in an emergency department with acute chest pain. J Gen Intern Med 1993; 8:231–235.
51. Ford D. The relationship of psychiatric illness to medically unexplained chest pain. Presented at Mental Disorders in General Health Care Settings: A Research Conference, Seattle, June 1987.
52. Walker EA, Katon WJ, Jemelka RP, Roy-Byrne PP. Comorbidity of gastrointestinal complaints, depression, and anxiety in the Epidemiologic Catchment Area (ECA) study. Am J Med 1992; 92(1A):265–305.
53. Kroenke K, Mangelsdorff AD. Common symptoms in ambulatory care: incidence, evaluation, therapy and outcome. Am J Med 1989; 86:262–266.
54. Karlson BS, Herlitz J, Pettersson P, Ekvall HE, Hjalmarson A. Patients admitted to the emergency room with symptoms indicative of acute myocardial infarction. J Intern Med 1991; 230:251–258.
55. Lee TH, Cook EF, Weissberg M, Sargent RK, Wilson C, Goldman L. Acute chest pain in the emergency room: identification and examination of low-risk patients. Arch Intern Med 1985; 145:65–69.

56. Mukerji V, Beitman BD, Alpert MA. Chest pain and angiographically normal coronary arteries: implications for treatment. Tex Heart Inst J 1993; 20(3):170–179.

57. Lavey EB, Winkle RA. Continuing disability of patients with chest pain and normal coronary arteriograms. J Chronic Dis 1979; 32:191–196.

58. Ockene JS, Shay MJ, Alpert JS, Weiner BH, Dolen JE. Unexplained chest pain in patients with normal coronary arteriograms. N Engl J Med 1980; 303:1249–1252.

59. Wielgosz AT, Fletcher RH, McCants CB, McKinnis RA, Haney TL, Williams RB. Unimproved chest pain in patients with minimal or no coronary disease: a behavioral phenomenon. Am Heart J 1984; 108: 67–72.

60. Katon W, Hall ML, Russo J, Cormier L, Hollifield M, Vitaliano PP. Beitman BD. Chest pain: relationship of psychiatric illness to coronary arteriographic results. Am J Med 1988; 84(1):1–9.

61. Bass C, Wade C, Hand D, Jackson G. Patients with angina with normal and near-normal coronary arteries: clinical and psychosocial state 12 months after angiography. Br Med J 1983; 287:1505–1085.

62. Beitman BD, Basha I, Flaker G, DeRosear L, Mukerji V, Trombka L, Katon W. Atypical or nonanginal chest pain: panic disorder or coronary artery disease? Arch Intern Med 1987; 147:1548–1552.

63. Cormier L, Katon W, Russo J, Hollifield M, Hall ML, Vitaliano PP. Chest pain with negative cardiac diagnostic studies: relationship to psychiatric illness. J Nerv Ment Dis 1988; 176:351–358.

64. Ballenger JC. Unrecognized prevalence of panic disorder in primary care, internal medicine, and cardiology. Am J Cardiol 1987; 60(suppl J):39J-47J.

65. Goldberg R, Morris P, Christian F, Badger J, Chabot S, Edlund M. Panic disorder in cardiac outpatients. Psychosomatics 1990; 31(2):168–173.

66. Chignon JM, Lepine JP, Ades J. Panic disorder in cardiac outpatients. Am J Psychiatry 1993; 150:780–785.

67. Goldberg R, Morris P, Christian F, Badger J, Chapot S, Edlund M. Panic disorder in cardiac outpatients. Psychosomatics 1990; 31:168–173.

68. Zaubler TS, Katon W. Panic disorder and medical comorbidity: a review of the medical and psychiatric literature. Bull Menninger Clinic 1996; 60:2(suppl A):A13–A38.

69. Kawachi I, Colditz GA, Ascherio A, Rimm EB, Giovannucci E, Stampfer MJ, Willett WC. A prospective study of phobic anxiety and risk of coronary heart disease in men. Circulation 1994; 89:1992–1997.

70. Kawachi I, Sparrow D, Vokonas PS, Weiss ST. Symptoms of anxiety and risk of coronary heart disease: the Normative Aging Study. Circulation 1994; 90:2225–2229.

71. Kawachi I, Sparrow D, Vokonas PS, Weiss ST. Decreased heart rate variability in men with phobic anxiety (data from the Normative Aging Study). Am J Cardiol 1995; 75:882–885.

72. Yeragani VK, Pohl R, Berger R, Balon R, Ramesh C, Glitz D, Srinivasan K, Weinberg P. Decreased heart rate variability in panic disorder patients: a study of power-spectral analysis of heart rate. Psychiatr Res 1993; 46:89–103.

73. Roy-Byrne PP, Schmidt P, Cannon RO, Diem H, Rubinow DR. Microvascular angina and panic disorder. Int J Psychiatry Med 1989; 19: 315–325.

74. Barsky AJ, Delamater BA, Clancy SA, Antman EM, Ahern DK. Somatized psychiatric disorder presenting as palpitations. Arch Intern Med 1996; 156:1102–1108.

75. Katon WJ, Von Korff, Lin E. Panic disorder: relationship to high medical utilization. Am J Med 1992; 92(suppl 1A):7S–11S.

76. Laraia MT. Blacks and whites presenting to a cardiac emergency room with negative cardiac test results: evaluation for panic disorder and other cormorbid health problems. UMI Dissertation Services. Ann Arbor, MI: Bell & Howell, 1996.

77. Carter C, Maddox R, Amsterdam E, McCormick S, Waters C, Billett J. Panic disorder and chest pain in the coronary care unit. Psychosomatics 1992; 33:302–310.

78. Beitman BD, Basha IM, Trombka LH, Jayartna MA, Russell B, Flaker J, Anderson S. Pharmacotherapeutic treatment of panic disorder patients presenting with chest pain. J Fam Pract 1989; 28:177–180.

79. Mayou R, Kilmer I, Peare J. Behavioral treatment of atypical chest pain. Presented at Treatment of Mental Disorders in General Health Care Settings: A Research Conference, Pittsburgh, June 15, 1988.

80. Weber BE, Kapoor WN. Evaluation and outcomes of patients with palpitations. Am J Med 1997; 103(1):86.

81. Barsky AJ, Cleary PD, Barnett MC, Christiansen CL, Ruskin JN. The clinical course of palpitations in medical outpatients. Arch Intern Med 1995; 155:1782–1788.

82. Ballenger JC, Gibson R, Peterson GA, Laraia M. Functional MVP in agoraphobia/panic disorder. Presented the 139th annual meeting of the American Psychiatric Association, Washington, DC, May 1986.

83. Alpert MA, Sabeti M, Kushner MG, Beitman BD, Russell JL, Thiele JR, Mukerji V. Frequency of isolated panic attacks and panic disorder in patients with the mitral valve prolapse syndrome. Am J Cardiol 1992; 69:1489–1490.

84. Margraff J, Ehlers A, Roth WT. Mitral valve prolapse and panic disorder: a review of their relationship. Psychosom Med 1988; 50:93–113.

85. Gorman JM, Goetz RR, Fyer M, King DL, Fyer AJ, Liebowitz MR, Klein DF. The mitral valve prolapse-panic disorder connection. Psychosom Med 1988; 50:114–122.

86. Gorman JM, Fyer AF, Gliklich J, King D, Klein DF. Effect of sodium lactate on patients with panic disorder and mitral valve prolapse. Am J Psychiatry 1981; 138:247–249.

87. Grunhaus L, Gloger S, Birmacher B. Clomipramine treatment for panic attacks in patients with mitral valve prolapse. J Clin Psychiatry 1984; 45:25–27.

88. White WB, Baker CH. Episodic hypertension secondary to panic disorder. Arch Intern Med 1986; 146:1129–1130.

89. Todd GP, Chadwick IG, Yeo WW, Jackson PR, Ramsay LE. Pressor effect of hyperventilation in healthy subjects. J Human Hypertens 1995; 9:119–122.

90. Ballenger JC, Peterson GA, Laraia M, Hucek A, Lake CR, Jimerson D, Cox DJ, Trockman C, Shipe JR, Wilkinson C. A study of plasma catecholamines in agoraphobia and the relationship of serum tricyclic levels to treatment response. In: Ballenger JC, ed. Biology of Agoraphobia. Washington, DC: American Psychiatric Association Press, 1984:27–63.

91. Balon R, Ortiz A, Pohl R, Yeragani VK. Heart rate and blood pressure during placebo-associated panic attacks. Psychsom Med 1988; 50:434–438.

92. Shear MK. Pathophysiology of panic: a review of pharmacologic provocative tests and naturalistic monitoring data. J Clin Psychiatry 1986; 47:18–26.

93. Stein PP, Black HR. A simplified diagnostic approach to pheochromocytoma: a review of the literature and report on one institution's experience. Medicine 1990; 70:46–66.

94. Lessmeier TJ, Gamperling D, Johnson-Liddon V, Fromm BS, Steinman

RT, Meissner MD, Lehmann MH. Unrecognized paroxysmal supraventricular tachycardia: potential for misdiagnosis as panic disorder. Arch Intern Med 1997; 157:537–543.

95. Pohl R, Yeragani VK, Balon R, Lycaki H, McBride R. Smoking in patients with panic disorder. Psychiatry Res 1992; 43:253–262.

96. Bajwa WK, Asnis GM, Sanderson WC, Irfan A, van Praag HM. High cholesterol levels in patients with panic disorder. Am J Psychiatry 1992; 149:376–378.

97. Noyes R, Cook B, Garvey M, Summers R. Reduction of gastrointestinal symptoms following treatment for panic disorder. Psychosomatics 1990; 31:75–79.

98. Yeragani VK, Pohl R, Balon R, Ramesh C, Glitz D, Sherwood P. Risk factors for cardiovascular illness in panic disorder patients. Neuropsychobiology 1990; 23:134–139.

99. Taylor CB, Hayward C, King R, Ehlers A, Margraf J, Maddock R, Clark D, Roth WT, Agras WS. Cardiovascular and symptomatic reduction of alprazolam and imipramine in patients with panic disorder: results of a double-blind, placebo-controlled trial. J Clin Psychopharmacol 1990; 10:112–118.

100. National Center for Health Statistics. Acute conditions: incidence and associated disability, United States, National Center for Health Statistics, Rockville, MD. Vital and Health Statistics, National Health Survey Series 10, no. 77. DHEW publication (HSM) 73–1503, 1972.

101. Linet MS, Stewart WF, Cenentano DD, Ziegler D, Sprecher M. An epidemiologic study of headache among adolescents and young adults. JAMA 1989; 261(15):2211–2216.

102. Stewart WF, Shechter A, Liberman J. Physician consultation for headache pain and history of panic: results from a population-based study. Am J Med 92(suppl 1a):355–405.

103. Merikangas KR, Angst J, Isler H. Migraine and psychopathology: results of the Zurich cohort study of young adults. Arch Gen Psychiatry 1990; 47:849–853.

104. Stewart WF, Linet MS, Cenentano DD. Migraine headaches and panic attacks. Psychosom Med 1989; 51:559–569.

105. Weissman MM, Markowitz JS, Ouellette R, Greenwald S, Kahn JP. Panic disorder and cardiovascular/cerebrovascular problems: results from a community survey. Am J Psychiatry 1990; 147:1504–1508.

106. George MS, Lydiard RB. Case report: inability to walk as a symptom of panic disorder. Neuropsychiatry Neuropsychol Behav Neurol 1989; 2(3):219–223.

107. Jacob RG, Moller MB, Turner SM, Wall C III. Otoneurological examination of panic disorder and agoraphobia with panic attacks: a pilot study. Am J Psychiatry 1985; 142:715–720.

108. Sklare DA, Stein MB, Pikus AM, Uhde TW. Dysequilibrium and audiovestibular function in panic disorder: symptom profiles and test findings. Am J Otol 1990; 11:338–341.

109. Swinson RP, Cox BJ, Rutka J, Mai M, Kerr S, Juch K. Otoneurological functioning in panic disorder patients with prominent dizziness. Comp Psychiatry 1993; 34:127–129.

110. Yardley L, Luxon L, Bird J, Lear S, Britton J. Vestibular and posturographic test results in people with symptoms of panic and agoraphobia. J Audiolog Med 1994; 3:48–65.

111. Yardley L, Britton J, Lear S, Bird J, Luxon LM. Relationship between balance system function and agoraphobic avoidance. Behav Res Ther 1995; 33:435–439.

112. Jacob RG, Furman JM, Durrant JD, Turner SM. Panic, agoraphobia, and vestibular dysfunction. Am J Psychiatry 1996; 153:503–512.

113. Margraf J, Taylor CB, Ehlers A, Roth WT, Agras WS. Panic attacks in the natural environment. J Nerv Ment Dis 1987; 175:558–565.

114. Drachman DA, Hart CW. An approach to the dizzy patients. Neurology 1982; 22:323–330.

115. Simpson RB, Nedzelski JM, Barber HD, Thomas MR. Psychiatric diagnosis in patients with psychogenic dizziness or severe tinnitus. J Otolaryngol 1988; 17:325–330.

116. Clark DB, Leslie MI, Jacob RG. Balance complaints and panic disorder: a clinical study of panic symptoms in members of a self-help group for balance disorders. J Anxiety Disord 1992; 6:47–53.

117. Frommberger UH, Tettenborn B, Buller R, Benkert O. Panic disorder in patients with dizziness. Arch Intern Med 1994; 154:590–591.

118. Linzer M, Divine GW, Estes NAM. Medically unexplained syncope: relationship to psychiatric illness. Am J Med 1992; 92 (suppl 1A):18S–25S.

119. Walker EA, Katon WJ, Jemelka RP, Roy-Bryne PP. Comorbidity of gastrointestinal complaints, depression, and anxiety in the Epidemiologic Catchment Area Study. Am J Med 1992; 92:S26–S30.

120. Lydiard RB, Greenwald S, Weissman MM, Johnson J, Drossman DA, Ballenger JC. Panic disorder and gastrointestinal symptoms: findings from the NIMH Epidemiologic Catchment Area Project. Am J Psychiatry 1994; 151:64–70.

121. Drossman DA, Sandler RS, McKee DC, Lovitz AJ. Bowel patterns

among subjects not seeking health care. Gastroenterology 1982; 83(3): 529–534.

122. Thompson WG, Heaton KW. Functional bowel disorders in apparently healthy people. Gastroenterology 1980; 79:283–288.

123. Ferguson A, Sircus W, Eastwood MA. Frequency of "functional" gastrointestinal disorders. Lancet 1977; ii:613–614

124. Fielding JF. A year in out-patients with the irritable bowel syndrome. Ir J Med Sci 1977; 146:162–166.

125. Lydiard RB, Laraia MT, Howell EF, Ballenger JC. Can panic disorder present as irritable bowel syndrome? J Clin Psychiatry 1986; 47:470–473.

126. American Psychiatry Association. Diagnostic and Statistical Manual of Mental Disorders. 3rd ed. Washington, DC: American Psychiatric Association Press, 1987.

127. Lydiard RB, Fossey MD, Marsh W, Ballenger JC. Prevalence of psychiatric disorders in patients with irritable bowel syndrome. Psychosomatics 1993; 34:229–234.

128. Walker EA, Roy-Byrne PP, Katon WJ. Irritable bowel syndrome and psychiatric illness. Am J Psychiatry 1990; 147:565–572.

129. Walker EA, Gelfand AN, Gelfand MD, Katon WJ. Psychiatric diagnoses, sexual and physical victimization, and disability in patients with irritable bowel syndrome or inflammatory bowel disease. Psycholog Med 1995; 25:1259–1267.

130. Kinsman RA, Luparello T, O'Banion K, Spector S. Multidimensional analysis of the subjective symptomatology of asthma. Psychosom Med 1973; 35:250–267.

131. Carr RE, Lehrer PM, Rausch L, Hochron SM. Anxiety sensitivity and panic attacks in an asthmatic population. Behav Res Ther 1994; 32: 411–418.

132. Shavitt RG, Gentil V, Mandetta R. The association of panic/agoraphobia and asthma: contributing factors and clinical implications. Gen Hosp Psychiatry 1992; 14:420–423.

133. Yellowlees PM, Alpers JH, Bowden JJ, Bryant GD, Ruffin RE. Psychiatric morbidity in patients with chronic airflow obstruction. Med J Australia 1987; 146:305–307.

134. Perna G, Bertani A, Politi E, Columbo G, Bellodi L. Asthma and panic attacks. Biolog Psychiatry 1997; 42:625–630.

135. Dirks JF, Kinsman RA, Jones NF, Spector SL, Davidson PT, Evans NW. Panic-fear: a personality dimension related to length of hospitalization in respiratory illness. J Asth Res 1977; 14:61–71.

136. Baron C, Marcotte JE. Experience and reason—briefly recorded. Pediatrics 1994; 94:108–110.

137. Karajgi B, Rifkin A, Doddi S, Kolli R. The prevalence of anxiety disorders in patients with chronic obstructive pulmonary disease. Am J Psychiatry 1990; 147:200–201.

138. Smoller JW, Pollack MH, Otto MW, Rosenbaum JF, Kradin RL. Panic, anxiety, dyspnea, and respiratory disease. Theoretical and clinical considerations. Am J Respiratory Crit Care Med 1996; 154:6–17.

139. Spinhoven P, Ros M, Westgeest A, Van Der Does AJ. The prevalence of respiratory disorders in panic disorder, major depressive disorder and V-code patients. Behav Res Ther 1994; 32:647–649.

140. Zandbergen J, Bright M, Pols H, Fernandez I, De Loof C, Griez EJL. Higher lifetime prevalence of respiratory diseases in panic disorder. Am J Psychiatry 1991; 148:1583–1585.

141. Pollack MH, Kradin R, Otto MW, Worthington J, Gould R, Sabatino SA, Rosenbaum JF. Prevalence of panic in patients referred for pulmonary function testing at a major medical center. Am J Psychiatry 1996; 153:110–113.

142. Mullaney JA, Trippett CJ . Alcohol dependence and phobias: clinical description and relevance. Br J Psychiatry 1979; 135:565–573.

143. Jensen CF, Cowley DS, Walker RD. Drug preferences of alcoholic polydrug abusers with and without panic. J Clin Psychiatry 1990; 61:189–191.

144. Kushner MG, Shear KJ, Beitman BD. The relation between alcohol problems and the anxiety disorders. Am J Psychiatry 1990; 147:685–695.

145. Hesselbrock MN, Meyer RE, Keener JJ. Psychopathology in hospitalized alcoholics. Arch Gen Psychiatry 1985; 42:1050–1055.

146. Weiss KJ, Rosenberg DJ. Prevalence of anxiety disorders among alcoholics. J Clin Psychiatry 1985; 46:3–5.

147. Johannessen DJ, Cowley DS, Walker RD, Jensen CF, Parker L. Prevalence, onset, and clinical recognition of panic states in hospitalized male alcoholics. Am J Psychiatry 1989; 146:1201–1203.

148. Cowley DS. Alcohol abuse, substance abuse, and panic disorder. Am J Med 1992; 92(suppl 1A):41S-47S.

149. Roy A, DeJong J, Lamparski, Adinoff B, George T, Moore V, Garrett D, Kerich M, Linnoila M. Mental disorders among alcoholics. Arch Gen Psychiatry 1991; 48:423–427.

150. Reich J, Chaudhry D. Personality of Panic disorder alcohol abusers. J Nerv Ment Dis 1987; 175:224–228.

151. Thyer BA, Parrish RT, Himle J, Cameron OG, Curtis GC, Nesse RM. Alcohol abuse among clinically anxious patients. Behav Res Ther 1986; 24:357–359.

152. Lepola U, Koponen H, Leinonen E. A naturalistic 6-year follow-up study of patients with panic disorder. Acta Psychiatr Scand 1996; 93: 181–183.

153. Kushner MG, Mackenzie TB, Fiszdon J, Valentiner DP, Foa E, Anderson N, Wagensteen D. The effects of alcohol consumption on laboratory-induced panic and state anxiety. Arch Gen Psychiatry 1996; 53: 264–270.

154. Anthony JC, Tien AY, Petronis KR. Epidemiologic evidence on cocaine use and panic attacks. Am J Epidemiol 1989; 129:543–549.

155. Lydiard RB, Brady KT, Howell EF, Malcolm R, Ballenger JC. Lifetime prevalence of anxiety and affective disorders in hospitalized alcoholics. Am J Addictions 1992; 1:325–331.

156. Brady KT, Lydiard RB. The treatment of alcoholics with anxiety disorders. Innovations Clin Pract 1992; 14:75–85.

157. Fava M, Pedrazzi F, Guaraldi GP, Romano G, Genazzani AR, Facchinetti AR, Facchinetti F. Comorbid anxiety and depression among patients with late luteal phase dysphoric disorder. J Anx Disord 1992; 6:325–335.

158. Deci PA, Lydiard RB, Santos AB, Arana GW. Oral contraceptives and panic disorder. J Clin Psychiatry 1992; 53:163–165.

159. Wagner KD, Berenson AB. Norplant-associated major depression and panic disorder. J Clin Psychiatry 1994; 55:478–480.

160. Villeponteaux VA, Lydiard RB, Laraia MT, Stuart GW, Ballenger JC. The effects of pregnancy on pre-existing panic disorder. J Clin Psychiatry 1992; 53:6:201–203.

161. Facchinetti F, Romano G, Fava M, Genaazzani AR. Lactate infusion induces panic attacks in patients with premenstrual syndrome. Psychosom Med 1992; 54:288–296.

162. Harrison WM, Sanberg DP, Gorman J, Fyer M, Nee J, Uy J, Edincott J. Provocation of panic with carbon dioxide inhalation in patients with premenstrual dysphoria. Psychiatry Res 1989; 27:183–192.

163. Smith S, Rinehart JS, Ruddock VE, Schiff I. Treatment of premenstrual syndrome with alprazolam: results of a double-blind, placebo-controlled, randomized crossover clinical trial. Obstet Gynecol 1987; 70: 37–43.

164. Ballenger JC, Burrows G, DuPont RL Jr., Lesser IM, Noyes R Jr., Pecknold JC, Rifkin A, Swinson RP. Alprazolam in panic disorder and ago-

raphobia: results from a multicenter trial. I. Efficacy in short term treatment. Arch Gen Psychiatry 1988; 45:413–422.

165. Taylor CB, Arnow B. The Nature and Treatment of Anxiety Disorders. New York: The Free Press, 1988.

166. Sheehan DV, Sheehan KH. The classification of anxiety and hysterical states. I. Historical review and empirical delineation. J Clin Psychopharmacol 1982; 1:235–244.

167. Liskow B, Othmer E, Penich EC. Briquet's syndrome: a heterogenous disorder? Am J Psychiatry 1986; 143:626–629.

168. Noyes R, Reich J. Clancey J, O'Gorman TW. Reduction in hypochondriasis with treatment of panic disorder. Br J Psychiatry 1986; 149: 631–635.

169. Fava GA, Kellner R, Zielezny M, Grandi S. Hypochondriacal fears and beliefs in agoraphobia. J Affect Disord 1988; 14:239–244.

170. Lesser IM, Rubin RT, Pecknold JC, Rifkin A, Swinson RP, Lydiard RB, Burrows GD, Noyes R Jr, Dupont RL Jr. Secondary depression in panic disorder and agoraphobia. I. Frequency, severity and response to treatment. Arch Gen Psychiatry 1988; 45:437–443.

171. Lesser IM, Rubin RT, Rifkin A, Swinson RP, Ballenger JC, Burrows GD, Dupont RL, Noyes R, Pecknold JC. Second depression in panic disorder and agoraphobia. II. Dimensions of depressive symptomatology and their response to treatment. J Affect Disord 1989; 16:49–58.

172. Ballenger JC. Comorbidity of panic and depression. Int Clin Psychopharmacol, 1997. In press.

173. Ballenger JC. Panic disorder in the medical setting. J Clin Psychiatry 1997; 58(suppl 2):13–17.

174. Boulenger JP, Uhde TW, Wolff EA, Post RM. Increased sensitivity to caffeine in patients with panic disorders. Gen Psychiatry 1984; 41: 1067–1071.

175. George DT, Zerby A, Nobel S, Nutt, DJ. Panic effects in alcohol withdrawal: can subjects differentiate the symptoms? Biolog Psychiatry 1988; 24:240–243.

176. Hillard JR, Viewig WVR. Marked sinus tachycardia resulting from the synergistic effects of marijuana and nortriptyline. Am J Psychiatry 1983; 140:626–627.

177. Beaconsfield P, Ginsberg J, Rainsbury R. Marijuana smoking: cardiovascular effects in man and possible mechanisms. N Engl J Med 1972; 287:209–212.

178. Aaronson TA, Craig TJ. Cocaine precipitation of panic disorder. Am J Psychiatry 1986; 143:643–645.
179. Lindemann CG, Zitrin CM, Klein DF. Thyroid dysfunction in phobic patients. Psychosomatics 1984; 25:603–606.
180. Beitman BD, Mukerji V, Russell JL, Grafing M. Panic disorder in cardiology patients: a review of the Missouri Panic/Cardiology Project. J Psychiatr Res 1993; 27(suppl 1):35–46.
181. Permutt MA. Is it really hypoglycemia? If so, what should you do? Medical Times 1980; 108:35–43.
182. Ford CV, Bray GA, Swerdloff RS. A psychiatric study of patients referred with a diagnosis of hypoglycemia. Am J Psychiatry 1976; 133: 290–294.
183. Klerman GL, Weissman MM, Ouellette R, Johnson J, Greenwald S. Panic attacks in the community: social morbidity and health care utilization. JAMA 1991; 265:742–746.
184. Pincus HA. Patient oriented models for linking primary care and mental health care. Gen Hosp Psychiatry 1987; 9:95–101.
185. Eisenberg L. Treating depression and anxiety in primary care: closing the gap between knowledge and practice. N Engl J Med 1992; 326: 1080–1084.
186. Sharfstein SS, Stoline AM, Goldman HH. Psychiatric care and health insurance reform. Am J Psychiatry 1993; 150:7–18.
187. Daniels ML, Linn LS, Ward N, Leake B. A study of physician preferences in the management of depression in the general medical setting. Gen Hosp Psychiatry 1986; 8:229–235.
188. Callahan CM, Nienaber NA, Hendrie HC, Tierney WM. Depression in elderly outpatients: primary care physicians attitudes and practice patterns. J Gen Intern Med 1992; 7(1):26–31.
189. Barlow DH, Craske MG. Mastery of Your Anxiety and Panic. Albany: State University of New York Press, 1992.
190. Anxiety Disorders of America, 6000 Executive Blvd, Rockville, MD.
191. Ballenger JC. Panic disorder: efficacy of current treatments. Psychopharmacol Bull 1993; 29:477–486.
192. Mavissakalian MR, Perel JM. Clinical experiments in maintenance and discontinuation of imipramine therapy in panic disorder with agoraphobia. Arch Gen Psychiatry 1992; 49(4):318–323.
193. Ballenger JC, Lydiard RB, Turner SM. Panic disorder and agoraphobia. In: Gabbard GO, ed. Treatments of Psychiatric Disorders. 2nd ed. Washington, DC: American Psychiatric Press, 1995; 1421–1452.

194. National Institute of Mental Health Panic Disorder Consensus Confer-
      ence. Washington, DC, Sept 25, 1991.
195. Taylor CB, Hayward C, King R, Ehlers A, Margraf PJ, Maddock R,
      Clark D, Roth WT, Agras S. Cardiovascular and symptomatic reduction
      effects of alprazolam and imipramine in patients with panic disorder:
      results of a double-blind, placebo-controlled trial. J Clin Psychophar-
      macol 1990; 10:112–118.

2

The Longitudinal Course of Panic Disorder

Mark H. Pollack

Massachusetts General Hospital
and Harvard Medical School
Boston, Massachusetts

INTRODUCTION

The ongoing development and application of a wide range of pharmacological and cognitive-behavioral interventions for the treatment of panic has underscored the importance of understanding the longitudinal course of the disorder. Knowledge about the course of panic disorder informs patients and clinicians regarding the likely acute and long-term response to treatment, potential for sustained recovery or relapse, and outcome after treatment discontinuation. Information on course may help in the rational development of targeted treatment strategies for different patient subtypes, highlight patients at particular risk for acute and long-term difficulties, identify those who might benefit from time-limited versus ongoing maintenance treatment, and contribute to our understanding of the impact of treatment on normative course and recovery. In this chapter, we review converging lines of evidence from a number of sources including early studies of the course of anxiety disorders, long-term follow-up of treated patients, and recent naturalistic, longitudinal studies examining the course of panic disorder. We then discuss a developmental model of panic disorder that provides a context for understanding the apparent chronic course of panic disorder experienced by many patients.

EARLY FOLLOW-UP STUDIES OF ANXIETY PATIENTS

A number of studies examined the long-term outcome of anxiety patients prior to the widespread use of pharmacological and behavioral treatments for panic disorder (1–8). These studies likely included many patients with panic disorder, although the diagnostic nomenclature predating the DSM-III criteria included terms such as "anxiety state" or "anxiety neurosis," making determination of the exact proportion of panic patients difficult. However, given this limitation, at follow-up of up to 20 years, a substantial proportion (41–59%) of the anxious patients followed remained symptomatic, consistent with later studies of panic patients utilizing more recent diagnostic categories.

FOLLOW-UP STUDIES IN THE TREATMENT OF PANIC DISORDER

Examination of studies reporting on the long-term outcome of patients treated for panic disorder are consistent with the notion that most patients, even if improved after initiating treatment, remain at least somewhat symptomatic. Roy-Byrne and Cowley (9) reviewed published studies examining the outcome of panic patients 6 months to 7 years after treatment initiation. Most of the studies reviewed reflect the use of tricyclic antidepressants (TCAs), monoamine oxidase inhibitors (MAOIs), or high-potency benzodiazepines for panic disorder, and predate the widespread application of selective serotonin-reuptake inhibitors (SSRIs) for this indication. In their review, the authors emphasized that assessment of panic disorder outcome depends, to a large extent, on the outcome measure examined. For instance, while panic-free rates at follow-up are in the range of 30 to 80%, response rates fall when other outcome domains (including phobic anxiety and avoidance, generalized anxiety, functional impairment, and global status) are examined. For instance, resolution of phobic avoidance occurs in only 31% of patients, with 50% of patients remaining functionally impaired.

Follow-up studies of patients receiving antidepressants, high-potency benzodiazepines, and cognitive-behavioral therapies are consistent with the assertion that panic disorder is frequently chronic; although most patients improve with treatment, relatively few are persistently fully well over the long term. In one study of patients receiving initial treatment with a TCA, two-thirds of patients discontinued their medication during the mean follow-up period of 2.5 years (range 1–4 years); half of the patients discontinuing their treatment did so because of side effects (10). At follow-up, two-thirds of patients were on some medication. Three-quarters of the patients had experienced at least moderate levels of improvement, but only 14% were free of symptoms. In another study, 59% of panic patients remained symptomatic 3 years after participation in a placebo-controlled trial of diazepam and alprazolam (11).

Similarly, a naturalistic study of patients participating in an 8-month placebo-controlled trial of alprazolam and imipramine reported that about half of the patients continued to receive medication at 2-year follow-up; initial treatment assignment to alprazolam, imipramine, or placebo was not differentially predictive of the likelihood of remaining on medication. Although 70% of patients treated naturalistically were panic-free when assessed at follow-up, other components of the panic disorder syndrome were not assessed (12).

Katschnig et al. (13) reported a 4-year (range 2–6 years) follow-up of 367 patients who participated in the Cross National Collaborative Panic Study of alprazolam and imipramine. At follow-up, 50% of the patients were still taking medication. Patient outcome varied, with 31% recovering and staying well, 50% achieving an intermediate response characterized by recurrent or mild to moderate symptomatology, and 19% experiencing a more severe, chronic course. Here again, the type of medication received during the initial treatment trial did not differentially predict outcome at follow-up.

Other follow-up studies report similar results. For instance, in a 1.5-year follow-up of patients treated in a placebo-controlled trial of alprazolam and clonazepam, 40% of patients remained symptomatic and 78% remained on medication (14). Similarly, 70% of patients receiving an initial 4-month trial of alprazolam and behavior therapy remained on medication at 2- to 3-year follow-up, as did 50% of patients treated in similar fashion with imipramine and behavior therapy (15,16). Forty-three to 61% of the alprazolam and imipramine-treated patients, respectively, were in remission at follow-up.

These studies, following benzodiazepine-treated patients over time, generally report a reduction in doses, allaying concerns about dose escalation. However, the fact that benzodiazepine doses remain the same—or are actually reduced—despite many patients' remaining at least somewhat symptomatic raises the question of whether continued dosing at acute levels or an increase in dose may have proved more beneficial for some patients.

Conversely, some follow-up studies of patients treated with TCAs suggest that robust responders to acute therapy with imipramine maintain benefit at lower doses over the maintenance period (16–18). However, in the study by Mavissakalian and Perel (17,18), reduction in imipramine dose occurred only after patients had achieved a rigorously defined state of remission. Comparable data addressing this issue for SSRI-treated patients are not currently available.

Although concern about discontinuation-related difficulties has centered on benzodiazepine therapy, in the study of imipramine-treated patients by Noyes and colleagues (19) more than half of the patients receiving a TCA who experienced at least moderate improvement during treatment relapsed when attempting discontinuation of the antidepressant; most relapses occurred within the first 2 months after discontinuation. Only a quarter of the patients who successfully discontinued antidepressant treatment remained in remission for 2 years or longer, underscoring the high rate of relapse following even successful acute antidepressant treatment for panic disorder and suggesting the need for long-term maintenance therapy for many patients.

Similarly, in a report by Nagy and colleagues (16), over half of panic patients attempting discontinuation of imipramine experienced increased anxiety during or after taper, and more than half were unable to discontinue the medication. The authors of this study note that patient expectations may have played a role in exacerbating discontinuation-related difficulties, as patients were not blind to their taper status. Previous reports of significant symptoms emerging during sham benzodiazepine withdrawal and during placebo discontinuation ("pseudo-withdrawal") (11,20) are consistent with the assertion that cognitive factors contribute to discontinuation difficulties and lend increased credence to reports of the usefulness of cognitive-behavioral strategies for facilitating benzodiazepine discontinuation (21,22).

FOLLOW-UP OF PATIENTS TREATED WITH COGNITIVE-BEHAVIORAL THERAPY

Although some data suggest a favorable long-term course of patients receiving acute treatment with cognitive-behavioral therapy (CBT) for panic disorder, other studies suggest that CBT-treated patients, although improved with treatment, may also experience recurrent symptomatology and the need for ongoing treatment.

Clark and colleagues (23) compared imipramine at a mean dose of 233 mg/day, cognitive therapy, and applied relaxation in which patients were seen weekly for the first 3 months. Imipramine was discontinued after the 6-month assessment, at which point cognitive therapy and imipramine-treated patients were both experiencing more relief than those who had received applied relaxation. However, at 15-month follow-up, fewer patients who had been treated acutely with cognitive therapy had relapsed, suggesting a longer duration of effect from the acute treatment trial of cognitive therapy compared to medication treatment. However, as patients are rarely treated with brief trials of antidepressant therapy for panic disorder prior to discontinuation, the relevance of this study for clinical practice is limited.

Other follow-up studies of CBT have reported that over three-quarters of patients remain panic-free at 1.5- to 2-year follow-up, but that 30–50% continue to have other symptoms of the panic disorder syndrome, including agoraphobia and functional impairment (23–25). Brown and Barlow (26) reported on a 2-year follow-up of patients receiving an acute CBT intervention; 75% of patients were panic-free and 57% exhibited high endstate functioning when assessed cross-sectionally over the follow-up period. However, they noted that assessment of outcome depends, in part, on the period of observation and criteria for evaluation. For instance, only 21% of patients maintained high endstate functioning and required no further treatment over a 2-year period following acute CBT treatment. The results of this follow-up study underscores the need for a longitudinal perspective in assessing patients' response to CBT, as well as pharmacotherapy. Although both treatment modalities are acutely effective, a relative minority of patients treated with either intervention experience sustained and complete remission without the need for additional treatment.

DISCONTINUATION OF PHARMACOTHERAPY

Discontinuation of antidepressants or benzodiazepine therapy for panic disorder is frequently associated with withdrawal symptomatology and relapse (10,15,16,27). Patients discontinuing benzodiazepines tend to have acute difficulties, with reported rates of panic-attack recurrence of 49–74% (28–30). In a study by Noyes et al. (28), almost two-thirds of patients on alprazolam were unsuccessful in discontinuing their medication, and over half reported anxiety symptoms that were as bad or worse during discontinuation than prior to treatment. Gradual taper and use of long half-life agents may reduce the discontinuation-associated difficulties of benzodiazepines in clinical practice (31–33). However, a study by Schweizer and colleagues (34) comparing gradual versus abrupt discontinuation of panic disorder patients on benzodiazepines reported that 32% of the patients treated with long half-life benzodiazepines and 42% of those on short half-life benzodiazepines were not able to complete discontinuation even with gradual taper. More severely ill patients at baseline (i.e., greater number of panic attacks and duration of illness) experienced more difficulty with benzodiazepine taper (12).

Although there are no definitive data that answer the question of whether patients who successfully discontinue treatment for panic disorder and later relapse will respond as well to the second or third course of treatment, a small study (35) suggests that patients who relapse after imipramine discontinuation can be successfully retreated, although it may take longer to achieve remission in the subsequent treatment trial than during the initial treatment episode. Cognitive-behavioral strategies that reduce withdrawal symptomatology and provide patients with alternative strategies to use if anxiety symptoms return either during or after discontinuation have demonstrated robust efficacy in reducing withdrawal-associated distress and may prevent relapse for some patients following discontinuation (22,36).

LONGITUDINAL STUDIES OF PANIC DISORDER

At least two systematic, prospective studies of panic disorder have reported information relevant to the understanding of the longitudinal course of illness. In the Harvard Anxiety Research Program (HARP) study, which followed patients with a variety of anxiety disorders treated naturalistically in different settings, panic patients had a 39% probability of achieving remission (at least 2 months symptom-free) at 1-year follow-up; those with panic disorder and agoraphobia had only a 17% likelihood of remission (37). Of those achieving remission, approximately one-third eventually relapsed. The HARP study also demonstrated undertreatment of anxiety patients with pharmacotherapy as well as the relatively low rate at which patients receive CBT (38). It should be noted, however, that most of the information derived from this study refers to the period before the widespread use of SSRIs for panic and other anxiety disorders; we would expect that the favorable side-effect profile of the SSRIs may make it easier for patients to achieve therapeutic doses in general clinical practice, although this hypothesis requires empirical validation. Overall, undertreatment with medication and lack of utilization of CBT may have contributed to the high rates of chronicity of panic disorder observed in this study and underscores the need for comprehensive and aggressive treatment of these disorders.

In the Massachusetts General Hospital Longitudinal Study of Panic Disorder (39), 40% of the 250 patients followed experienced at least one period of remission (2 months symptom-free); however, close to 60% of those remitting experienced relapse during a 2-year period. Predictors of relapse included measures of increased severity (i.e., panic attacks, phobic avoidance, and global severity of illness) as well as anxiety sensitivity. Consistent with other reports (23), patients receiving CBT appeared to sustain remission for relatively longer periods of time (40).

In both the longitudinal studies cited above, the duration of illness prior to intake was more than 10 years, and findings for the studies were consistent with the assertion that the typical course of panic disorder is characterized by prolonged periods of illness and frequent relapse following remission. However, naturalistic studies do not control treatment intensity or duration, making it difficult to assess the impact of treatment intensity on maintenance of remission. For instance, patients who do not achieve acute benefit with standard doses of treatment may have their dose raised by their clinician; this may then lead to the impression from naturalistic observation that higher doses of pharmacotherapy are associated with poorer response to treatment. A relatively small study by Mavissakalian and Perel (17) suggested that longer-term treatment (18 months versus 6 months) following remission in patients treated with antidepressants resulted in a lower rate of relapse after discontinuation, although the follow-up period following discontinuation was only 6 months. A follow-up study of patients treated with the SSRI paroxetine reported a sixfold increase in relapse for patients discontinued after 6 months of treatment, compared to those who remained on the SSRI (30% vs. 5%) (41).

In another study by Mavissakalian and Perel (18), a group of patients who remitted during a 6-month trial of imipramine (mean dose 168 mg/day) remained well during a 1-year maintenance phase in which doses were reduced by 50%, suggesting that lower-dose TCA therapy may be adequate to maintain remission in patients responding robustly to acute full-dose therapy. However, it is important to emphasize that patients in this study met strict criteria for remission prior to dose reductions. Similar data addressing this issue do not currently exist for SSRIs, the antidepressant agents now most commonly used as first-line treatments for panic disorder.

Different aspects of the panic disorder syndrome may require varying time periods for response. In one study of patient treated with TCAs (42), panic attacks remitted over a 3- to 9-month period, while 1.5 to 2 years was necessary for patients to become free of anticipatory anxiety. In a report from a placebo-controlled trial of imipramine and alprazolam in patients with panic disorder and comorbid depression (43), the degree of phobic avoidance was a negative predictor of response at 4, but not 16 weeks, suggesting that phobic avoidance may require months to respond fully. Resolution of anticipatory anxiety, phobic anxiety, and avoidance may occur only after patients test the protective antipanic effects of medication and other interventions while exposing themselves to feared situations. Consistent with this hypothesis, CBT and even self-directed exposure instructions enhance the effect of antidepressants for panic disorder (44).

A DEVELOPMENTAL MODEL OF PANIC DISORDER

While most patients remain at least somewhat symptomatic after acute and follow-up treatment, some do experience sustained benefit following treatment discontinuation. Consistent with this hypothesis, the degree of symptomatology at follow-up in some studies is not related to whether patients remained on medication (12,15,16). Differences in outcome may, to some extent, reflect differences in patient characteristics and the natural course of the illness. Patients whose course of illness is characterized by time-limited episodes of panic and more enduring remissions may remain panic-free following medication discontinuation after successful acute treatment. Those whose course involves frequent relapses may suffer from a more chronic form of illness requiring ongoing medication treatment to sustain benefits. Patients with an anxiety diathesis, characterized in part by inhibited temperament or frank anxiety disorders in childhood, may be most likely to experience a chronic form of panic disorder. Supporting this assertion, patients with a childhood history of anxiety difficulties are more likely to experience higher rates of phobic avoidance, anxiety sensitivity, and mood and anxiety comorbidity, characteristics associated with chronicity and relapse in panic disorder patients (45).

Review of treatment follow-up studies and longitudinal examinations of the course of panic disorder are consistent with the notion that panic disorder is chronic for many affected patients who thus may require ongoing maintenance therapy to maintain benefit. A diathesis model for panic disorder positing a constitutional predisposition for anxiety manifesting early in childhood and variably expressed over time provides a useful perspective in understanding the apparent chronicity of the disorder demonstrated in longitudinal studies. A variety of patient characteristics associated with early expression of anxiety difficulties—including degree of agoraphobia, anxiety sensitivity, and presence of comorbid anxiety and affective and personality disorders—all confer a poorer treatment response and increased chronicity in affected panic disorder patients (45). Converging lines of evidence suggest that panic disorder in adulthood may represent one manifestation of an underlying constitutional vulnerability or diathesis for anxiety that is familial, related to both genetic and environmental factors, expressed early in life in the form of fearful and inhibited temperament or childhood anxiety disorders, and variably expressed over the life cycle.

The assertion that panic disorder is familial is supported by family and twin studies of the disorder (46,57). Studies demonstrate elevated rates of anxiety disorders in the children of adult patients with anxiety disorders (48,49) and the parents of children with anxiety disorders (50,51). However, whether the familial transmission is for a specific disorder or for a general predisposition to pathological anxiety remains unresolved. In a twin study examining over 1000 female twin pairs, concordance for panic disorder was twice that in monozygotic, as compared to dizygotic twins, consistent with a genetic contribution to the familial transmission of panic disorder (52). Of interest, however, further analysis from this study revealed that genetic factors accounted for only 30–40% of the familial transmission of panic, with much of the other variance being due to nongenetic, including presumably environmental, factors. The importance of genetics in the transmission of panic across generations may be similar to that described for depression by Kendler and colleagues (53), who noted that genetic factors may make individuals more sensitive to the negative impact of stressful life events and other environmental factors and influence the nature of pathological reactions to these stressors.

A large proportion of patients with panic disorder report a significant life event in the year prior to onset of panic (54), consistent with the notion that genetically vulnerable individuals may have onset of disorder triggered by stressful environmental factors. In one report (55), panic disorder patients with a childhood history of multiple childhood anxiety disorders were significantly more likely to report a negative life event antecedent to the onset of their panic disorder than individuals without evidence of early anxiety difficulties. Vulnerable individuals manifesting early difficulties with anxiety may be particularly reactive to the adverse impact of stressful life events. However, whether anxiety-prone individuals are actually more likely to experience adverse environmental events, or just more likely to react negatively to events that do occur, remains unclear.

Many patients with panic disorder report that their parents were physically overprotective and yet emotionally distant (56,57); such a parenting style may predispose to the development of agoraphobia in vulnerable children by reinforcing phobic patterns of avoidance, and failing to provide the emotional support and nurturing necessary to face feared situations. Whether this type of parenting truly characterizes the upbringing of many children who later develop panic disorder awaits prospective study, but this conceptualization does provide support for early intervention strategies aimed at teaching the parents of at-risk children how to appropriately manage their anxious offspring, and identifies themes that may be fruitfully explored in therapy.

TEMPERAMENT AND THE DEVELOPMENT OF PATHOLOGICAL ANXIETY

Animal models, including work with primates, are useful in exploring the relative and interactive contributions of genetics and environmental factors to the development and persistence of pathological anxiety. For example, consistent with a heritable component to anxiety, Suomi (58) identified a subgroup of rhesus monkeys characterized by fearful temperament and hyperreactivity who gave birth to similarly affected offspring. Primates reared under conditions of separation, insecurity, and stress manifest persistent anxiety (59,60). Adverse developmental experiences during infancy may have long-term effects on central noradrenergic and serotonergic systems, setting the stage for the subsequent development of anxiety and affective disorders, and altering pharmacological responsivity (61). These animal studies support the idea that an interaction between genetic and environmental factors influences the development of anxiety disorders.

A parallel line of investigation in humans has examined behavior-

ally inhibited temperament in children, including focus on the presentation and course of children at risk (i.e., the offspring of adult anxiety
patients) (62,63). Behavioral inhibition (BI) is a laboratory-based temperamental construct characterized by irritability and colic in infancy
and shyness, fearfulness, and the tendency to constrict behavior in
novel or unfamiliar situations during childhood (64). Inhibited children
develop higher rates of anxiety disorders than nonfearful children, with
rates increasing with age, consistent with the notion of an underlying
anxiety diathesis with increasing expression over time (65). Behaviorally inhibited children also experience higher rates of non-anxiety disorders, suggesting that the early expression of this fearful temperament
may reflect a generalized vulnerability to the development of psychopathology (66).

Children of parents with anxiety disorders are more likely to manifest behavioral inhibition (63), and parents of BI children have increased rates of childhood and adult anxiety disorders (particularly
panic disorder and social phobia), consistent with the notion that BI in
children is linked to a familial predisposition to anxiety disorders.
While the definitive establishment of a link between BI in childhood
and expression of panic disorder in adulthood awaits long-term, prospective studies, the data available to date do strongly suggest this link.
However, not all children identified as behaviorally inhibited early on
remain so over time (67). In one study, 70% of BI children were free
of anxiety disorders at follow-up (68), suggesting that other factors
may influence the emergence of pathological anxiety through time. The
primate work cited earlier (58–60), as well as reports of increased rates
of adverse life stressors in panic patients in general (54) and those with
early anxiety difficulties in particular (55), point to the potential importance of early developmental experiences in shaping neural substrates
and the presentation of symptomatology throughout the life cycle in
individuals genetically predisposed to anxiety. Behavioral inhibition
and other manifestations of fearful temperament expressed early in life
may reflect a general predisposition to anxiety, with a variety of genetic, familial, psychosocial, and psychological factors determining
whether an individual develops pathological anxiety and the way in
which this anxiety is expressed.

Retrospective reports by adult anxiety patients also support a link between childhood and adult psychopathology. Between 20 and 40% of patients with panic disorder report that they had their first panic attack before age 20 (69–71), with up to 11% reporting the onset of panic before the age of 10 (70,71). While earlier reports suggested a specific link between separation anxiety in childhood and adult panic disorder (72), this concept has since been broadened to include a more general link between pathological anxiety during childhood and adulthood (48,73–75). Although there is relatively limited information on how a childhood history of anxiety affects the latter course of anxiety disorders, a number of studies (48, 76,77) report that adult patients with panic disorder and agoraphobia with a childhood history of anxiety disorders tend to have an earlier age of symptom onset and more severe presentation.

In the Massachusetts General Hospital Longitudinal Study of Panic Disorder (39,78), over half of adult panic patients reported having had at least one anxiety disorder during childhood. A history of childhood anxiety (including separation anxiety, overanxious disorder, social phobia, and avoidant disorder) was associated with increased rates of comorbid adult anxiety disorders, personality disorders, and affective disorders, particularly depression, and anxiety sensitivity. These factors were generally associated with a more chronic course of panic disorder in adulthood. For instance, 68% of patients with comorbid anxiety disorders had a history of childhood anxiety. Adult disorders tended to be manifestations of persistent childhood difficulties (25). Patients with childhood anxiety experienced more agoraphobia as adults, suggesting that early anxiety experience contributed to patterns of avoidance through adulthood. Examination of the longitudinal course of naturalistically treated panic patients suggests that a history of childhood anxiety disorders does not independently affect the likelihood of remission in patients naturalistically treated over time, but is linked to increased agoraphobic avoidance and comorbidity, which are critical determinants of chronicity (45). Thus, early intervention efforts in children with anxiety disorders directed at the reduction of avoidance and prevention of comorbidity may improve the course of anxiety in adulthood.

In summary, a growing body of evidence supports the hypothesis that some individuals with panic disorder have an underlying anxiety diathesis, often first expressed in childhood and leading to an increased risk of comorbid disorders, phobic avoidance, and chronic course of illness during adulthood. This model may help explain the persistence of symptoms and chronicity observed in longitudinal studies of panic disorder patients and the high rates of relapse seen after treatment. The developmental model of panic disorder suggests the importance of early identification of individuals predisposed to anxiety and the possibility that early intervention and treatment of affected individuals in childhood may improve the longitudinal course of illness.

REFERENCES

1. Marks IM, Lader M. Anxiety states (anxiety neurosis): a review. J Nerv Ment Dis 1973; 156:3–18.
2. Blair R, Gilroy JM, Pilkington F. Some observations on outpatient psychotherapy: follow-up on 235 cases. Br Med J 1957; 1:318–321.
3. Eitinger L. Studies in neurosis. Acta Psychiatrica et Neurologica Scandinavica 1955; 30(suppl 101):5–47.
4. Ernst K. Die Propouse der Neurosen. Berlin: Springer-Verlag, 1959.
5. Greer S, Crawley RH. Some observations on the natural history of neurotic illness (Archdall Medical Monograph 3). Sydney: Australian Medical Publishing, 1966.
6. Harris A. The prognosis of anxiety states. Br Med J 1938; 2:649–654.
7. Miles HHW, Barrabes EL, Finesinger JE. Evaluation of psychotherapy: with a follow-up study of 62 cases of anxiety neurosis. Psychosom Med 1951; 13:83–105.
8. Wheeler EO, White PD, Reed EW, et al. Neurocirculatory asthenia (anxiety neurosis, effort syndrome, neurasthenia): a twenty year follow-up study of one hundred and seventy-three patients. JAMA 1950; 142:878–889.
9. Roy-Byrne PP, Cowley DS. Course and outcome in panic disorder: a review of recent follow-up studies. Anxiety 1995; 1:151–160.
10. Noyes R, Garvey M, Cook B. Follow up study of patients with panic attacks treated with tricyclic antidepressants. J Affect Disord 1989; 16: 249–257.
11. Noyes R, Reich J, Christiansen J, Suelzer M, Pfohl B, Coryell WB. Out-

come of panic disorder: relationship to diagnostic subtypes and comorbidity. Arch Gen Psychiatry 1990; 47:809–818.

12. Rickels K, Schweizer E, Weiss S, Zavodnick S. Maintenance drug treatment for panic disorder. II. Short- and long-term outcome after drug taper. Arch Gen Psychiatry 1993; 50:61–68.

13. Katschnig H, Stolk J, Klerman GL. Long-term follow-up of panic disorder. I. Clinical outcome of a large group of patients participating in an international multicenter clinical drug trial. Presented at the 27th Annual Meeting of the American College of Neuropsychopharmacology, San Juan, PR, 1989.

14. Pollack MH, Otto MW, Tesar GE, Cohen LS, Meltzer-Brody S, Rosenbaum JF. Long-term outcome after acute treatment with clonazepam and alprazolam for panic disorder. J Clin Psychopharmacol 1993; 13:257–263.

15. Nagy LM, Krystal JH, Woods SW, Charney DS. Clinical and medication outcome after short-term alprazolam and behavioral group treatment of panic disorder: 2.5 year naturalistic follow-up study. Arch Gen Psychiatry 1989; 46:993–999.

16. Nagy LM, Krystal JH, Charney DS, Merikangas KR, Woods SW. Long-term outcome of panic disorder after short-term imipramine and behavioral group treatment: 2.9 year naturalistic follow-up study. J Clin Psychopharmacol 1993; 13:16–24.

17. Mavissakalian MR, Perel JM. Clinical experiments in maintenance and discontinuation of imipramine therapy in panic disoder with agoraphobia. Arch Gen Psychiatry 1992; 49:318–323.

18. Mavissakalian MR, Perel JM. Protective effects of imipramine maintenance treatment in panic disorder with agoraphobia. Am J Psychiatry 1992; 149:1053–1057.

19. Noyes R, Garvey MJ, Cook BL, Samuelson L. Problems with tricyclic antidepressant use in patients with panic disorder or agoraphobia: results of a naturalistic follow-up study. J Clin Psychiatry 1989; 50:163–169.

20. Tyrer P, Casey P, Gall J. The relationship between neurosis and personality disorder. Br J Psychiatry 1983; 142:404–408.

21. Otto MW, Pollack MH, Meltzer-Brody S, Rosenbaum JF. Cognitive-behavioral therapy for benzodiazepine discontinuation in panic disorder patients. Psychopharmacol Bull 1992; 28:123–130.

22. Spiegel DA, Bruce TJ, Gregg SF, Nuzzarello A. Does cognitive-behavior therapy assist slow-taper alprazolam discontinuation in panic disorder? Am J Psychiatry 1994; 151:876–881.

23. Clark DM, Salkovskis PM, Hackmann A, Middleton H, Anastasiades P, Gelder M. A comparison of cognitive therapy, applied relaxation and imipramine in the treatment of panic disorder. Br J Psychiatry 1994; 164:759–769.

24. Craske MG, Brown TA, Barlow DH. Behavioral treatment of panic: a two-year follow-up. Behav Ther 1991; 22:289–304.

25. Otto MW, Pollack MH, Rosenbaum JF, Sachs GS, Asher RH. Childhood history of anxiety in adults with panic disorder: association with anxiety sensitivity and comorbidity. Harvard Rev Psychiatry 1994; 1:288–293.

26. Brown TA, Barlow DH. Long-term outcome in cognitive-behavioral treatment of panic disorder: Clinical predictors and alternative strategies for assessment. J Consult Clin Psychol 1995; 63:754–765.

27. Noyes R, Garvey MJ, Cook BL, Perry PJ. Benzodiazepine withdrawal: a review of the evidence. J Clin Psychiatry 1988; 40:382–389.

28. Noyes R, Garvey MJ, Cook B, Suelzer M. Controlled discontinuation of benzodiazepine treatment for patients with panic disorder. Am J Psychiatry 1991; 148:517–523.

29. Dupont R, Pecknold J. Alprazolam withdrawal in panic disorder patients. Presented at the 138th Annual Meeting of the American Psychiatric Association, Washington, DC, 1985.

30. Fyer A, Leibowitz M, Gorman J. Discontinuation of alprazolam treatment in panic patients. Am J Psychiatry 1987; 144:303–308.

31. Mellman T, Uhde T. Withdrawal syndrome with gradual tapering of alprazolam. Am J Psychiatry 1986; 143:1464–1466.

32. Pecknold JC, Swinson RP, Kuch K, Lewis CP. Alprazolam in panic disorder and agoraphobia: results from a multicenter trial. III. Discontinuation effects. Arch Gen Psychiatry 1988; 45:429–436.

33. Pollack MH, Otto MW. Long-term phamacological treatment of panic disorder. Psychiatric Ann 1994; 24:291–298.

34. Schweizer E, Rickels K, Case WG, Greenblatt DJ. Long-term therapeutic use of benzodiazepines: effects of gradual taper. Arch Gen Psychiatry 1990; 47: 908–915.

35. Mavissakalian MR, Perel JM, deGroot C. Imipramine treatment of panic disorder with agoraphobia: the second time around. J Psychiatr Res 1993; 27:61–68.

36. Otto MW, Pollack MH, Sachs GS, Reiter SR, Meltzer-Brody S, Rosenbaum JF. Discontinuation of benzodiazepine treatment: efficacy of cognitive-behavioral therapy for patients with panic disorder. Am J Psychiatry 1993; 150:1485–1490.

37. Keller MB, Yonkers KA, Warshaw MG, Pratt LA. Remission and re-

lapse in subjects with panic disorder and panic with agoraphobia: a prospective short-interval naturalistic follow-up. J Nerv Ment Dis 1994; 182:290–296.

38. Goisman RM, Rogers MP, Steketee GS, Warshaw MG, Cuneo P, Keller MB. Utilization of behavioral methods in a multicenter anxiety disorders study. J Clin Psychiatry 1993; 54:213–218.

39. Pollack MH, Otto MW, Rosenbaum JF, Sachs GS, O'Neil C, Asher R, Meltzer-Brody S. Longitudinal course of panic disorder: findings from the Massachusetts General Hospital Naturalistic Study. J Clin Psychiatry 1990; 51:12–16.

40. Otto MW, Pollack MH, Sabatino SA. Maintenance of remission following cognitive-behavior therapy for panic disorder: possible deleterious effects of concurrent medication treatment. Behav Ther 1996; 27:473–482.

41. Burnham DB, Steiner MX, Gergel IP, Oakes R, Bailer DC, Wheadon DE. Paroxetine long-term safety and efficacy in panic disorder and prevention of relapse: a double-blind study. Presented at the American College of Neuropsychopharmacology Meeting, San Juan, PR, Dec 1995.

42. Muskin PR, Fyer AJ. Treatment of panic disorder. J Clin Psychopharmacol 1981; 1:81–90.

43. Pollack MH, Otto MW, Sachs GS, Leon A, Shear MK, Deltito JA, Keller MB, Rosenbaum JF. Anxiety psychopathology predictive of outcome in patients with panic disorder treated with imipramine, alprazolam, and placebo. J Affect Disord 1994; 30:273–281.

44. Mavissakalian MR. Sequential combination of imipramine and self-directed exposure in the treatment of panic disorder with agoraphobia. J Clin Psychiatry 1990; 51:184–188.

45. Pollack MH, Otto MW, Majcher D, Worthington JJ, Sabatino S, Rosenbaum JF. Relationship of childhood anxiety to adult panic disorder: correlates and influence on course. Am J Psychiatry 1996; 153:376–381.

46. Crowe RR, Noyes R, Pauls DL, Slymen D. A family study of panic disorder. Arch Gen Psychiatry 1983; 40:1065–1069.

47. Torgersen S. Genetic factors in anxiety disorders. Arch Gen Psychiatry 1983; 40:1085–1089.

48. Berg I. School phobia in the children of agoraphobic women. Br J Psychiatry 1976; 128:86–89.

49. Weissman MM, Leckman JF, Merikangas KR, Gammon GD, Prosoff BA. Depression and anxiety disorders in parents and children: results from the Yale family study. Arch Gen Psychiatry 1984; 41:845–852.

50. Gittelman-Klein R. Psychiatric characteristics of the relatives of school

phobic children. In: Sanker DVS, eds. Mental Health in Children. New York: PJD, 1975.

51. Last CG, Phillips JE, Statfeld A. Childhood anxiety disorders in mothers and their children. Child Psychiatry Hum Dev 1987; 18:103–112.

52. Kendler KS, Neale MC, Kessler RC, Heath AC, Eaves LJ. Panic disorder in women: a population-based twin study. Psycholog Med 1993; 23: 397–406.

53. Kendler KS, Kessler RC, Walters EE, MacLean C, Neale MC, Heath AC, Eaves LJ. Stressful life events, genetic liability and onset of an episode of major depression in women. Am J Psychiatry 1995; 152:833–842.

54. Roy-Byrne PP, Geraci M, Uhde T. Life events and the onset of panic disorder. Am J Psychiatry 1986; 143:1424–1427.

55. Manfro GG, Otto MW, McArdle ET, Worthington JJ, Rosenbaum JF, Pollack MH. Relationship of antecedent stressful life events to childhood and family history of anxiety and the course of panic disorder. J Affect Disord 1996; 41:135–139.

56. Tucker WI. Diagnosis and treatment of the phobic reaction. Am J Psychiatry 1956; 112:825–830.

57. Perris C, Jacobbson L, Lindström H, von Knorring L, Perris H. Development of a new inventory for assessing memories of parental rearing behavior. Acta Psychiatr Scand 1980; 61:265–274.

58. Suomi SJ. Anxiety-like disorder in young nonhuman primates. In: Gittelman R, eds. Anxiety Disorders in Childhood. New York: Guilford Press, 1986:1–23.

59. Coplan JD, Rosenblum LA, Friedman S, Bassoff JB, Gorman JM. Behavioral effects of oral yohimbine in differentially reared nonhuman primates. Neuropsychopharmacology 1992; 6:31–37.

60. Rosenblum LA, Paully GS. The effects of varying environmental demands on maternal and infant behavior. Child Dev 1984; 55:305–314.

61. Rosenblum LA, Coplan JD, Friedman S. Adverse early experiences affect noradrenergic and serotonergic functioning in adult primates. Biolog Psychiatry 1993; 35:221–227.

62. Kagan J, Reznick JS, Gibbons J. Inhibited and unihibited types of children. Child Dev 1989; 60:838–845.

63. Rosenbaum JF, Biederman J, Gersten M, Hirshfeld Dr, Meminger SR, Herman JB, Kagan J, Reznick JS, Snidman N. Behavioral inhibition in children of parents with panic disorder and agoraphobia: a controlled study. Arch Gen Psychiatry 1988; 45:463–470.

64. Kagan J, Reznick JS, Snidman N. Biological bases of childhood shyness. Science 1988; 240:167–171.

65. Biederman J, Rosenbaum JF, Bolduc-Murphy EA, Faraone SV, Chaloff J, Hirshfeld DR, Kagan J. A three-year follow-up of children with and without behavioral inhibition. J Am Acad Child Adolesc Psychiatry 1993; 32:814–821.

66. Rosenbaum JF, Biederman J, Bolduc-Murphy EA, Faraone SV. Behavioral inhibition in childhood: a risk factor for anxiety disorders. Harvard Rev Psychiatry 1993; 1:2–16.

67. Hirshfeld DR, Rosenbaum JF, Biederman JF, Bolduc EA, Faraone SV, Snidman N, Reznick JS, Kagan J. Stable behavioral inhibition and its association with anxiety disorder. J Am Acad Child Adolesc Psychiatry 1992; 31:103–111.

68. Biederman J, Rosenbaum JF, Hirshfeld DR, Faraone SV, Bolduc EA, Gersten M, Meminger SR, Kagan J, Snidman N, Reznick JS. Psychiatric correlates of behavioral inhibition in young children of parents with and without psychiatric disorders. Arch Gen Psychiatry 1990; 47:21–26.

69. Breier A, Charney DS, Heninger GR. Major depression in patients with agoraphobia and panic disorder. Arch Gen Psychiatry 1984; 41:1129–1135.

70. Thyer BA, Parrish RT, Curtis GC, Nesse RM, Cameron GG. Ages of onset of DSM-III anxiety disorders. Compr Psychiatry 1985; 26:113–122.

71. von Korff MR, Eaton WW, Keyl PM. The epidemiology of panic attacks and panic disorder: results of three community surveys. Am J Hum Epidemiol 1985; 122:970–981.

72. Klein DF. Delineation of two drug responsive anxiety syndromes. Psychopharmacologia 1964; 5:397–408.

73. Aronson T, Logue C. On the longitudinal course of panic disorder: developmental history and predictors of phobic complications. Compr Psychiatry 1987; 28:344–355.

74. Berg I, Marks I, McGuire R, Lipsedge, M. School phobia and agoraphobia. Psycholog Med 1974; 4:428–434.

75. Otto MW, Gould R, Pollack MH. Cognitive-behavioral treatment of panic disorder: considerations of the treatment of patients over the long-term. Psychiatr Ann 1994; 24:299–306.

76. Perugi G, Deltito J, Soriani A, Musetti L, Petracca A, Nisita C, Marenimani I, Cassano GB. Relationships between panic disorder and separation anxiety with school phobia. Compr Psychiatry 1988; 29:98–107.

77. Ayuso JL, Alfonso S, Rivera A. Childhood separation anxiety and panic

disorder: a comparative study. Prog Neuropsychopharmacol Biolog Psychiatry 1989; 13:665–671.

78. Pollack MH, Otto MW, Rosenbaum JF, Sachs GS. Personality disorders in patients with panic disorder: association with childhood anxiety disorders, early trauma, comorbidity and chronicity. Compr Psychiatry 1992; 33:78–83.

Neurobiology of Panic Disorder

Andrew W. Goddard
Yale University School of Medicine
New Haven, Connecticut

Jack M. Gorman
Columbia University
and New York State Psychiatric Institute
New York, New York

Dennis S. Charney
Yale University School of Medicine
and Yale Mental Health Clinical Research Center
New Haven, Connecticut

INTRODUCTION

Biological perspectives on the pathogenesis of panic disorder have rapidly evolved over the past two decades. Particular clinical characteristics of the panic syndrome—including its spontaneous and episodic nature, the occurrence of nocturnal panics, the presence of autonomic symptomatology, its familiality, and its response to select pharmacotherapies—have inspired the search for underlying neurobiological abnormalities. Efforts to elucidate the biological bases of panic have been revitalized by recent developments in neuroimaging and molecular genetics. The clinical application of these powerful new research tools promises to provide new insights into abnormal brain function in human anxiety disorders. In this chapter we review the current evidence implicating neurochemical, neurophysiological, and functional neuroanatomical abnormalities in the pathogenesis of panic disorder. We discuss the clinical relevance of these findings, including implications for successful treatment. Future research directions are also discussed.

NEUROCHEMICAL ABNORMALITIES IN PANIC DISORDER

Noradrenergic Dysfunction

Preclinical Overview

The norepinephrine (NE) transmitter system has long been associated with stress responses in animals and humans, and therefore has been a logical candidate system to study in relation to human panic disorder. Some workers have thought of the NE system as a mediator of fear responses (1). Others, however, have conceptualized the role of the NE system in stress responses as involving enhancement of attentional processes that in turn contribute to adaptive fear responses (2). The NE system has the necessary anatomical connections to assist in the implementation of fear responses to threatening stimuli. Specifically, the locus ceruleus (LC), the major NE-containing nucleus in the mammalian brain, receives afferent information from the sensory systems that monitor the internal and external environments (3) and also sends efferents to multiple brain target areas implicated in anxiety and fear behaviors, such as the amygdala, hippocampus, hypothalamus, cortex, and spinal cord. Furthermore, a link between the NE system and fear behaviors has been established by physiological studies in animals. Electrical stimulation of the LC produced fearlike behaviors in monkeys, while bilateral destructive lesions of this structure were associated with reductions in these behaviors (1). Other studies of NE function in animals indicate that the NE system is stress-responsive, as evidenced by dramatic increases in LC firing following exposure of freely moving cats to dangerous or threatening situations (4). The NE system has also been implicated in other neurophysiological processes such as behavioral sensitization to stress (5) and fear conditioning (6). These properties of the NE system may be highly relevant to understanding aspects of the pathogenesis of panic disorder.

Clinical Studies

There is considerable clinical evidence implicating NE system hyperactivity in the pathophysiology of panic disorder. For example, panic patients are abnormally sensitive to pharmacological challenge with the α_2-adrenoreceptor antagonist yohimbine, with up to two-thirds experiencing panic attacks accompanied by increases in plasma levels of the NE metabolite 3-methoxy-4-hydroxyphenethyleneglycol (MHPG) (7–9). Yohimbine sensitivity is well replicated (10,11) and appears to be a relatively specific biological marker of active panic disorder, the one exception being posttraumatic stress disorder (12). Panic patients also have abnormal responses to challenge with the α_2-agonist clonidine, exhibiting greater hypotension, decreases in plasma MHPG, and less sedation than controls in response to clonidine (13,14). Taken together, these findings implicate presynaptic α_2-receptor dysregulation in the pathophysiology of panic. A hyperadrenergic state in panic disorder is also suggested by the observation of blunted responses of growth hormone (GH) to clonidine (15). It has been postulated that subsensitivity of postsynaptic α_2-receptor occurs secondary to NE hyperactivity in the presynaptic portion of the neuron (16). However, this abnormality is not specific to panic disorder (17). Examining other dimensions of NE function, investigators have found panic patients to be sensitive to isoproterenol challenge, and accordingly have proposed a hypothesis of increased peripheral β-adrenoreceptor sensitivity of panic (18). Another aspect of NE function of potential relevance to fear behaviors is neuropeptide Y (NPY) activity. NPY is colocalized with NE in LC neurons and may act as a neuromodulator of NE function (19). Recent clinical data suggest that plasma NPY levels are abnormally elevated in panic patients, perhaps reflecting a compensatory response to NE system overactivity (20). Another group, however, did not replicate this finding (21).

Clinical Implications

The NE hypothesis of panic disorder provides a useful framework within which to consider a number of clinical issues. The mean age of onset—in the late teens to early 20s—coincides with the estimated completion of neurodevelopment of the brain NE system (22). It has been hypothesized that defects or delays in maturation of the NE system could account for the emergence of symptoms at this time (16). The fact that episodes of panic disorder are commonly triggered by stressful life events (23) is also consistent with what we know about the physiology of the NE system (i.e., that it is a stress-responsive neurotransmitter system). Furthermore, the evolution of agoraphobic symptoms in over 50% of patients with panic might be the result of fear conditioning processes that are partly NE-mediated. The sensitivity of actively panicking patients to psychostimulants (including caffeine), and also to the initiation of tricyclic antidepressants (TCAs), is consistent with the presence of a hyperadrenergic state in panic patients. Also, the age-related "burnout" of clinical symptoms has been postulated to be due to loss of LC/NE neurons with age (24). Another important clinical observation about panic patients is their hypervigilance to internal and external cues that could contribute to panic attacks. This phenomenon may be explained by the NE system's role in attentional processes, as mentioned earlier, and could also be due to the occurrence of parallel activation of the central and peripheral NE systems (25) described in the preclinical literature.

The NE system has also been implicated in the response to successful treatment of panic patients with TCAs and monoamine oxidase inhibitors (MAOIs), agents that directly modulate NE functioning (reviewed in Ref. 16). There is also evidence that other effective antipanic treatments such as benzodiazepines (BZDs) (26) may partly mediate their therapeutic effects by regulating NE system functioning. However, in one study, cognitive-behavioral treatment of panic did not appear to alter one index of abnormal NE function, namely, the blunted GH response to clonidine (27).

While the NE hypothesis of panic has considerable merit, in that it is well grounded in preclinical neuroscience and has led to the identification of specific clues to possible pathogenic mechanisms in patients, it has limitations. For instance, studies of panic patients undergoing phobic exposure (28) and lactate-induced panic protocols (29) detected no significant change in plasma levels of the NE metabolite MHPG. Also, clonidine administration only partially blocked lactate-induced panic (30), suggesting that other pathological mechanisms beyond the NE system account for lactate sensitivity. Further, chronic treatment with the antipanic agent imipramine, which significantly decreases NE function, did not block yohimbine-induced panic (31). Finally, genetic linkage of the $\alpha_{1,2}$- and $\beta_{1,2}$-adrenoreceptors to panic disorder has not been established (32).

5-HT Dysfunction

Preclinical Overview

The serotonin (5-HT) neuronal system originates primarily from two groups of brainstem nuclei: the median and dorsal raphe nuclei (33). There are extensive cortical and subcortical projections from these nuclei. Earlier thinking that 5-HT neurons might mediate fear responses in a unitarian fashion has been rejected. In general, the recent animal literature suggests that the 5-HT system responds acutely to threat with increases in 5-HT function. This pattern of response to stress by the 5-HT system (particularly in cortical areas) has been postulated to lead to enhancement of information processing concerning the threatening stimulus (34). There is also evidence that 5-HT neurons may have a restraining effect on brainstem structures implicated in panic responses (e.g., the periaqueductal gray area) (reviewed in Ref. 35). Disruption of this restraining influence may precipitate a panic episode. Another important characteristic of the 5-HT system is the many 5-HT-receptor types now known to exist. Several of these (5-HT$_3$, 5-HT$_{1A}$, and 5-HT$_{2A}$) have been closely implicated in fear behaviors in animals and, as a consequence, have been the target for recent anxiolytic drug development efforts (36).

Clinical Studies

There have been a number of clinical studies of 5-HT function in panic disorder, which have produced mixed results. The 5-HT-releasing agent fenfluramine is anxiogenic in panic patients, but tends to increase generalized or anticipatory anxiety rather than true panic (37). Examination of postsynaptic 5-HT-receptor function in panic disorder with the mixed 5-HT agonist/antagonist m-chlorophenylpiperazine (m-CPP) has produced equivocal results (38,39). Thus, the status of postsynaptic 5-HT-receptor sensitivity in panic disorder needs further clarification.

In addition, acute up- (40) or down- (41) modulation of presynaptic function did not provoke anxiety symptoms in panic patients, consistent with normal presynaptic 5-HT function in panic. Other work, with the selective 5-HT$_{1A}$ partial agonist ipsapirone, has implicated 5-H$_{1A}$-receptor subsensitivity in the disorder (42). In conclusion, there is currently no well-replicated abnormality in 5-HT function that constitutes a biological marker for panic disorder.

Clinical Implications

While the role of the 5-HT system in the pathophysiology of panic requires further elucidation, the role of 5-HT in the treatment of the disorder is well established. The antipanic efficacy of the selective serotonin-reuptake inhibitors (SSRIs) has been consistently reported in the worldwide literature over the last decade (43). There is some evidence that the SSRIs may even be superior to other standard antipanic medications, including the TCA imipramine and the BZD alprazolam (44). The therapeutic mechanisms of SSRIs in panic have been closely examined in recent years. Chronic SSRI administration is thought to result in a net increase in 5-HT neurotransmission via desensitization of the somatodendritic and terminal autoreceptors (45–47). Abnormalities in 5-HT regulation in panic disorder are presumably stabilized or controlled by this mechanism. Empirical data also support the notion that SSRIs may exert part of their therapeutic action by 5-HT/NE (48,49) or 5-HT/CCK interactions (50), or augmented 5-HT control of a brainstem suffocation-alarm mechanism (51). Following up on the outstanding success of SSRIs in controlling pathological anxiety, one group recently reported that trait-anxiety in humans was partially related to a polymorphism in the 5-HT transporter gene regulatory region (52). It will be of interest in the future to see if genes coding for the 5-HT transporter or receptors are specifically abnormal in panic disorder.

Lactate and CO_2 Metabolism and Panic

Overview

The literature in this area evolved from early observations by Cohen and White (53) that neurotic patients had exaggerated plasma lactate responses to exercise and were also sensitive to exposure to 4% CO_2. Follow-up clinical studies demonstrated that sodium lactate was panicogenic when administered to anxious patients (54), as was 5% CO_2 inhalation (55). The biochemical mechanisms responsible for these effects have been elusive. Metabolic alkalosis induced by administration of lactate or sodium bicarbonate (56) may contribute to panicogenesis. However, acidosis secondary to CO_2 inhalation also appears to produce similar effects in panickers. Alternatively, respiratory alkalosis, brought on by voluntary hyperventilation, has been reported by some groups to trigger panic episodes in panic patients (57). CO_2 fluctuations and pH alterations may elicit panic by activating a suffocation false-alarm response in patients that have a pre-existing hypersensitivity of their suffocation-alarm mechanism (58). The neural basis of such a mechanism remains undetermined. Candidate structures might include brainstem structures such as ventral medullary chemoreceptors, the periaqueductal gray area (59), and the parabrachial nucleus (60).

Clinical Studies

Lactate-induced panic is an extremely well-replicated phenomenon, relatively specific to panic disorder, and attenuated by a wide array of effective antipanic therapies, including imipramine (61), phenelzine (62), alprazolam (29), and cognitive-behavioral therapy (63). Approximately two-thirds of all patients with a history of panic will be lactate-sensitive (64). There is some debate as to whether lactate acts peripherally or centrally. Recent animal data (65) and MRS data in humans (66), however, indicate that increases in brain lactate levels parallel increases in plasma levels. Panic patients are sensitive to both D- and L-isomers of lactate, suggesting that further metabolism of lactate is not required for panic provocation to occur (67). As already mentioned, acute CO_2 administration can also precipitate panic in patients. Acute hypercapnia, produced by rebreathing a 5% CO_2 mixture, is panicogenic (55,68), as is a single (69) or brief inhalation of 35% CO_2 (70).

Clinical Implications

The relationship between respiration and panic is highly relevant clinically. Many panickers have hyperventilation or suffocation sensations as prominent symptoms of their panics, and hyperventilation, in turn, produces more physical sensations, thereby intensifying the experience of panic. While hyperventilation is now thought to be neither necessary nor sufficient to cause naturalistic panic, breathing retraining methods have proved to be an important behavioral strategy in the clinical treatment of panic patients (71). In addition to the dramatic hyperventilation seen in acute panic, there is not infrequently a more chronic pattern of irregular, shallow breathing in panic patients; this can be targeted with breathing retraining. Examination of the respiratory mechanisms in panic may yield some explanation for the observation that panic-prone females tend to have exacerbation of their panic symptoms premenstrually and during the postpartum period. It has been suggested that, since progesterone is a respiratory stimulant, rapid withdrawal of progesterone at these times may lead to rising CO_2 levels, which in turn trigger a sensitive suffocation-alarm system (58). LeDoux (72) has hypothesized a role for CO_2 in the acquisition of situational panic attacks. Neurons in the lower brainstem sensitive to CO_2 fluctuations project to the amygdala (73). Fear-conditioning mechanisms at the level of the amgygdala may then be activated by these afferents so that future CO_2 fluctuations serve as a cue for panicky responses. In this scheme, after arousal has been triggered in this way, explicit memory systems (retrieving information about past panics) in the hippocampus and neocortex may feed back to the amygdala, further elaborating the panic response.

BZD/GABA Dysfunction

Preclinical Overview

The gamma-aminobutyric acid (GABA) neuronal system, the brain's major inhibitory transmitter system (74), is an extensive network of interneurons. Via this network, the GABA system is able to modulate neuronal excitation in most brain regions. BZD-receptor agonists—medications that target the GABA system—produce neuronal inhibition via BZD-receptor modulation of the $GABA_A$-receptor mechanism, leading to a variety of pharmacological effects including anxiolysis, muscle relaxation, and sedation in both animals and humans (75). Conversely, BZD inverse agonists such as certain β-carbolines (β-CCE and FG-7142) are anxiogenic and proconvulsant. These results have generated much interest in the role of the BZD/GABA$_A$-receptor complex and the GABA neuronal system in the pathophysiology of human stress and anxiety disorders (76). Animal studies of exposure to chronic inescapable stress (a potential model for human panic) have detected regional (frontal cortex, hippocampus, hypothalamus) reductions in BZD-receptor binding (77–79). Recently, an intriguing animal model of panic disorder has been created by means of a biochemically induced GABA-level deficit in the dorsomedial hypothalamus (80). Rats with this lesion had a panic-like reaction when challenged with a sodium lactate infusion, a standard panic-provocation maneuver in humans. Another animal model, in which mice displayed neophobic behavior reminiscent of human agoraphobia, was created by a gene knockdown of the γ_2-GABA$_A$ subunit (81). Based on these data, a thorough search for potential dysfunction of the GABA neuronal system in humans with panic disorder is indicated.

Clinical Studies

Several groups looking for abnormalities in BZD-receptor function in panic have reported positive findings. One group (82) observed that panic patients had less slowing of saccadic eye-movement velocity after diazepam administration than did healthy controls, consistent with subsensitivity of BZD receptors in panic. However, this group also recently reported a similar finding in patients with obsessive-compulsive disorder (83). Also, the BZD antagonist flumazenil was reported to be panicogenic in panic patients but not healthy controls (84), consistent with an intrinsic BZD-receptor abnormality or a deficit of an endogenous anxiolytic agent in the disorder. This finding, while intriguing, remains to be replicated. A recent candidate gene study (85) did not link 8/13 GABA$_A$-receptor subunit genes to the diagnosis of panic disorder, an important piece of evidence against hypotheses of instrinsic GABAA-receptor abnormalities in panic. Direct, in vivo assessment of BZD-receptor status in panic disorder by single-photon emission computed tomography (SPECT) neuroreceptor imaging techniques has been performed by several groups, with evidence of reduction in BZD binding in some brain regions (for a summary, see the section "Neuro-imaging in Panic Disorder" below). Reliable evidence of specific de-fects in GABA functioning in panic disorder is currently lacking. Plasma (86,87) and CSF (88) GABA levels in panic patients appear normal. However, in the CSF study, a low baseline plasma-GABA level predicted poorer response to treatment with alprazolam or imipramine. In vivo assessment of cortical GABA levels in panic patients by mag-netic resonance spectroscopy (MRS) techniques is currently in prog-ress.

Clinical Implications

Perhaps the most compelling, albeit indirect, evidence favoring BZD/ GABA hypotheses of panic disorder is the robust and rapid clinical response of patients to BZD agonists. High-potency BZDs, such as alprazolam and clonazepam, are considered standard pharmacothera-pies for panic disorder (89,90). The antipanic benefits of these agents also appear to be maintained over the intermediate and long term (91). Other effective antipanic treatments, such as valproic acid (92) and the MAOI drug phenelzine (93), tend to increase brain GABA levels. It is therefore conceivable that enhancement of GABA function is a com-mon characteristic of effective treatment strategies for panic.

Cholecystokinin and Panic

Preclinical Overview

There is an now an exciting body of literature indicating involvement in panic of the neuropeptide cholecystokinin (CCK). Brain CCK (mainly sulphated CCK octapeptide, CCK-8s) is located in high concentrations in regions implicated in fear responses such as the cerebral cortex, hip-pocampus, and amygdala (94). The two major CCK-receptor subtypes (A and B) are present in the brain, but the CCK_B subtype is predominant and the one linked to fear behaviors (95). Preclinical studies have con-sistently reported fear-related behavioral changes following exogenous administration of CCK agonists (96,97). Conversely, administration of selective CCK_B-receptor antagonists such as CI-988 and L-365,260 to rats produced anxiolytic effects as measured by the elevated plus maze paradigm (98). At present, the anatomical location (central vs. peripheral) of the mechanisms involved in CCK-induced behavioral responses remains controversial.

Clinical Studies

A number of clinical studies have also implicated the CCK system in the genesis of human anxiety. Panic patients were observed to be abnormally sensitive to the anxiogenic effects of CCK-4 (99), with a 25-μg i.v. bolus dose triggering panic attacks in 91% of patients compared to similar reactions in only 17% of controls. The anxiety behavioral response to CCK-4 is dose-dependent (100), very similar to that in naturalistic panic, and has been well replicated (101). Panic patients are also hypersensitive to challenge with the mixed CCK agonist pentagastrin (a synthetic pentapeptide) (102,103). Blockade of CCK-4-induced anxiety in panic patients has been reported following pretreatment with a single oral dose of 50 mg of the selective CCK_B antagonist L-365,260 (104). Overall, these findings implicate CCK_B-receptor hypersensitivity in the pathophysiology of panic. Observations that panic patients have abnormally low concentrations of CSF (105) and lymphocyte (106) CCK-8s suggest a primary underproduction of CCK-8 in panic with compensatory CCK-receptor supersensitivity. The mechanism of CCK panic in humans is the focus of ongoing research, because other systems, such as the NE and 5-HT, may also be involved.

Clinical Implications

The CCK research findings have led to clinical trials testing the antipanic efficacy of CCK_B antagonists. Unfortunately, the results to date have been disappointing, due partly to the poor bioavailability of this class of compounds (107). However, chronic administration of other known effective treatments for panic, such as imipramine (108) and fluvoxamine (50), attenuate CCK-induced panic, implicating NE/CCK and 5-HT/CCK neuronal interactions in their therapeutic actions. Other anxiety disorders (to a lesser extent) appear to share abnormalities in CCK function with panic, notably generalized anxiety disorder (109).

Interestingly, females with late luteal phase dysphoric disorder are also sensitive to CCK's anxiogenic effects (110). Thus, it is unclear at this point to what extent the CCK abnormalities discussed are a marker of acute illness vs a trait marker. Candidate gene studies focusing on the CCK_B receptor should be of value in determining the contribution of the CCK system toward a panic diathesis. The close similarity of CCK-4 panic to naturalistic panic, together with the brevity of its effect (typically less than 2 minutes), suggests that CCK release could be an important factor initiating clinical panic, with other systems (perhaps NE, 5-HT, BZD/GABA) being responsible for maintaining or amplifying panic responses.

HPA-Axis Dysregulation

Preclinical Overview

The hypothalamic-pituitary-adrenal (HPA) axis plays a major role in coordinating responses to physiological and behavioral stressors and is therefore of considerable interest to anxiety disorder researchers. In the more recent preclinical literature, corticotropin-releasing factor (CRF) has emerged as an important mediator of stress responses in animals (111). CRF-containing neurons have wide projections to other CNS systems implicated in fear behaviors (e.g., LC, amygdala, hippocampus). CRF is anxiogenic when injected into the LC (112). In addition, intraventricular administration of CRF in animals also produces profound fear responses (113). Primates (114) exposed to early variable psychosocial deprivation were observed to have elevated CRF levels. These observations are of particular relevance to our understanding of the potential biological impact of environment events such as trauma and the role they might play as antecedent factors in the pathogenesis of panic.

Clinical Studies

In general, the clinical research literature indicates mild HPA-axis dysfunction in panic disorder. In contrast to the reports of elevated CSF levels of CRF in depression (115) and posttraumatic stress disorder

(PTSD) (116), these levels were normal in unmedicated panic patients (117). However, a possible role for CRF in initiating panic responses is not ruled out by the negative CSF data. Two of three CRF-stimulation studies (118,119, but not 120) with panic patients reported blunted ACTH responses following acute CRF infusion, suggestive of down-regulation of CRF receptors in the pituitary secondary to episodic hypersecretion of CRF. Studies examining the pituitary/adrenal portion of the HPA axis with the dexamethsaone-suppression test have produced variable results. In one recent study (121), panic patients tended to have overnight hypercortisolemia and more frequent ultradian secretory bursts compared to controls. The replicated finding of blunted GH responses to GH-releasing factor in panic patients also implicates HPA-axis abnormalities in the pathophysiology of the disorder (122,123).

Clinical Implications

The available research data suggest that there may be subtle abnormalities in HPA-axis regulation in panic disorder. Patients with greater functional impairment, high panic-attack frequency, and comorbidity may be more likely to manifest persistent HPA-axis dysregulation, while patients with milder illness may tend to exhibit acute HPA-axis dysfunction only in the context of acute psychosocial stressors (121). It may also be that HPA activation contributes more to anticipatory anxiety than to true panic. Another significant clinical issue is that of trauma as a risk factor for subsequent panic disorder. A community survey (123) of those meeting a panic disorder diagnosis indicated a very high rate (approximately 60%) of traumatic life events in females. Also, the rates of antecedent traumatic events (prior to first onset of panic symptoms) in a large cohort of over 300 panic patients from a multisite clinical trial were approximately 30% (Goddard and Woods et al., unpublished data). Very few patients had comorbid PTSD in this sample. In light of the preclinical data reviewed, it is plausible that the traumatized panic patient subgroup might be biologically distinct from nontraumatized patients, with persistent HPA-axis dysfunction implicated as a predisposing illness factor. It is conceivable that a trauma history together with panic disorder has different prognostic implications (perhaps more treatment resistance or tendency toward recurrence) than those of uncomplicated panic.

CLINICAL NEUROPHYSIOLOGY IN PANIC DISORDER

Startle Studies

Preclinical Overview

There is now considerable evidence that the amygdala is an important structure involved in anxiety and fear behaviors (125,126). Lesions of the central nucleus of the amygdala in rats block fear expression, while electrical stimulation of this structure elicits fear behaviors (127). The central nucleus has strong anatomical connections to the hypothalamus and brainstem regions, which are responsible for many of the signs and symptoms of fear. The amygdala has been implicated in neurobehavioral processes such as fear conditioning and contextual conditioning. Fear conditioning (cue-specific fear) provides a useful preclinical model of specific phobias, while contextual conditioning (generalization of fear responses to multiple cues present during a threat condition) may provide a model for more complex anxiety disorders such as panic disorder and PTSD (60). To assess central nucleus functioning during fear states, a number of investigators have developed paradigms of fear conditoning across a variety of animal species. One such paradigm involves conditioning of acoustic startle response in rats (128). In this model, acoustic startle responses are increased under stressful conditions (e.g., threat of shock). The N-methyl-D-aspartate (NMDA) antagonist AP5 blocked extinction of fear-potentiated startle responses in this paradigm (129). In addition, NMDA antagonists were able to block acquisition of conditioned fear (130). In conclusion, NMDA/glutamate systems seem to be involved in learning processes relevant to fear and anxiety. These neural events appear to be coordinated via the amygdala, particularly the central nucleus.

Clinical Studies

There have been few studies examining fear conditioning in anxiety patients. Clinical studies using the fear-potentiated startle paradigm have been conducted in healthy controls, panic patients, and PTSD patients. Interestingly, panic patients and controls were found to have similar baseline startle and fear-potentiated startle responses (131). However, a subgroup of younger panic patients (<40 years old) exhibited elevated baseline startle with no increase in fear-potentiated startle, consistent with fear to the experimental context. Structures other than the amygdala are implicated in contextual fear mechanisms, including the hippocampus and the bed nucleus of the stria terminalis (132). It is possible that dysfunction in these structures could contribute to the pathogenesis of panic disorder. Studies are currently underway to test whether panic patients with agoraphobia perform differently in the potentiated startle paradigm than those without agoraphobia.

Clinical Implications

It is conceivable that panic patients more readily acquire conditioned fears or alternatively have a deficit in their ability to terminate fear responses. Either or both of these processes could contribute to the development of agoraphobia following the onset of spontaneous panics. Specific behavior therapies (exposure therapies) are frequently used in panic patients to facilitate the extinction of phobic learning. In the future, medications that down-modulate glutamate function, such as the metabotropic glutamate agonists (133), may become additional therapeutic strategies for the prevention of phobia acquisition or facilitation of phobia extinction.

EEG Studies

Clinical Studies

There is evidence of EEG abnormalities in panic disorder, further implicating biological mechanisms in its pathogenesis. In one study (134), almost 30% of patients (total $n = 120$) had minor EEG abnormalities. Furthermore, in this subgroup, there was an unusually high rate (61%) of follow-up MRI abnormalities, many in the septohippocampal area. There are some genetic data linking panic disorder to a heritable EEG trait (low-voltage alpha) that maps to chromosome 20q (135), and other data indicating that alcoholics with anxiety disorders are 10 times more likely than controls to exhibit this trait (136). Other investigators (137) have observed in panic patients abnormally increased absolute power in EEG delta, theta, and alpha bands, and decreased beta power. This group (138) also noted that panickers failed to activate theta and alpha EEG waves during relaxation procedures, a finding consistent with increased baseline arousal. In another EEG study (139), temporal-lobe EEG traces were abnormal in panic patients at baseline and following EEG activation (the stimulus was the presentation of an odor). In addition, within the patient group, different baseline and activation EEG patterns were found in patients with—versus those without—dissociative symptoms. Sleep EEG studies (140–142) have generally found that panic disorder is dissimilar to major depression in that there is no evidence of reduced REM latency. These authors otherwise reported mild reduction in sleep efficiency or relatively normal sleep associated with panic. Sleep panics, when they occurred, tended to appear during stage 3, non-REM sleep (140). The EEG data, overall, further support the biological dissection of panic disorder from mood disorders. They also suggest that further neuropsychiatric assessment of temporal lobe and limbic function in panic is likely to be a fruitful research approach.

Clinical Implications

The possible relationship between seizure disorders and panic disorder is an intriguing one at both a clinical and a theoretical level. Temporal-lobe seizure disorder can present with panic attacks (143), and both panic and temporal-lobe seizure patients appear to experience a significant overlap in the psychological symptoms they report (144). With respect to therapeutics, panic and seizure patients respond to some of the same medications, such as BZDs and valproic acid, suggesting the possibility of shared pathophysiological processes. Whether panic disorder lies on a biological spectrum with some seizure disorders remains to be seen. However, given these findings, clinicians should not hesitate to refer patients with atypical panic attacks (e.g., attacks with syncopal symptoms or alterations in conscious state) for neurological consultation and work-up. Another clinical application of the research findings reviewed above is inquiry about sleep panic. This can often help the clinician decide whether the patient has ever experienced a true spontaneous panic, an essential component of the panic diagnosis.

Cardiovascular Physiology and Panic

Clinical Studies

Subtle abnormalities in cardiovascular regulation may occur in panic disorder. In an ambulatory EKG monitoring study (145), panic patients were found to have normal heart rate and rhythm between panics. Follow-up studies therefore investigated responsivity of panic patients to physiological and psychological stressors. One group found no patient/control difference in physiological responses to a cognitive stressor, cold stress, and CO_2 challenge (146). In other work, panic patients had more pronounced heart-rate increases to an orthostatic challenge compared to controls, consistent with abnormally increased sympathetic or decreased vagal control of cardiac responses (147). A number of studies have examined aspects of heart-rate variability in panic disorder. Briefly, time series data from simple EKGs can be transformed into frequency data by a mathematical function known as Fourier transformation. In the normal individual there is a substantial heart-rate variability (beat-to-beat variation), particularly due to high-frequency (HF) elements. This HF component is thought to reflect respiratory sinus arrhythmia, a phenomenon primarily under vagal control. Many studies in panic disorder have found reductions in heart-rate variability (148–150) due to either loss of the HF power or a relative increase in mid-frequency (MF) power (a measure that reflects both sympathetic and vagal inputs). Panicogenic agents such as lactate (151) and isoproterenol (152) exaggerate reductions in heart-rate variability in panic patients, while successful treatment (with either cognitive-behavioral therapy or imipramine) was associated with normalization of patterns of heart-rate variability (153). Thus, a potential mechanism of panicogenesis in patients with active disease may be decreases in vagal tone permitting a predominance of sympathetic activation of cardiac function. Vagal afferents feeding back to brainstem areas implicated in panic might contribute to elaboration of the panic episode. Follow-up studies of panic patients who subsequently undergo vagotomies for GI indications would be of interest, to test whether vagal mechanisms are necessary for panic to occur.

Clinical Implications

Cardiovascular and autonomic symptoms are key symptoms of typical panic attacks. Most patients have palpitations with their panic episodes. The data reviewed suggest that panic patients may tend to be hyperreactive to some stressors because of subtle alterations in cardiac regulation. It is unclear what the long-term health effects of such reactivity might be. There is some evidence that panic patients (particularly males) are more prone to cardiovascular disorders such as hypertension and ischemic heart disease (154), although this is still controversial. Also, in general medical populations, abnormalities in heart-rate variability are robust predictors of cardiac morbidity (155). Thus, timely and appropriate treatment of panic symptoms may prevent serious medical complications.

NEUROIMAGING IN PANIC DISORDER

There is accumulating evidence of structural and functional neuroanatomical abnormalities in panic. These findings and their potential clinical significance are summarized in Table 1 (adapted from Ref. 156). Thus far, frontal, temporal, and limbic/hippocampal areas appear to be implicated in panic disorder. However, the specificity of these findings needs to be established. For example, some brain regions, such as the anterior cingulate gyrus (157,158), may mediate phenomena present in both pathological and normal anxiety states. Animal (159) and recent healthy-human data (160) suggest a role for the medial frontal cortex and orbitofrontal cortex in extinction processes, and processes that limit fear reactions. In addition, fMRI data in healthy humans suggest amygdalocortical activation during fear conditioning (161). Imaging studies of these regions in panic patients are clearly warranted. At present, PET blood-flow studies are in progress with panic patients to determine whether amygdala activation occurs during CO_2-induced panic.

CONCLUSIONS

A substantial body of evidence indicates dysfunction of brain monoamine (NE, 5-HT), neuropeptide, and BZD/GABA systems in panic disorder. Panic patients have abnormal sensitivity to fluctuations in brain CO_2 and pH levels, possibly due to a sensitive suffocation-alarm mechanism. There may be subtle EEG abnormalities, particularly in temporal lobe areas, further consistent with disrupted brain function in panic disorder. The data indicate subtle cardiovascular dysregulation in panic in the form of reduced heart-rate variability. Neuroimaging investigations have uncovered evidence of frontal, temporal, and hippocampal dysfunction in panic patients. Although diverse hypotheses involving these biological systems have been advanced to account for the pathophysiology of panic disorder, it is clear that no one lesion in a given system is sufficient to account for the majority of cases or the variety of clinical phenomena that are manifest during different phases of the illness (e.g., anticipatory anxiety, situational panic attacks, dissociative symptoms, nocturnal attacks, comorbid depressive symptoms, phobic avoidance, and hypochondriasis). The research to date suggests that either there are a number of biological subtypes of panic or there are multiple biological abnormalities in a given individual that result in the expression of panic.

Competing psychological (cognitive-behavioral) accounts of the pathogenesis of panic disorder do not fully explain the biological data presented in this review. As an example, several challenge paradigms (including TRH infusion and insulin induction of hypoglycemia) (reviewed in Ref. 171) that provoke intense physical symptoms in panic patients are not panicogenic. We believe that newer neuronal models of panic may assist in the reconciliation of these diverging perspectives on panic. Several models of this kind propose a central coordinating role for the amygdala in panicogenesis (60,72). The amygdala has extensive afferent and efferent connections to many other fear-relevant neuronal structures. These models are generating new hypotheses concerning the pathophysiology and treatment of panic. Older research strategies (neurochemical and neurophysiological approaches) are now being fruitfully combined with new technologies (functional neuroimaging) to test these hypotheses.

Table 1   Neuroimaging in Panic Disorder

Technique	Finding	Neurochemistry	Clinical significance
MRI	More right medial temporal lobe abnormalities in lactate-sensitive panic patients than in controls (162). Septohippocampal abnormalities in panic patients (134).	Possible HPA-axis hyperactivity	There is an indication for head MRI in atypical presentations. Structural changes could also be the result of chronic illness. Chronic HPA overactivity might cause hippocampal cell damage.
PET-rCBF (blood flow)	Right parahippocampal gyrus rCBF increased at rest in lactate-sensitive panickers vs. controls (163).		Trait overactivity in limbic structures could predispose to spontaneous panics.
PET-FDG (glucose metabolism)	Right > left hippocampal, decreased left inferior parietal and anterior cingulate glucose metabolism during an auditory discrimination task in panic patients vs. controls (164).		Abnormal information processing of sensory stimuli may lead to abnormal cognition in patients.

Table 1 Continued

Technique	Finding	Neurochemistry	Clinical significance
SPECT-rCBF	Bilateral fronto-cortical reductions in rCBF following yohimbine-induced panic in patients vs. controls (165).	NE system hyperactivity	During panics, altered frontal lobe functioning may impair normal executive abilities.
SPECT-rCBF	Resting blood flow defects in hippocampi, increased rCBF in right > left inferior frontal cortex and left occipital cortex in lactage-sensitive, drug-naive panickers vs. controls (166)	NE hyperactivity, 5-HT dysregulation	Memory dysfunction a possible early manifestation of panic disorder. May predispose to agoraphobia.
SPECT (BZD) receptor binding)	Left lateral temporal lobe decrease in iomazenil tracer activity in panic patients vs. dysthymics (167). Decreased frontal and temporal lobe BDZ binding in panic patients vs. epileptics (168).	BZD/GABA system subsensitivity	May contribute to abnormal stimulus processing in panic patients. BZD agonists used in treatment may compensate for these processing errors.

Table 1 Continued

Technique	Finding	Neurochemistry	Clinical significance
	Asymmetry of prefrontal cortical BZD binding in panic disorder vs. controls (169). Decreased left hippocampal BZD binding in panic disorder vs controls (170).		
MRS (spectroscopy)	Abnormal brain lactate increases provoked by hyperventilation in panic disorder (66).	Respiratory ph/ CO_2 chemoreceptor hypersensitivity or suffocation-alarm hypersensitivity	Chronic or intermittent hyperventilation in panic disorder may elevate CNS lactate levels, which in turn trigger further spontaneous panics.

Source: Adapted from Ref. 156.

REFERENCES

1. Redmond DE Jr, Huang YH, Snyder DR, et al. Behavioral effects of stimulation of the locus coeruleus in the stumptail monkey (*Macaca arctoides*). Brain Res 1976; 116:502–510.
2. Aston-Jones G, Chiang C, Alexinsky T. Discharge of noardrenergetic locus coeruleu neurons in behaving rats and monkeys suggests a role in vigilance. Prog Brain Res 1991; 88:501–520.

3. Fillenz M. Noradrenergic Neurons. Cambridge, England: Cambridge University Press; 1990.
4. Abercrombie ED, Jacobs BL. Single-unit response of noradrenergic neurons in the locus coeruleus of freely moving cats. I. Acutely presented stressful and nonstressful stimuli. J Neurosci 1987; 7:2837–2843.
5. Nisenbaum LK, Zigmund MJ, Sved AF, Abercrombie ED. Prior exposure to chronic stress results in enhanced synthesis and release of hippocampal norepinephrine in response to a novel stressor. J Neurosci 1991; 11:1478–1484.
6. Rasmussen K, Jacobs BL. Single unit activity of the locus coeruleus in the freely moving cat. I. During naturalistic behaviors and in response to simple and complex stimuli. Brain Res 1986; 371:324–334.
7. Charney DS, Heninger GR, Breier A. Noradrenergic function in panic anxiety: effects of yohimbine in healthy subjects and patients with agoraphobia and panic disorder. Arch Gen Psychiatry 1984; 41:751–763.
8. Charney DS, Woods SW, Goodman WK, et al. Neurobiological mechanisms of panic anxiety: biochemical and behavioral correlates of yohimbine-induced panic attacks. Am J Psychiatry 1987; 144:1030–1036.
9. Charney DS, Woods SW, Krystal JH, et al. Noradrenergic neuronal dysregulation in panic disorder: the effects of intravenous yohimbine and clonidine in panic disorder patients. Acta Psychiatr Scand 1992; 86:273–282.
10. Gurguis GNM, Uhde TW. Plasma 3-methoxy-4-hydroxyphenylethylene glycol (MHPG) and growth hormone responses to yohimbine in panic disorder patients and normal controls. Psychoneuroendocrinology 1990; 15:217–224.
11. Albus M, Zahn TP, Breier A. Anxiogenic properties of yohimbine. I. Behavioral, physiological and biochemical measures. Eur Arch Psychiatry Clin Neurosci 1992; 241:337–344.
12. Southwick SM, Krystal J, Morgan CA, et al. Abnormal noradrenergic function in posttraumatic stress disorder. Arch Gen Psychiatry 1993; 50:266–274.
13. Charney DS, Heninger GR. Abnormal regulation of noradrenergic function in panic disorders: effects of clonidine in healthy subjects and patients with agoraphobia and panic disorders. Arch Gen Psychiatry 1986; 43:1042–1054.
14. Nutt DJ. Altered alpha-2-adrenoceptor sensitivity in panic disorder. Arch Gen Psychiatry 1989; 46:165–169.
15. Uhde TW, Vittone BJ, Siever LJ, et al. Blunted growth hormone re-

sponse to clonidine in panic disorder patients. Biolog Psychiatry 1986; 21:1077–1081.

16. Charney DS, Woods SW, Nagy LM, Southwick SM, Krystal JH, Heninger GR. Noradrenergic function in panic disorder. J Clin Psychiatry 1990; 51(suppl A):5–11.

17. Abelson JL, Glitz D, Cameron OG, et al. Blunted growth hormone response to clonidine in patients with generalized anxiety disorder. Arch Gen Psychiatry 1991; 48:157–162.

18. Pohl R, Yeragani VK, Balon R, et al. Isoproterenol-induced panic attacks. Biolog Psychiatry 1988; 24:891–902.

19. Wahlestedt C, Pich EM, Koob GF, Yee F, Heilig M. Modulation of anxiety and neuropeptide Y-Y$_1$ receptors by antisense oligodeoxy-nucleotides. Science 1993; 259:528–531.

20. Boulenger J, Jerabek I, Jolicoeur FB, et al. Elevated plasma levels of neuropeptide Y in patients with panic disorder. Am J Psychiatry 1996; 153:114–116.

21. Stein MB, Hauger RL, Dhalla KS, Chartier MJ, Asmundson GJG. Plasma neuropeptide Y in anxiety disorders: finding in panic disorder and social phobia. Psychiatry Res 1996; 59:183–188.

22. Kimura F, Nakamura S. Postnatal development of α-adrenoceptor-mediated autoinhibition in the locus coeruleus. Dev Brain Res 1987; 35: 21–26.

23. Rapee RM, Litwin EM, Barlow DH. Impact of life events on subjects with panic disorder and on comparison subjects. Am J Psychiatry 1990; 147:640–644.

24. Bondareff W, Mountjoy CQ. Number of neurons in nucleus locus ceruleus in demented and non-demented patients: rapid estimation and correlated parameters. Neurobiol Aging 1986; 7:397–300.

25. Svensson TH. Peripheral autonomic regulation of locus coeruleus neurons in the brain: putative implications for psychiatry and psychopharmacology. Psychopharmacology 1987; 92:1–7.

26. Charney DS, Heninger GR. Noradrenergic function and the mechanism of action of antianxiety treatment. I. The effect of long-term alprazolam treatment. Arch Gen Psychiatry 1985; 42:458–467.

27. Middleton HC. An enhanced hypotensive response to clonidine can still be found in panic patients despite psychological treatment. J Anx Disord 1990; 4:213–219.

28. Woods SW, Charney DS, McPherson CA, et al. Situational panic attacks: behavioral, physiological, and biochemical characterization. Arch Gen Psychiatry 1987; 44:365–375.

29. Carr D, Sheehan DV, Surman OS, et al. Neuroendocrine correlates of lactate-induced anxiety and their response to chronic alprazolam therapy. Am J Psychiatry 1986; 143:483–494.
30. Coplan JD, Liebowitz MR, Gorman JM, et al. Noradrenergic function in panic disorder: effects of intravenous clonidine pretreatment on lactate induced panic. Biolog Psychiatry 1992; 31:135–146.
31. Charney DS, Heninger GR. Noradrenergic function and the mechanism of action of antianxiety treatment. II. The effect of long-term imipramine treatment. Arch Gen Psychiatry 1985; 42:473–481.
32. Wang ZW, Crowe RR, Noyes R Jr. Adrenergic receptor genes as candidate genes for panic disorder: a linkage study. Am J Psychiatry 1992; 149:470–474.
33. Azmitia EF, Whitaker-Azmitia PM. Anatomy, cell biology, and plasticity of the serotonic system: neuropsychopharmacological implications for the actions of psychotrophic drugs. In: Bloom FE, Kupfer DJ, eds. Psychopharmacology: The Fourth Generation of Progress. New York: Raven Press, 1995:443–449.
34. Handley SL. 5-hydroxytryptamine pathways in anxiety and its treatment. Pharmacol Ther 1995; 66:103–148.
35. Grove G, Coplan JD, Hollander E. The neuroanatomy of 5-HT dysregulation and panic disorder. J Neuropsychiatry Clin Neurosci 1997; 9: 198–207.
36. Lucki I. Serotonin receptor specificity in anxiety disorders. J Clin Psychiatry 1996; 57(suppl 6):5–10.
37. Targum SD, Marshall LE. Fenfluramine provocation of anxiety in patients with panic disorder. Psychiatry Res 1988; 28:295–306.
38. Charney DS, Woods SW, Goodman WK, Heninger GR. Serotonin function in anxiety. II. Effects of the serotonin agonist MCPP in panic disorder patients and healthy subjects. Psychopharmacology 1987; 92: 14–24.
39. Kahn RS, Wetzler S, van Praag HM, et al. Behavioral indications for serotonin receptor hypersensitivity in panic disorder. Psychiatry Res 1988; 25:101–104.
40. Charney DS, Heninger GR. Serotonin function in panic disorders: the effects of intravenous tryptophan in healthy subjects and panic disorder patients before and during alprazolam treatment. Arch Gen Psychiatry 1986; 43:1059–1065.
41. Goddard AW, Sholomskas DE, Augeri FM, Walton KE, Charney DS, Heninger GR, Goodman WK, Price LH. Effects of tryptophan depletion in panic disorder. Biolog Psychiatry 1994; 36:775–777.

42. Lesch KP, Wiesmann M, Hoh A, et al. 5-HT1A receptor-effector system responsivity in panic disorder. Psychopharmacology 1992; 106: 111–117.

43. Sheehan DV, Harnett-Sheehan K. The role of SSRIs in panic disorder. J Clin Psychiatry 1996; 10:51–58.

44. Boyer W. Serotonin reuptake inibitors are superior to imipramine and alprazolam in alleviating panic attacks: a meta-analysis. Int Clin Psychopharmacol 1995; 10:45–49.

45. Blier P, de Montigny C, Chaput Y. Modifications of the serotonin system by antidepressant treatments: implications for the therapeutic response in major depression. J Clin Psychopharmacol 1987; 7(suppl 6): 24S–35S.

46. DeMontigny C, Chaput Y, Blier P. Modification of serotonergic neuron properties by long-term treatment with serotonin reuptake blockers. J Clin Psychiatry 1990; 51(12, suppl B).

47. Pineyro G, Blier P, Dennis T, de Montigny D. Desensitization of the neuronal 5-HT carrier following its long-term blockade. J Neurosci 1994; 14:3036–3047.

48. Goddard AW, Woods SW, Sholomskas DE, et al. Effects of the serotonin reuptake inhibitor fluvoxamine on noradrenergic function in panic disorder. Psychiatry Res 1993; 48:119–133.

49. Coplan JD, Papp LA, Pine DS, Martinez J, Cooper T, Rosenblum LA, Klein DF, Gorman JM. Clinical improvement with fluoxetine therapy and noradrenergic function in patients with panic disorder. Arch Gen Psychiatry 1997; 54:643–648.

50. van Megen H, Westenberg H, den Boer J. Effects of the selective serotonin reuptake inhibitor fluvoxamine of CCK-4 induced panic attacks. Psychopharmacology 1997; 10(suppl 3):12S.

51. Pols HJ, Hauzer RC, Meijer JA, Verburg K, Griez EJ. Fluvoxamine attenuates panic induced by 35% CO_2 challenge. J Clin Psychiatry 1996; 57:539–542.

52. Lesch KP, Bengel D, Heils A, Sabol SZ, Greenberg BD, Petri S, Benjamin J, Muller CR, Hamer DH, Murphy DL. Association of anxiety-related traits with a polymorphism in the serotonin transporter gene regulatory region. Science 1996; 274:1527.

53. Cohen ME, White PD. Life situations, emotions and neurocirculatory asthenia. Psychosom Med 1951; 13:335–357.

54. Pitts FN, McClure JN. Lactate metabolism in anxiety neurosis. N Engl J Med 1967; 277:1329–1336.

55. Gorman JM, Askanazi J, Liebowitz, MR, et al. Response to hyperventi-

lation in a group of patients with panic disorder. Am J Psychiatry 1984; 141:857–861.

56. Gorman JM, Battista D, Goetz R, et al. A comparison of sodium bicarbonate and sodium lactate infusion in the induction of panic attacks. Arch Gen Psychiatry 1989; 46:145–150.

57. Bass C, Kartsounis L, Lelliott P. Hyperventilation and its relation to anxiety and panic. Integrative Psychiatry 1987; 5:274–272.

58. Klein DF. False suffocation alarms, spontaneous panics and related conditions: an integrative hypothesis. Arch Gen Psychiatry 1993; 50: 306–317.

59. Jenke F, Moreau JL, Martin JR. Dorsal periaqueductal gray–induced aversion as a simulation of panic anxiety: elements of face and predictive validity. Psychiatry Res 1995; 57:181–191.

60. Charney DS, Deutsch A. A functional neuroanatomy of anxiety and fear: implications for the pathophysiology and treatment of anxiety disorders. Crit Rev Neurobiol 1996; 10(3/4):419–446.

61. Rifkin A, Klein DF, Dillon D, et al. Blockade by imipramine or desipramine of panic induced by sodium lactate. Am J Psychiatry 1981; 138: 676–677.

62. Kelly D, Mitchell-Heggs N, Shean D. Anxiety and the effects of sodium lactate assessed clinically and physiologically. Br J Psychiatry 1974; 119:129–141.

63. Shear MK, Fryer AJ, Baill G, et al. Vulnerability to sodium lactate in panic disorder patients given cognitive-behavioral therapy. Am J Psychiatry 1991; 148:795–797.

64. Liebowitz MR, Fryer AJ, Gorman JM. Lactate provocation of panic attacks. 1. Clinical and behavioral findings. Arch Gen Psychiatry 1984; 41:764–770.

65. Dager SR, Rainey JM, Kenny MA, et al. Central nervous system effects of lactate infusion in primates. Biolog Psychiatry 1990; 27:193–204.

66. Dager SR, Strauss WL, Marro KI, et al. Proton magnetic resonance spectroscopy investigation of hyperventilation in subjects with panic disorder and comparison subjects. Am J Psychiatry 1995; 152:666–672.

67. Gorman JM, Goetz RR, Dillon D, et al. Sodium D-lactate infusion in panic disorder patients. Neuropsychopharmacology 1990; 3:181–189.

68. Woods SW, Charney DS, Lake J, et al. Carbon dioxide sensitivity in panic anxiety. Arch Gen Psychiatry 1986; 43:900–909.

69. Greiz E, Zandbergen J, Pols H, de Loof C. Response to 35% CO_2, as

a marker of panic in severe anxiety. Am J Psychiatry 1990; 147:796–807.

70. Papp LA, Kline DF, Martinez JM, Schneier F, Cole R, Liebowitz MR, Hollander E, Fyer AJ, Jordan F, Gorman JM. Diagnostic,substance specificity of carbon dioxide-induced panic. Am J Psychiatry 1993; 150:250–257.

71. Salkovskis P, Jones DRO, Clark DM. Respiratory control in the treatment of panic attacks: replication and extension with concurrent measurement of behavior and PCO_2 Br J Psychiatry 1986; 148:526–553.

72. LeDoux J. The Emotional Brain. New York: Simon and Schuster, 1996.

73. Ruggerio DA, Gomez RE, Cravo SL, Anwar M, Reis DJ. The rostral ventrolateral medulla: anatomical substrates of cardiopulmonary intergration. In: Koepchen H-P, Huopaniemi T, eds. Cardiorespiratory and Motor Coordination. New York: Springer, 1991:89–102.

74. Cooper JR, Bloom FE, Roth RH. The Biochemical Basis of Neuropharmacology. 7th ed. New York: Oxford University Press, 1996.

75. Paul S. GABA and glycine. In: Bloom FE, Kupfer DJ, eds. Psychopharmacology: The Fourth Gereration of Progress. New York: Raven Press, 1995:87–94.

76. Zorumski CF, Isenberg KE. Insights into the structure and function of GABA-benzodiazepine receptors: ion channels and psychiatry. Am J Psychiatry 1991; 148:162–173.

77. Drugan RC, Morrow AL, Weizman R, Weizman A, Deutsch SI, Crawley JN, Paul SM. Stress-induced behavioral depression in the rat is associated with a decrease in GABA receptor-mediated chloride ion flux and brain benzodiazepine receptor occupancy. Brain Res 1989; 487:45–51.

78. Weizman R, Weizman A, Kook KA, Vocci F, Deutsch SI, Paul SM. Repeated swim stress alters brain benzodiazepine receptors measured in vivo. J Pharmacol Exp Ther 1989; 249:701–707.

79. Wiezman R, Weizman A, Kook KA, Vocci F, Deutsch SI, Paul SM. Adrenalectomy prevents the stresss-induced decrease in in vivo [3H]Ro15-1788 binding to GABAA benzodiazepine receptors in the mouse. Brain Res 1990; 519:347–350.

80. Shekhar A, Keim S, Simon JR, McBride WJ. Dorsomedial hypothalamic GABA dysfunction produces physiological arousal following sodium lactate infusions. Pharmacol Biochem Behav 1996; 55:249–256.

81. Crestani F, Benke D, Reyes G, Fritschy JM, Lusher B, Mohler H. Impairment of $GABA_A$ receptor function by subunit gene targeting in mice results in neophobia [abstr 327.2]. Soc Neurosci Abstr 1996; 22.

82. Roy-Byrne PP, Cowley DS, Greenblatt DJ, et al. Reduced benzodiazepine senitivity in panic disorder. Arch Gen Psychiatry 1990; 47:534–538.

83. Roy-Bryne P, Wingerson DK, Radant A, Greenblatt DJ, Cowley DS. Reduced sensitivity in patients with panic disorder: comparison with patients with obsessive-compulsive disorder and normal subjects. Am J Psychiatry 1996; 153:1444–1449.

84. Nutt DJ, Glue P, Lawson CW, et al. Flumazenil provocation of panic attacks: evidence for altered benzodiazepine sensitivity in panic disorder. Arch Gen Psychiatry 1990; 47:917–925.

85. Crowe RR, Wang ZW, Noyes R, Albrecht BE, Darlison MG, Bailey M, Johnson KJ, Zoega T. Candidate gene study of eight GABA$_A$ receptor subunits in panic disorder. Am J Psychiatry 1997; 154:1096–1100.

86. Roy-Byrne PP, Cowley DS, Hommer D, et al. Effect of acute and chronic benzodiazepines on plasma GABA in anxious patients and controls. Psychopharmacology 1992; 109:153–156.

87. Goddard AW, Narayan M, Woods SW, Germine M, Kramer GL, Davis LL, Petty F. Plasma levels of GABA and panic disorder. Psychiatry Res 1996; 63:223–225.

88. Rimon R, Lepola U, Jolkkonen J, Halonen T, Reikkien P. Cerebrospinal fluid gamma-aminobutyric acid in patients with panic disorder. Biolog Psychiatry 38:737–741.

89. Ballenger JC, Burrows GD, DuPont R Jr, Lessre IM, Noyes R Jr, Pecknold JC, Rifkin A, Swinson RP. Alprazolam in panic disorder and agoraphobia: results from a multicenter trial. I. Efficacy in short-term treatment. Arch Gen Psychiatry 1988; 45:413–422.

90. Tesar GE, Rosenbaum JF, Pollack MH, Otto MW, Sachs GS, Herman JB, Cohen LS, Spier SA. Doubled-blind, placebo-controlled comparison of clonazepam and alparazolam for panic disorder. J Clin Psychiatry 1991; 52:69–76.

91. Nagy LM, Krystal JH, Woods SW, Charney DS. Long-term efficacy of alprazolam in panic disorder: a 2.5 year follow-up study. Arch Gen Psychiatry 1990; 46:993–999.

92. Loscher W. Valproate induced changes in GABA metabolism at the subcellular level. Biochem Pharmacol 1981; 30:1364–1366.

93. Paslawski T, Treit D, Baker GB, George M, Coutts RT. The antidepressant drug phenelzine produces antianxiety effects in the plus-maze and increases in rat brain GABA. Psychopharmacology 1996; 127:19–24.

94. Crawley JN. Comparative distribution of cholecystokinin and other neuropeptides. Ann NY Acad Sci 1995; 448:1–8.

95. Harro J, Vasar E, Bradwejn J. Cholecystokinin in animal and human research on anxiety. TiPS 1993; 14:244–249.
96. Fekete M, Lengyel A, Hegedus B, Penke B, Zarandy M, Toth GK, Telegdy G. Further analysis of the effects of cholecystokinin octapeptide on avoidance in rats. Eur J Pharmacol 1984; 98:79–91.
97. Singh L, Lewis AS, Field MJ, Hughes J, Woodruff GN. Evidence for an involvement of the brain cholecystokinin B receptor in anxiety. Proc Natl Acad Sci USA 1991; 88:1130–1133.
98. Woodruff GN, Huges J. Cholecystokinin antagonists. Ann Rev Pharmocol Toxicol 31:469–501.
99. Bradwejn J, Koszycki D, Shriqui C. Enhanced sensitivity to cholecystokinin tetrapeptide in panic disorder. Arch Gen Psychiatry 1991; 48: 603–610.
100. Bradwejn J, Koszycki D. Annable L, Couetoux du Tertre A, Reines S, Karkanias C. A dose- ranging study of the behavioral and cardiovascular effects of CCK-tetrapeptide in PD. Biolog Psychiatry 1992; 32:903–912.
101. Bradwejn J, Koszycki D, Payeur R, Bourin M, Borthwick H. Study of the replication of action of cholecystokinin in panic disorders. Am J Psychiatry 1992; 149:962–964.
102. van Megen HJGM, Westenberg HGM, den Boer JA, Haigh JRM, Traub M. Pentagastrin induced panic attacks: enhanced sensitivity in panic disorder patients. Psychopharmacology 1994; 114:449–455.
103. Abelson JL, Nesse RM. Pentagastrin infusions in patients with panic disorder. I. Symptoms and cardiovascular responses. Biolog Psychiatry 1991; 36:73–83.
104. Bradwejn J, Koszycki D, Couetoux du Tetre A, van Megen H, den Boer J, Westenberg H, Annable L. The panicogenic effects of cholecystokinin-tetrapeptide are antagonized by L-365,260, a central cholecystokinin receptor antagonist, in patients with panic disorder. Arch Gen Psychiatry 1994; 51:486–493.
105. Lydiard RB, Ballenger JC, Laraia MT, Fossey MD, Beinfeld MC. CSF cholecystokinin concentrations in patients with panic disorder and normal comparison subjects. Am J Psychiatry 1992; 149:691–693.
106. Brambilla F, Bellodi L, Perna G, Garberi A, Sacerdote P. Lymphocyte cholecystokinin concentrations in panic disorder. Am J Psychiatry 1993; 150:1111–1113.
107. Kramer MS, et al. A placebo-controlled trial of L-365-260, a CCKB antagonist, in panic disorder. Biolog Psychiatry 1995; 37:462–466.
108. Bradwejn J, Koszycki D. Imipramine antagonism of the panicogenic

effects of cholecystokinin tetrapeptide in panic disorder patients. Am J Psychiatry 1994; 151:261–263.

109. Brawman-Minzter O, et al. Effects of cholecystokinin agonist pentagastrin in patients with generalized anxiety disorder. Am J Psychiatry 1997; 154:700–702.

110. Le Melledo J-M, et al. Premenstrual dysphoric disorder and response to cholecystokinin-tetrapeptide. Arch Gen Psychiatry 1995; 52:605–605.

111. Dunn AJ, Berridge CW. Physiological and behavioral reponses to corticotropin-releasing factor administration: is CRF a mediator of anxiety or stress responses? Brain Res Rev 1990; 15:71–100.

112. Butler PD, Weiss JM, Stout JC,Nemeroff CB. Corticotropin-releasing factor produces fear-enhancing and behavioral activating effects following infusion into the locus coeruleus. J Neurosci 1990; 10:176–183.

113. Sutton RE, Koob GF, LeMoal M, et al. Corticotropin releasing factor produces behavioral activation in rats. Nature 1982; 297:331.

114. Coplan JD, Andrews MW, Rosenblum LA, Owens MJ, Freidman S, Gorman JM, Nemeroff CB. Persistent elevations of cerebrospinal fluid concentrations of corticotropin-releasing factor in adult nonhuman primates exposed to early-life stressors: implications for the pathophysiology of mood and anxiety disorders. Proc Natl Acad Sci USA 1996; 93: 1619–1623.

115. Nemeroff CB, Widerlov E, Bissette G, et al. Elevated concentrations of CSF corticotropin-releasing factor-like immunoreactivity in depressed patients. Science 1984; 226:1342.

116. Bremner JD, Licinio J, Darnell A, Krystal JH, Owens MJ, Southwick SM, Nemeroff CB, Charney DS. Elevated CSF cortocotropin-releasing factor concentrations in posttraumatic stress disorder. Am J Psychiatry 1997; 154:624–629.

117. Jolkkonen J, Lepola U, Bissette G, et al. CSF corticotropin-releasing factor is not affected in panic disorder. Biolog Psychiatry 1993; 33: 136–138.

118. Roy-Byrne PP, Uhde TW, Post RM, et al. The corticotropin-releasing hormone stimulation test in patients with panic disorder. Am J Psychiatry 1986; 143:896.

119. Holsboer F, von Bardeleben U, Buller R, Heuser I, Steiger A. Stimulation response to corticotropin-releasing hormone (CRH) in patients with depression, alcoholism, and panic disorder. Horm Metab Res 1987; 16(suppl):80–81.

120. Rappaport MH, Risch SC, Golsham S, Gillin JC. Neuroendocrine effects of ovine corticotropin-releasing hormone in panic disorder patients. Psychiatry 1989; 26:344–348.

121. Abelson JL, Curtis GC. Hypothalamic-pituitary-adrenal axis activity in panic disorder. Arch Gen Psychiatry 1996; 53:323–331.

122. Rapapport MH, Risch SC, Gilliin JC, Janowsky DS. Blunted growth hormone response to peripheral infusion of human growth hormone-releasing factor in patients with panic disorder. Am J Psychiatry 1989; 146:92–95.

123. Tancer ME, Stein MB, Black B, Uhde TW. Blunted growth hormone responses to growth hormone releasing factor and to clonidine in panic disorder. Am J Psychiatry 1993; 150:336–337.

124. Stein MB, Walker JR, Anderson G, Hazen AL, Ross CA, Eldridge G, Forde DR. Childhood physical and sexual abuse in patients with anxiety disorders and in a community sample. Am J Psychiatry 1996; 153:275–277.

125. Davis M. The role of the amygdala in fear and anxiety. Am Rev Neurosci 1992; 15:353–375.

126. LeDoux JE. Emotion and the amygdala. In: Aggleton JP, ed. The Amygdala: Neurobiological Aspects of Emotion, Memory and Mental Dysfunction. New York: Wiley-Liss, 1992:339–352.

127. Kaada BR. Stimulation and regional ablation of the amygdaloid complex with reference to functional representations. In: Eleftheriou BE, ed. The Neurobiology of the Amygdala. New York: Plenum Press, 1972:205–281.

128. Davis M. Animal models of anxiety based upon classical conditioning: the conditioned emotional response and fear potentiated startle effect. Pharmacol Ther 1990; 47:147–165.

129. Falls WA, Miserendino MJ, Davis M. Extinxtion of fear-potentiated startle: blockade by infusion of an NMDA antagonist into the amygdala. J Neurosci 1992; 12:854–863.

130. Miserendino MJD, Sananes CB, Melia KR, Davis M. Blocking of acquisition but not expression of conditioned fear-potentiated startle by NMDA antagonists in the amygdala. Nature 1990; 345:716–718.

131. Grillon C, Amelli R, Goddard AW, Woods SW, Davis M. Fear-potentiated startle in panic disorder patients. Biolog Psychiatry 1994; 35(7): 775–777.

132. Phillips RG, LeDoux JE. Differential contribution of amygdala and hippocampus to cued and contextual fear conditioning. Behav Neurosci 1992; 106:274–285.

133. Vandergriff JL, Rasmussen K. The selective AMPA antagonist, LY300168, suppresses morphine withdrawal-induced activation of locus coeruleus neurons and behavioral signs of morphine withdrawal [abstr 478.2]. 27th Annual Meeting of the Society for Neuroscience, New Orleans, Oct 25–30, 1997.

134. Dantendorfer K, Prayer D, Kramer J, Amering M, Baischer W, Berger P, Schoder M, Steinberger K, Windhaber J, Imhof H, Katschnig H. High frequency of EEG and MRI brain abnormalities in panic disorder. Psychiatry Res 1996; 68:41–53.

135. Knowles JA, Fyer AJ, Vieland VJ, Heiman GA, Rassnick H, Fine LD,Woodley KA, Das K, Adams PB, Hodge SE, Ott J, Klien DF, Weissman MM, Gilliam TC. Suggestion of genetic linkage of panic disorder to chromosome 20q 13.2–13.3, 1994. Submitted.

136. Enoch M, Rorbaugh JW, Davis EZ, Harris CR, Ellingsom RJ, Andreason P, Moore V, Varner JL, Brown GL, Eckardt MJ, et al. Relationship of genetically transmitted alpha EEG traits to anxiety disorders and alcoholism. Am J Med Genet 1995; 60:400–408.

137. Knott VJ, Bakish D, Lusk S, Barkely J, Perugini M. Quantitative EEG correlates of panic disorder. Psychiatry Res 1996; 68:31–39.

138. Knott VJ, Bakish D, Lusk S, Barkely J. Relaxation-induced EEG alterations in panic disorder. J Anx Disord 1997; 11:365–376.

139. Locatelli M, Bellodi L, Perna G, Scarone S. EEG power modifications in panic disorder during a temporolimbic activation task: relationships with temporal lobe clinical symptomatology. J Neuropsychiatry Clin Neurosci 1993; 5:409–414.

140. Mellman TA, Uhde TW. Electroencephalographic sleep in panic disorder. Arch Gen Psychiatry 1989; 46:178–184.

141. Stein MB, Enns MW, Kryger MH. Sleep in nondepressed patients with panic disorder. II. Polysomnographic assessment of sleep architecture and sleep continuity. J Affect Disord 1993; 28:1–6.

142. Arriaga F, Paiva T, Matos-Pires A, Cavaglia F, Lara E, Bastos L. The sleep of non-depressed patients with panic disorder: a comparison with normal controls. Acta Psychiatr Scand 1996; 93:191–194.

143. Young GB, Chandarana PC, Blume WT, McLachlan RS, Munoz DG, Girvin JP. Mesial temporal lobe seizures presenting as anxiety disorders. J Neuropsychiatry Clin Neurosci 1995; 7:352–357.

144. Toni C, Cassano GB, Perugi G, Murri L, Mancino M, Petracca A, Akiskal H, Roth SM. Psychosensorial and related phenomena in panic disorder and in temporal lobe epilepsy. Compr Psychiatry 1996; 37: 125–133.

145. Freedman RR, Ianni P, Ettedgui E, Puthezhath N. Ambulatory monitor-
      ing of panic disorder. Arch Gen Psychiatry 1985; 42:244–248.
146. Roth WT, Margraf J, Ethers A, Taylor CB, Maddock RJ, Davies S,
      Agras WS. Stress test reactivity in panic disorder. Arch Gen Psychiatry
      1992; 49:301–310.
147. Stein MB, Tracer ME, Uhde TW. Heart rate and plasma norepinephrine
      responsivity to orthostatic challenge in anxiety disorders. Arch Gen
      Psychiatry 1992; 49:311–317.
148. Yeragani VK, Phol R, Berger R, Balon R, Ramesh C, Glitz D, Sriniva-
      san K, Weinberg P. Decreased heart rate variabilty in panic disorder
      patients: a study of power-spectral analysis of heart rate. Psychiatry
      Res 1993; 46:89–103.
149. Rechlin T, Weis M, Spitzer A, Kaschka WP. Are affective disorders
      asscociated with alterations of heart rate variability? J Affect Disord
      1994; 32:271–275.
150. Klein E, Cnaani E, Harel T, Braun S, Ben-Haim SA. Altered heart rate
      variability in panic disorder patients. Biolog Psychiatry 1995; 37:18–
      24.
151. Yeragani VK, Srinivasan K, Balon R, Ramesh C, Berchou R. Lactate
      sensitivity and cardiac cholinergic function in panic disorder. Am J
      Psychiatry 1994; 151:1226–1228.
152. Yeragani VK, Pohl R, Srinivasan K, Balon R, Ramesh C, Berchou R.
      Effects of isoproterenol infusions on heart rate variability in patients
      with panic disorder. Psychiatry Res 1995; 56:289–293.
153. Middleton HC, Ashby M. Clinical recovery from panic disorder is asso-
      ciated with evidence of changes in cardiovascular regulation. Acta
      Psychiatr Scand 1995; 91:108–113.
154. Weissman MM, Markowitz JS, Ouelette R, Greenwald S, Kahn
      JP. Panic disorder and cardiovascular/cerebrovascular problems:
      results from a community survey. Am J Psychiatry 1990; 147:1504–
      1508.
155. Malik M, Camm AJ. Heart rate variability. Clin Cardiol 1990; 13:570–
      576.
156. Goddard AW, Charney DS. Toward an integrated neurobiology of
      panic disorder. J Clin Psychiatry 1997; 58(suppl 2):4–11.
157. Benkelfat C, Bradwejn J, Meyer E, et al. Functional neuroanatomy of
      CCK-4-induced anxiety in normal healthy volunteers. Am J Psychiatry
      1995; 152:1180–1184.
158. Rauch SL, Savage CR, Albert NM, et al. A positron emission tomo-

graphic study of simple phobic symptom provocation. Arch Gen Psychiatry 1995; 52:20–28.

159. Thorpe SJ, Rolls ET, Maddison S. The orbitofrontal cortex: neuronal activity in the behaving monkey. Exp Brain Res 1983; 49:93–115.

160. Jayanmard J, Shlik SH, Kennedy FJ, Vaccarino J, Bradwejn C. Positron emission tomography study of cholecystokinin-4-induced panic attacks in healthy volunteers[abstr 714.2]. 27th Annual Meeting of the Society for Neuroscience, New Orleans, Oct 25–30, 1997.

161. LaBar KS, Gatenby JC, Gore JC, LeDoux JE, Phelps EA. Amygdalocortical activation during conditioned fear acquisition and extinction: a mixed-trial MRI study [abstr 553.11]. 27th Annual Meeting of the Society for Neuroscience, New Orleans, Oct 25–30, 1997.

162. Ontiveros A, Fontaine R, Breton G, et al. Correlation of severity of panic disorder and neuroanatomical changes on magnetic resonance imaging. J Neuropsychiatry Clin Neurosci 1989; 1:404–408.

163. Reiman EM, Raichle ME, Butler FK, et al. A focal brain abnormality in panic disorder, a severe form of anxiety. Nature 1984; 310:683–685.

164. Nordahl TE, Semple WE, Gross M, et al. Cerebral glucose metabolic differences in patients with panic disorder. Neuropsychopharmacology 1990; 3:261–272.

165. Woods SW, Koster K, Krystal JK, et al. Yohimbine alters regional cerebral blood flow in panic disorder. Lancet 1988; ii:678.

166. DeCristofaro MR, Sessarego A, Pupi A, et al. Brain perfusion abnormalities in drug naive, lactate-sensitive panic patients. Biolog Psychiatry 1993; 33:505–512.

167. Kaschka W, Feistel H, Ebert D. Reduced benzodiazepine receptor binding in panic disorders measured by iomazenil SPECT. J Psychiatr Res 1995; 29:427–434.

168. Schlegel S, Steinert H, Bockisch A, Hahn K, Schloesser R, Benkert O. Decreased benzodiazepine receptor binding in panic disorder measured by IOMAZENIL-SPECT: a preliminary report. Eur Arch Psychiatry Clin Neurosci 1994; 244:49–51.

169. Kuikka JT, Pitkanen A, Lepola U, Partanen K, Vainio P, Bergstrom KA, Wieler HJ, Kaiser KP, Mittelbach L, Koponen H, et al. Abnormal regional benzodiazepine receptor uptake in the prefrontal cortex in patients with panic disorder. Nucl Med Commun 1995; 16:273–280.

170. Bremner DJ, Innis RB, White T, Masahiro F, Silbersweig D, Goddard AW, Staib L, Cappiello A, Woods SW, Baldwin R. Charney DS. SPECT [I-123] measurement of the benzodiazepine receptor in panic

disorder [abstr]. 36th Annual Meeting of the American College of Neuropsychopharmacology, Waikoloa, Hawaii, Dec 1997.

171.   Price LH, Goddard AW, Barr, L, Goodman WK. Pharmacologic chal-
       lenges in anxiety disorders. In: Bloom FE, Kupfer DJ, eds. Psychophar-
       macology: The Fourth Generation of Progress. New York: Raven Press,
       1995:1311–1325.

4

Early Antecedents of Panic Disorder

Genes, Childhood, and the Environment

Dina R. Hirshfeld and Jerrold F. Rosenbaum
Massachusetts General Hospital
and Harvard Medical School
Boston, Massachusetts

Jordan W. Smoller, Steffany J. Fredman, and Maria T. Bulzacchelli
Massachusetts General Hospital
Boston, Massachusetts

The field of developmental psychopathology has emphasized the identification of specific risk and protective factors that confer vulnerability
or resiliency to psychopathology at various ages. The study of such
antecedents is relevant to clinicians because it aids both in understanding the mechanisms by which disorders develop and in identifying specific individuals at risk. The better we understand the precursors of
panic disorder, the more accurately we can identify individuals to target
for preventive interventions. The more clearly we elucidate the mechanisms by which these vulnerability factors interact to bring about disorder, the more empirically founded and efficient these interventions
can be.

In this chapter, we review what is known about the genetic,
temperamental, childhood, familial, and environmental risk factors for

panic disorder. While the number of studies addressing these topics has multiplied over the past decade, research in this area is still in its early stages. Studies of the genetics of panic disorder have just begun to move beyond family and twin studies into molecular-genetic analyses. With respect to other risk factors, no study to date has actually followed individuals at high risk for panic disorder from infancy through the period of risk. Our sources instead represent a combination of retrospective studies of adults already affected and cross-sectional and prospective studies of children at heightened risk for panic disorder (e.g., offspring of adults with panic disorder, or children with anxiety disorders or behavioral inhibition). The most compelling evidence comes from areas in which retrospective findings in adults with panic disorder converge with prospective findings in young children at risk. Therefore, in each section, we review both types of studies, present hypotheses about early antecedents, and point out areas for future research. Since the work in this area is limited, particularly with regard to factors predisposing specifically to panic disorder among the anxiety disorders, in some sections we broaden our focus to discuss risk factors for onset of anxiety disorders in general, or factors hypothesized to predispose to the onset of panic. In the final section, we discuss the ways in which our preliminary knowledge about early precursors of panic disorder can inform clinical and preventive practice.

GENETIC INFLUENCES

Well before the diagnoses of "panic disorder" and "agoraphobia" were introduced into the standard nosology by DSM-III, there was evidence from family history studies that pathological anxiety can run in families (1–3). In the past two decades, more sophisticated study designs have been applied to determine the familial and genetic basis of panic disorder. As we discuss below, family studies have consistently demonstrated that panic disorder can be familial, although the relative contribution of genes and environment to that familiality has been harder to establish. Encouraged by evidence that panic disorder may be heritable and exploiting recent dramatic advances in molecular genetics, investigations are currently underway to map genes that influence panic anxiety. At the time of this writing, however, no genetic loci influencing panic disorder have been conclusively identified. In this section, we briefly review the evidence that genetic factors influence the panic disorder phenotype.

Family and Twin Studies

Since the introduction of panic disorder as a diagnostic entity in 1980 with the publication of DSM-III, at least five family history studies (4–8) and seven direct-interview family studies (9–18) have been reported. Every one of these studies has documented an excess risk of panic disorder among the relatives of affected probands. Because agoraphobia is considered an associated condition, several of the studies have reported rates of panic disorder with and without agoraphobia. Table 1 summarizes the direct-interview family studies. Overall, these studies have found that first-degree relatives of probands with panic disorder have about a three- to 17-fold higher lifetime risk of panic disorder compared to relatives of unaffected probands.

Early-onset panic disorder may represent a more genetically influenced subtype (8,19). In a large family study, Goldstein and colleagues (19) found that relatives of probands who developed panic disorder before age 20 had a 17-fold higher risk of panic disorder compared to relatives of normal controls, while relatives of probands with later-onset panic disorder had a sixfold increased risk compared to relatives of controls. Relatives of the early-onset panic probands had higher rates of agoraphobia but did not differ from the relatives of later-onset panic probands in age of onset of panic or in symptom profiles.

Several segregation analyses, in which inheritance patterns (e.g., recessive, dominant, polygenic) are tested statistically to determine whether they fit the data obtained in a family study, have been performed for panic disorder (9,20–22). All these analyses failed to reject the possibility that a single major gene (either an incompletely penetrant dominant gene or a recessive gene) influences panic disorder. However, the limitations of these analyses must be understood. A segregation analysis may indicate that the pattern of cases in a set of pedigrees could be explained by single major locus inheritance, but it cannot prove that this model is accurate. Other models may

Table 1 Direct-Interview Family Studies of Panic Disorder and Agoraphobia

Study	Probands	Relative risk to first-degree relatives of ill vs. control probands			
		PD with or without AG	PD without AG	PD with AG	AG
Crowe et al. (1983)	PD	10.7	—	—	—
	PD + AG	13.7	—	—	—
Noyes et al. (1986)	PD without AG	—	4.1	—	0.45
	AG	—	2.0	—	2.8
Mendlewicz et al. (1993)	PD without AG	—	14.7	—	0.53
Maier et al. (1993)	PD with or without AG	3.4	3.6	2.9	—
	PD without AG	3.3	4.3	2.2	—
	PD with AG	3.6	2.9	3.8	—
Goldstein et al. (1994)	PD without MDD[a]	8.77 (2.28–33.8)	9.48 (0.97–92.4)	8.28 (1.53–44.7)	13.73 (1.38–137.0)
Horwath et al. (1995)	PD with MDD[a]	5.66 (1.51–21.2)	7.51 (0.81–70.0)	4.25 (0.80–22.4)	5.39 (0.55–53.3)

Study		Estimate		
Goldstein et al. (1997)	Early-onset PD (≤20 years old)[a]	16.9 (4.4–64.3)	—	—
	Later-onset PD (>20 years old)[a]	5.6 (1.5–20.8)	—	—
Mannuzza et al. (1994, 1995)	PD without MDD	2.8	—	—
	PD with MDD	4.1	—	—
Fyer et al. (1995, 1996)	PD with or without AG	3.3	—	—
	PD with AG	3.0	3.0 (1.0–8.7)	—
	PD with social phobia	3.0	—	—

[a] Estimates are hazard ratios adjusted for age, sex, interview status, and proband ascertainment source. 95% confidence intervals, where available, are given in parentheses.

PD = panic disorder; AG = agoraphobia; MDD = major depressive disorder.

Table 2 Twin Studies of Panic Disorder

Study	Diagnosis	Number of twin pairs	Concordance (%)	
			MZ	DZ
Clinical samples				
Torgersen (1983)	Anxiety disorder with panic attacks	85	31	0
Skre et al. (1993)	Panic disorder	81	42	17
Population-based				
Kendler et al.	Panic disorder	1033	23.9	10.9
(1992, 1993)	Agoraphobia		23.2	15.3
Perna et al. (1997)	Panic/agoraphobia	60	73	0
	Sporadic panic attacks		57	43

also provide an adequate "fit." For example, the only study that examined a multifactorial polygenic model (9) was unable to reject it. Definitive evidence that genes contribute to the etiology of a disorder requires the isolation of the specific genes involved by molecular-genetic analysis.

Although estimates of risk have varied, the weight of evidence from family studies clearly supports the view that panic disorder and agoraphobia are familial. However, because members of a family share environments as well as genes, a disorder may run in families for reasons that have little to do with genetics. How influential are genetic factors in the familiality of panic disorder? By parsing the contributions of genes and environment, twin studies can help answer this question. While numerous twin studies have examined the heritability of anxiety traits and symptoms, only a few have looked at concordance rates for categorical diagnoses of panic disorder with or without agoraphobia (23–27) (see Table 2).

In the first of these studies, Torgersen (23) interviewed 299 same-sex twin pairs ascertained as part of a nationwide survey of twins treated for neurotic disorders in Norway. The diagnoses were made primarily on the basis of computer coding of the results of an interview with the Present State Examination according to DSM-III criteria. Thirty-two identical (MZ) and 53 fraternal (DZ) probands were found to have an anxiety disorder as their primary diagnosis. Probandwise concordance rates for MZ twins were higher than for DZ twins for all anxiety disorders except generalized anxiety disorder (GAD), but the differences were not statistically significant because of the limited number of cases. However, when panic disorder, possible panic disorder (fewer than five attacks in a 1-month period), and agoraphobia with panic attacks were combined into the category "anxiety disorder with panic attacks," a significant difference emerged, with 31% of MZ twins and 0% of DZ twins concordant. It should be noted, however, that there were no MZ twin pairs in which both twins had the same specific anxiety disorder. Also, given the familiality of panic disorder, the low concordance rate for DZ twins is difficult to explain. The other clinical sample of twins was ascertained from an outpatient clinic and from records of inpatient admissions to Norwegian psychiatric hospitals. Eighty-one same-sex twin pairs were interviewed using the Structured Clinical Interview for DSM-III (SCID), and diagnoses were recoded according to DSM-III-R criteria. Forty-nine of the probands met criteria for at least one anxiety disorder; of these, 61% had panic disorder (73% of these had agoraphobia), and another 6% had agoraphobia without panic disorder. Of probands with panic disorder, 5/12 (42%) of MZ twins were concordant compared with 3/18 (17%) of DZ twins, although this difference did not reach statistical significance.

The largest twin study of panic disorder involved 1033 female twin pairs from the population-based Virginia Twin Registry (24,26) and used the SCID to make DSM-III-R diagnoses. For clinical diagnoses, two levels of affected status were defined: clinician-narrow, which included only "definite" and "probable" cases, and clinician-broad, which also included "possible" cases. Probandwise concordance rates were higher for MZ than DZ twins for both the "narrow" (23.9% vs. 10.9%) and "broad" (23.2% vs. 5.7%) diagnoses of panic disorder. Model-fitting of genetic and environmental components of variance indicated that the liability to panic was due primarily to additive genetic and individual-specific environmental effects rather than to family environment. Depending on the diagnostic criteria, the estimated heritability of panic disorder ranged from 32 to 46%. It is important to note, however, that heritability estimates depend on the population being studied and might differ in other samples.

Most recently, Perna and colleagues (27) reported on a population-based volunteer sample of 60 twin pairs who were diagnosed according to DSM-IV criteria based on a nonstructured psychiatric interview. Of the twin pairs in which a proband had panic disorder, eight of 11 (73%) of MZ twin pairs were concordant for panic disorder compared to none of the six DZ pairs. They also found that concordance rates for subsyndromal spontaneous panic attacks were nonsignificantly higher in MZ (57%) than in DZ (43%) pairs. Again, the small sample size raises questions about the precision of these concordance estimates.

In general, twin studies are consistent with the hypothesis that genetic factors influence the liability to panic disorder but that environmental factors explain a larger portion of the variance. The interpretability of these studies is limited by the small number of affected twins in these samples.

Molecular-Genetic Analyses

A variety of molecular-genetic analyses now exist for disease gene mapping (see Ref. 28 for review). Classically, linkage between a genetic marker of known chromosomal location and a disease phenotype is evaluated with a "lod score" statistic. The lod score (logarithm of the odds ratio of linkage) compares the likelihood that two loci are linked with the likelihood that they are not linked given the observed data. Conventionally, a lod score of ≥ 3 is taken to indicate linkage between two loci while a lod score of ≤ -2 is taken to exclude linkage, although different thresholds have been proposed for the study of complex disorders (29). Several issues complicate the use of classic (or "parametric") lod score linkage analysis for an entity such as panic disorder. First of all, the analysis requires the specification of parameters (e.g., mode of inheritance, penetrance) that are unknown in the case of most psychiatric disorders. Second, it may be that panic disorder is influenced by multiple genes of modest effect rather than the single major genes that are more readily identified by lod score linkage analyses. As a result, alternative methods that can overcome such obstacles are being increasingly utilized. These include "nonparametric" methods that examine the sharing of chromosomal segments by affected members of a pedigree (e.g., affected-sibling pair analysis) and association and linkage disequilibrium methods that can detect loci exerting modest effects on complex phenotypes (30).

Several groups have undertaken molecular-genetic studies to search for loci that may be linked to or associated with the panic disorder phenotype. In the first linkage study of panic disorder, Crowe and colleagues (31) reported a lod score of 2.26 for the α-haptoglobin gene on chromosome 16. However, they subsequently excluded close linkage to this locus by examining additional pedigrees. Several "genome scans" are currently underway. In this approach, genetic markers spaced at relatively short intervals across the entire genome are evaluated to determine whether any are linked to the phenotype. Thus far, preliminary reports from these ongoing efforts have not identified any loci linked to panic disorder (32,33).

Disease gene identification can sometimes be accelerated by evaluating specific "candidate genes" that code for proteins suspected to play a role in the pathogenesis of the disorder. Alternatively, if close linkage is not found between the disorder phenotype and a specific candidate gene, that candidate can be ruled out as a genetic cause of the disorder (at least in the pedigrees in which it was evaluated). To date, several candidate genes, including a variety of neurotransmitter and neuropeptide receptor genes, have been tested and failed to show linkage to or association with the panic disorder phenotype (31, 34–40).

Given the evidence that panic disorder is familial and heritable, why has it proved difficult to map susceptibility genes for panic disorder? Molecular-genetic studies of panic disorder face the formidable obstacles that complicate all efforts to map genes for psychiatric disorders. Like other psychiatric disorders, panic disorder is a "complex disorder" that does not seem to follow typical Mendelian inheritance patterns (i.e., dominant, recessive, or sex-linked) (28). The genetic component of panic disorder may be due to several genes (oligogenic) or many genes (polygenic), each exerting a small effect. It might be that the genetic susceptibility to panic disorder requires interactions among different genetic loci (epistasis) or between genetic loci and the environment (multifactorial inheritance). Each of these possibilities can complicate linkage studies. Another threat to linkage studies is the potential for misclassifying affected status due, for example, to incomplete penetrance (not all individuals with the disease genotype express the disease phenotype) or the existence of phenocopies (nongenetic cases of the disorder). It is clear, then, that efforts to establish or even exclude genetic factors in panic disorder will be difficult.

However, the most formidable challenge to identifying genes influencing panic disorder may be the problem of how to define the phenotype (41). The boundaries between psychiatric disorders are often difficult to draw. The diagnostic criteria found in DSM-IV were not designed for genetic studies, and it would be rather surprising if they captured only the elements of panic disorder that are under genetic influence. In a linkage or association study, however, one must decide whether each subject is ''affected'' or not, and phenotypic misclassification can dramatically reduce the power of genetic studies. Unfortunately, the optimal phenotype definition for panic disorder remains uncertain.

For example, questions remain about the genetic relationship between panic disorder and other psychiatric disorders. The clinical features and treatment of panic disorder overlap with those of other anxiety disorders and depression. Are these disorders genetically distinct, or are they influenced in part by common genetic factors? Evidence from family studies suggests that the familial risk of panic disorder is distinguishable from the risk for social phobia, simple phobia, and GAD (11,12,18,42). However, evidence from a large twin study indicated that panic disorder and phobias have shared genetic influences (43). As we discuss below, family studies of anxious temperament (''behavioral inhibition to the unfamiliar'') also provide evidence for a shared genetic diathesis underlying panic and phobic disorders (44). The familial/genetic relationship between panic disorder and major depression has been somewhat controversial. Most family studies examining relatives of panic disorder probands have not found an increased familial risk of major depression (9,11,12,15,17,45), although there have been conflicting reports (14). Comorbid panic disorder and major depression in probands has been associated in some studies with elevated risk of depression, panic disorder, and comorbid panic disorder and depression among first-degree relatives (14–17). However, panic that occurs exclusively within depressive episodes does not appear to be associated with an increased familial risk of panic disorder (46,47).

Like depression, alcoholism frequently affects individuals with panic disorder (48). Does this represent a shared diathesis, "self-medication" of anxiety, or simply the co-occurrence of two common disorders? Several family studies have documented elevated rates of alcoholism in first-degree relatives of probands with panic disorder or agoraphobia (10,11,13,49–53), but others have not (7,9,12,16,46). However, twin studies suggest that if a familial association does exist between panic disorder and alcoholism, it does not appear to be due to a shared genetic diathesis (25,54).

Summary of Genetic Factors

Although the genetic bases of panic disorder are not well understood at this time, several points are worth noting. First, the evidence for the heritability of panic disorder allows us to consider offspring of parents with panic disorder as individuals at high risk for the disorder. This means that prospective longitudinal studies of such children can aid in identifying potential childhood precursors to panic disorder. Second, estimates of heritability suggest that both genetic and environmental factors (especially those that are individual-specific) contribute to the risk for panic disorder. Thus, a full study of the antecedents of panic disorder will need to address environmental and experiential factors as well. Finally, both the genetic and environmental bases of panic disorder may be multifactorial; therefore, there may well be substantial heterogeneity among children at risk for panic disorder. For example, if a large number of etiological factors were known to be associated with panic disorder (e.g., several different mutations, several types of adversity), and a subset were required for its development, then there would be considerable heterogeneity among individuals at risk (55). Some cases might be determined mainly by genetic factors, others primarily by specific environmental factors. Similarly, children at risk for panic disorder might well be both clinically (phenotypically) and neurobio-

Table 3 Summary of Genetic Epidemiology of Panic Disorder

Panic disorder is a familial phenotype (~3- to 17-fold excess risk to first-degree relatives).

Twin studies support a genetic component: heritability was ~30–45% in a large population-based study of female twins.

The mode of inheritance (e.g., single major gene vs. polygenic) has not been established.

Panic disorder and agoraphobia may share genetic determinants, but there have been conflicting data about the relationship of panic disorder to phobic disorders and depression.

To date, no specific genetic loci have been convincingly associated with the panic disorder phenotype.

logically heterogeneous. Table 3 summarizes current information about the genetic epidemiology of panic disorder.

CHILDHOOD PRECURSORS

Retrospective studies of adults and children affected with panic disorder, as well as prospective studies of offspring of parents with panic disorder, have identified a number of potential childhood precursors to panic disorder. These include childhood anxiety disorders, the temperamental style known as "behavioral inhibition to the unfamiliar," and, to some degree, certain physiological markers.

Childhood Anxiety Disorders

Retrospective childhood histories of adults with panic disorder have suggested that anxiety disorders in childhood commonly precede the onset of panic disorder. At first it was thought that childhood separation anxiety disorder in particular was associated with later panic disorder and agoraphobia (56–59, 107). Investigators compared the adult agoraphobic's need for a familiar companion with the child's fear of being apart from his or her parent, and observed that similar neurotransmitter systems were associated with both disorders, evident in the discovery that imipramine treated both successfully (57). However, recent studies have found that other childhood disorders, such as avoidant disorder (or social phobia) and overanxious disorder, are also common in childhood histories of adults with panic disorder (61,62). For example, Otto and colleagues (61) found that of 100 adults with panic disorder, 55% met criteria for at least one childhood anxiety disorder based on structured retrospective interviews. The most frequent disorders diagnosed were social phobia (36%) and overanxious disorder (28%).

Interestingly, it is the more severe cases of adult panic disorder that appear to be harbingered by childhood anxiety disorders. Thus, Otto and Pollack found that adults with panic disorder who had been affected by childhood anxiety disorders were more likely than others to develop agoraphobia, to show earlier onset of panic attacks and phobic avoidance, and to have comorbid anxiety and mood disorders as adults (61,63). Another retrospective study found that childhood separation anxiety disorder conferred a risk for comorbidity of anxiety disorders in adulthood (59,64).

Childhood anxiety disorders appear to precede the onset of panic disorder in youths as well. Biederman and colleagues (65) assessed 472 unselected, clinically referred children and adolescents using structured diagnostic interviews and found that the youngsters with panic disorder with or without agoraphobia showed elevated rates of all anxiety and depressive disorders compared with the psychiatric comparison children. When the mean ages at onset of these comorbid disorders were examined, the authors found that, among the youths with agoraphobia, the earliest anxiety disorder to emerge was simple phobia, followed by avoidant and separation anxiety disorder, followed by agoraphobia. Social phobia, overanxious disorder, and obsessive-compulsive disorder (OCD) tended to follow onset of agoraphobia. Youths with panic disorder showed a similar course, but they had slightly later ages of onset for all the disorders. Interestingly, in the 65% of panic-disordered youngsters who also had agoraphobia, onset of panic disorder tended to follow onset of agoraphobia. This observation contrasts with explanations of the etiology of agoraphobia as a conditioned avoidance response to settings in which panic attacks have occurred. However, it should be noted that children can experience intense anxiety (or limited symptom attacks) without meeting full criteria for panic disorder. This study suggests that some sort of ''anxiety-proneness,'' reflected in a tendency to develop childhood anxiety disorders, may precede the onset of panic disorder.

These findings from retrospective assessments are consistent with cross-sectional and prospective studies of children at risk for panic disorder. A growing number of studies have suggested that young offspring of parents with panic disorder are at increased risk for a spectrum of childhood anxiety disorders. For example, in Weissman and colleagues' classic study (66), children of parents with major depressive disorder who also had panic disorder or agoraphobia were found to have an increased rate of anxiety disorders compared with children of parents with major depression only or without psychiatric disorders (22% vs. 0% vs 2.3%, respectively). In another study, children of adults with panic disorder were found to have higher rates of DSM-III childhood anxiety disorders than children of normal controls, but not those of depressed parents (67). Similarly, children of parents with panic disorder and agoraphobia, with or without comorbid depression, were more likely than normal controls (but not offspring of parents with depression only) to have elevated rates of multiple childhood anxiety disorders (that is, two or more DSM-III childhood anxiety disorders in the same individual) (45). Another group found higher rates of (DSM-III-R) separation anxiety disorder in the offspring of parents with panic disorder plus major depression than in children of normal controls (68). Most recently, children of parents with anxiety disorders (the majority of whom had panic disorder) were found to have higher rates of anxiety disorders than children of normal controls but not than children of parents with depression (69). A 20-year follow-up of individuals who had been treated for school phobia with separation anxiety in childhood found that these individuals had a higher rate of panic disorder with agoraphobia compared with community controls (70).

It is important to note that several studies have suggested that anxiety disorders often precede the development of major depression (71–74) or other affective disorders (75) as well. Thus, the specificity of the association between childhood anxiety disorders and panic disorder requires further study.

It is not known exactly why childhood anxiety disorders are associated with later panic disorder. One possibility is that childhood anxiety disorders reflect a constitutional anxiety-proneness that manifests in different syndromes at different points in development. Another possibility is that children who learn maladaptive (e.g., avoidant) strategies for coping with anxiety in childhood use them later to cope with panic attacks, thereby triggering agoraphobia (61). Given the likelihood that the pathway to panic disorder is multifactorial, each of these explanations may apply to different cases.

Temperament

The idea that childhood anxiety syndromes prefigure adult panic disorder leads naturally to the question of whether there are qualities observable early in life that predispose to anxiety. The study of child temperament and its relation to adjustment and to later personality characteristics has increasingly attracted the attention of developmental researchers over the past few decades. With regard to panic disorder, the best-studied temperamental construct is "behavioral inhibition to the unfamiliar," described by Jerome Kagan and colleagues (76–88). This temperamental trait, observable in laboratory protocols as early as in toddlerhood, consists of a stable tendency to be cautious, quiet, and behaviorally restrained in situations of novelty, and is estimated to occur in 10 to 15% of children. Behavioral inhibition manifests differently at different developmental periods: affected children tend to be irritable and reactive as infants, shy and fearful as toddlers, and cautious, quiet, and introverted when they reach school age. In contrast, about 20% of children display an opposing "uninhibited" profile characterized by bold, gregarious behavior and imperturbability to novelty.

Since the early 1980s, Kagan and colleagues have followed two independent cohorts of children, classified at 21 or 31 months of age as either behaviorally inhibited or uninhibited. To minimize variability and phenocopies produced by stress (e.g., associated with low socioeconomic status), the study included only Caucasian, middle-class children. The children were classified on the basis of behaviors displayed in the laboratory when exposed to unfamiliar settings, people, and toys. Differences in behavior among children in these two categories were substantially preserved from infancy to later assessments at ages 4, 5.5, and 7.5 years (76–80). Correlations between indices of inhibition at the various ages ranged from 0.39 to 0.67, and 70% of inhibited children retained their classification as inhibited at age 7.5 years. These data suggest that the tendency to approach or to withdraw from novelty is an enduring trait. A study of an independent sample of 100 children who showed varying degrees of initial inhibition confirmed that behavioral inhibition remained stable from 14 to 48 months, but only among the 20% of children who were most extremely inhibited (88). This has led Kagan to conceptualize behavioral inhibition as a categorical construct, not a dimensional one. Other researchers have also confirmed the stability of inhibited behavior over the school-age years (89–91).

Several studies have suggested that behavioral inhibition in children has a significant genetic contribution. Matheny (92) found that at ages 18 and 30 months, monozygotic twin pairs were more concordant for inhibited behaviors than dizygotic twins. Moreover, the changes in these behaviors as the children grew older were similar in monozygotic but not dizygotic twin pairs. Robinson and colleagues (93) reported that the estimated heritabilities (h^2) of behavioral inhibition in over 150 twin pairs were 0.53, 0.42, and 0.51 at ages 14, 20, and 24 months, respectively. DiLalla, Kagan, and Reznick (94) reported that at age 24 months, monozygotic twins were more concordant for inhibited behaviors than dizygotic twins (intraclass correlations of aggregate indices of observed inhibited behaviors were 0.82 vs. 0.47, respectively). In this study, the estimated heritability of inhibited behavior was especially high for children rated as extreme in inhibition, supporting Kagan's view that children extreme in inhibition represent a distinct subtype of children.

Behavioral inhibition itself has precursors observable in early infancy. Kagan and Snidman (86,88) have found that about 20% of healthy, middle-class 16-week-old infants become both motorically active and distressed in response to a variety of stimuli that include brightly colored toys moved back and forth in front of their faces and tape recordings of a woman speaking brief sentences. They have termed these children ''high-reactive.'' In turn, about two-thirds of high-reactive infants go on in toddlerhood to become behaviorally inhibited when they encounter unfamiliar people, events, and situations. The association between high reactivity (high negative affect and irritability in early infancy) and inhibition in toddlerhood has been independently confirmed (95). Thus, some, but not all, inhibited children (a little over half) begin life as high-reactive infants (88).

Kagan has theorized that inhibited, compared with uninhibited, children inherit a neurochemistry that produces a low threshold of excitability in the amygdala and its projections to the ventral striatum, hypothalamus, anterior cingulate, central gray, medulla, and sympathetic nervous system (79,88,96). Consistent with this hypothesis, several studies have documented evidence of autonomic arousal among inhibited children. Even before birth, high-reactive infants were found to have higher fetal heart rates, and they maintained higher heart rates at 2 weeks of age while sleeping and being held erect by their mother (88). Older inhibited children, compared with uninhibited ones, consistently showed a greater acceleration of heart rate to a change in posture or when presented with events requiring effortful assimilation or cognitive work (82,97). This increased acceleration contrasts with that in noninhibited children, who tend to habituate to stress. At age 5, in response to mild cognitive stress, inhibited children were more likely to have increased laryngeal muscle tension, pupillary dilation, and higher levels of urinary MHPG, a metabolite of norepinephrine (88). From ages 4 to 8 years, inhibited children exhibited a greater increase in diastolic blood pressure when their posture changed from a sitting to a standing position, suggesting increased noradrenergic tone. In addition, inhibited children had higher salivary cortisol at age 5 but not at age 7 (88). Other physiological differences noted more frequently in inhibited children included greater activation of the anterior area of the right compared with left cerebral hemisphere (88), lower left frontal activation in young children (98,99), and higher potentiated startle in adolescents (88). However, it should be noted that not all inhibited children show these physiological differences. Nonetheless, the combination of behavioral responses of retreat and avoidance and increased arousal in the limbic-sympathetic axes converge with current hypotheses about the neurobiological bases of panic disorder (100–102). These similarities suggest that behavioral inhibition may serve as a marker of anxiety-proneness in young children.

Behavioral inhibition in response to novel stimuli has been observed in other mammalian species as well, including rats, cats (103), dogs, and monkeys (104–106, 108–110). Suomi and colleagues (104–106, 108–110) have noted that some environmental stressors, such as repeated separations, generate persistent "anxiety-like" behaviors in certain rhesus monkeys. These anxiety-like syndromes are much more easily generated in some monkeys than in others; Suomi calls these monkey "high-reactive." The factors that best predict which monkeys will display persisting anxiety to separation are under genetic control and include characteristics similar to those of behaviorally inhibited children, such as diminished exploration and retreat in novel situations, and markers of increased limbic-sympathetic arousal. The existence of behavioral inhibition to novelty in other species is consistent with hypotheses that would link behavioral inhibition to structures that developed relatively early during the evolution of the human central nervous system.

The similarity between Kagan's descriptions of inhibited children at school age and reports from agoraphobic adults about their own childhood (56,111, 113) prompted Rosenbaum and Biederman and colleagues to hypothesize that behavioral inhibition might be an early marker of anxiety disorder, and as such might be observable in the offspring of parents with panic disorder.

Table 4 summarizes the evidence from these pilot studies linking behavioral inhibition to parental and child anxiety disorders. First, behavioral inhibition was assessed in children of parents with panic disorder with agoraphobia (114) and in comparison groups consisting of offspring of parents with major depression and other psychiatric disorders (total $N = 56$). The rates of behavioral inhibition in children of probands with panic disorder and agoraphobia, with or without comorbid major depressive disorder (70% and 85%, respectively), were significantly higher than in children of parents in the psychiatric comparison group without panic disorder with agoraphobia or major depressive disorder (15.4%). Children of parents with major depressive disorder alone had a rate of behavioral inhibition (50%) that could not be differentiated statistically from the rates in either of the other groups. The elevated rate of behavioral inhibition among children of parents with panic disorder has been supported by data from other research groups (115,116).

Rosenbaum, Biederman, Hirshfeld, Faraone, Kagan, Snidman, and colleagues are currently seeking to replicate their earlier findings, using a large sample of children from over 200 families of parents with and without panic disorder, of more varied racial and socioeconomic background, and including both normal comparison subjects and a design involving repeated assessments of behavioral inhibition. Preliminary results from this project confirm the original suggestion that behavioral inhibition is higher among offspring of panic disorder patients than among offspring of normal parents.

Studies have also revealed that children with behavioral inhibition were themselves more likely than others to develop childhood anxiety disorders (117,118). These studies assessed children from two samples: 1) children from the Rosenbaum (114) study who were the offspring of patients with and without panic disorder at the Massachusetts General Hospital (MGH sample) and 2) children from one of Kagan's longitudinal cohorts who had originally been identified at 21 months of age as being inhibited or uninhibited (76). Inhibited children from the MGH sample were significantly more likely than normal controls to have four or more disorders per child (27.8% vs. 0%), two or more anxiety disorders per child (22.2% vs. 0%; $p = 0.04$), and oppositional disorder (33.3% vs. 5.0%; $p = 0.04$). In the Kagan sample, the inhibited children had a substantially higher rate of two or more anxiety disorders when compared with uninhibited children, but this difference fell short of statistical significance (18.2% vs. 0%, Fisher's Exact Test; $p = 0.07$). Taken together, the findings from both samples suggest that behavioral inhibition is associated with anxiety disorders in children. In children at risk for panic disorder, behavioral inhibition may be associated with other psychiatric disorders as well.

If indeed temperamental behavioral inhibition is associated with childhood anxiety disorders, children who remain most consistently inhibited over time ought to be at highest risk for anxiety disorders. To test this hypothesis, children from the Kagan sample who had originally been classified as inhibited at 21 months were stratified into those who remained inhibited at ages 4.0 years, 5.5 years, and 7.5 years and those who did not remain inhibited at all of these assessments (119). As predicted, stably inhibited children had significantly higher rates of any (at least one) anxiety disorder (66.7% vs. 20.7%; $p < 0.05$), multiple (two or more) anxiety disorders (33.0% vs. 0%; $p < 0.05$), and phobic disorders (50.0% vs. 6.9%; $p < 0.05$).

In a 3-year follow-up study (118), significant differences were found between all inhibited and all not-inhibited children in the rates of multiple (four or more) psychiatric disorders, multiple (two or more)

Table 4 Summary of Evidence Linking Behavioral Inhibition to Vulnerability for Anxiety Disorders

Study	Sample	Results
Behavioral inhibition (BI) is observed in offspring patients with panic disorder.		
Rosenbaum et al. (1988)	2–7-year-old children of parents with PDAG with or without comorbid MDD and children of depressed or other psychiatric controls ($N = 56$)	Offspring of parents with PDAG, with or without comorbid MDD, had significantly higher rates of BI compared with psychiatric controls.
Mannassis et al. (1995)	18–59-month-old children of mothers with anxiety disorders (mostly PD) ($N = 20$)	Rate of BI in children of anxious mothers was 65%.
Battaglia et al. (in press)	Young children (mean age 5.8 years) of parents with PD with or without AG and children of controls without PD ($N = 35$)	Children of PD parents had significantly longer latency to first spontaneous comment in a novel laboratory situation (an index of BI).
Children with BI are observed to exhibit or develop childhood anxiety disorders.		
Biederman et al. (1990)	Same as Rosenbaum et al. (1988) and 7–8-year-old children from Kagan et al.'s longitudinal sample (Garcia-Coll et al., 1984) originally selected at age 21 months as extremely BI or uninhibited ($N = 41$)	Children with BI in both samples had higher rates of anxiety disorders than children without BI.
Biederman et al. (1993)	Same as above, re-examined at 3-year follow-up (when children ranged in age from 4 to 11 years)	Children with BI had higher rates of anxiety disorders and of new onset of anxiety disorders than children without BI.

Children who are stably BI over time account for the elevated rates of anxiety disorders.

Hirshfeld et al. (1992)	Kagan et al.'s longitudinal nonclinical sample stratified into children who were BI at all assessments (at age 21 months and 4, 5, and 7 years old) vs. children who were not stably inhibited.	Children with stable BI had significantly higher rates of any anxiety, multiple (≥ 2) anxiety, and phobic disorders. Stably inhibited children had parents with higher rates of multiple childhood anxiety, continuing anxiety, and avoidant disorders.
Biederman et al. (1993)	See above	At 3-year follow-up, stably inhibited children had higher rates of all anxiety disorders assessed, particularly multiple anxiety disorders and avoidant disorder.

Parents of BI children from a nonclinical cohort have higher rates of anxiety disorders.

Rosenbaum et al. (1991)	Kagan and colleagues' longitudinal nonclinical sample (used in Biederman et al., 1990)	Significantly higher rates of social phobia, any childhood anxiety, avoidant, overanxious, and continuing anxiety disorder were found in parents of children with BI.

PD = panic disorder; AG = agoraphobia; MDD = major depressive disorder; BI = behavioral inhibition.

anxiety disorders, avoidant disorder, separation anxiety disorder, and agoraphobia. Three-quarters of those who had separation anxiety at baseline were found to have agoraphobia at follow-up. Moreover, the probabilities of new onsets of anxiety disorders were greater for the inhibited children. Rates of disorder were greatest among children who had stable behavioral inhibition.

These studies converge with other studies that have suggested that an early tendency to exhibit anxiety, shyness, or social withdrawal predicts later anxiety syndromes or difficulties during childhood. For example, in a 5-year prospective study (120), Richman et al. found that 3-year-olds whose mothers described them as exhibiting excessive anxiety were likely to develop "neurotic disorders" (anxiety and depressive disorders) by age 8. This association appeared specific, since no other factor from age 3 predicted neurotic disorders, nor did anxiety at age 3 predict any other type of psychopathology.

Finally, Rosenbaum and colleagues (44) examined rates of anxiety disorders in the parents and siblings of the inhibited children from the Kagan longitudinal cohort (a "bottom-up" approach). When compared to parents of uninhibited and normal comparison children, parents of inhibited children had significantly higher rates of social phobia, any (one or more) childhood anxiety disorder, avoidant and overanxious disorders, and a history of an anxiety disorder that continued from childhood to adulthood. Although the number of siblings meeting criteria for anxiety disorder was small, siblings of inhibited children had higher rates of phobias than comparison children. In this study too, focusing on the children who were most stably and consistently inhibited strengthened the association (119). The finding that behavioral inhibition predicted increased rates of anxiety disorders in biological relatives strengthened the belief that this characteristic of children is linked to the familial predisposition to anxiety disorders. However, it did not suggest a specific link between behavioral inhibition and panic disorder with agoraphobia.

While no studies to date have followed children at high risk for panic disorder through the age of risk, two studies address the issue of whether childhood behavioral inhibition predicts panic disorder in adulthood (112, 121). Reznick et al. (121) developed a retrospective self-report instrument to be administered to adults to assess characteristics of behavioral inhibition in the elementary-school years. When it was administered to adult patients who had been treated successfully for either panic disorder or depression, both groups were found to have significantly higher behavioral inhibition scores than control adults who had never been diagnosed with depression or panic. The second study is a prospective study by Caspi and colleagues (112), who followed to age 21 a sample recruited in early childhood. They found that children who had been inhibited (socially reticent, fearful, and having difficulty concentrating with an unfamiliar examiner) at age 3 had higher rates of any psychiatric disorder and of multiple disorders compared with children rated as well-adjusted at age 3. Although these individuals had elevated rates of depression, they did not have higher rates of anxiety disorders. The idea that adult panic disorder patients often show premorbid trait anxiety (for the most part assessed by self-report in early adulthood) has been noted in several prospective or retrospective community studies (122).

These studies underscore that the specificity of behavioral inhibition as a predictor of panic disorder has not been demonstrated. As noted above, in the Kagan cohort social phobia was more common among parents of inhibited child probands than panic disorder (44). In addition, rates of behavioral inhibition appear to be elevated among offspring of depressed patients (114,123). It may be that behavioral inhibition puts individuals at higher risk for a broad spectrum of anxiety and depressive disorders. Alternatively, as a marker of difficulty coping with novelty or uncertainty, behavioral inhibition may identify children who are more susceptible to stressors that might precipitate the development of psychopathology for which they have a genetic predisposition. These possibilities require further study.

Despite these uncertainties, the evidence available so far does support the hypothesis that among the offspring of parents with panic disorder, behavioral inhibition identifies children at highest risk for developing anxiety disorders. Our group has hypothesized that these children may show a developmental trajectory marked by high-reactive behavior and irritability in infancy; behavioral inhibition from toddlerhood; avoidant, phobic disorders or overanxious disorder in middle childhood; separation anxiety followed by agoraphobia in later childhood; social phobia in early adolescence; and panic disorder in adolescence or young adulthood (124,125). This hypothesis can be tested through longitudinal follow-up of large controlled samples of children at risk for panic disorder such as the one currently under study at our center.

Physiological Differences

While behavioral inhibition to the unfamiliar has psychophysiological correlates, the correspondence between these features and the behavioral markers of inhibition is not always consistent, paralleling the inconsistencies noted in anxious adults between subjective accounts of anxiety and concurrent physiological measures. Another approach to identifying physiological precursors to panic disorder is to compare physiological measures directly between children at risk for panic disorder (usually the offspring of panic patients) and children of controls. Several research groups have conducted such studies, with mixed results.

Reichler and colleagues (126) examined mitral valve prolapse, lactate after exercise, 24-hour urinary catecholamines, and platelet monoamine oxidase (MAO) activity in offspring of panic disorder patients. They found a trend toward higher catecholamines and MAO activity, but the differences did not reach statistical significance. Kagan and colleagues' study of young (2- to 7-year-old) offspring of panic disorder and other patients found that more panic than control offspring showed an acceleratory trend in heart rate over a cognitive battery, but the difference just missed statistical significance (97). Acceleratory trend in heart rate was more closely related to the child's inhibition (indexed by long latencies to spontaneous comments and few comments) than to parental panic disorder. Battaglia and colleagues (116) found that 4- to 8-year-old children of panic disorder patients exhibited higher heart rates than children of nonpsychiatrically disordered controls in response to anxiogenic films. The two groups did not differ in respiration rate, autonomic modulation, or cortisol secretion at home or in the unfamiliar or anxiogenic lab situations. Grillon and colleagues (127) assessed startle reflex in 10- to 17-year-old children of parents with anxiety disorders (panic disorder or social phobia) with or without alcoholism. They found that offspring of anxiety patients had increased startle responsivity compared with controls; this difference remained significant even when the child's diagnosis was controlled for. The authors note that it is not clear whether the increase in magnitude of startle was a trait-like disposition in these children or whether the increased responsivity is state-related, reflecting a tendency to be anxious in response to the test procedure or situation. A small body of literature has documented other physiological markers observed in children who have themselves developed anxiety disorders (125,128,129). However, at this point, it appears that behavioral markers and childhood anxiety disorders diagnosed based on structured diagnostic interviews are more reliable than strictly physiological measures for identifying youngsters who might be at risk for later panic disorder. Naturally, it could be hypothesized that children identified in this manner who also showed physiological signs would be at higher risk for later panic disorder.

COGNITIVE VULNERABILITY FACTORS

When developmental psychopathologists speak of vulnerability factors, they often mean inherited constitutional factors or inborn temperamental biases. It is important to note, however, that a variety of cognitive or behavioral tendencies, regardless of whether they are predominantly hereditary or learned in origin, can make an individual more vulnerable to later psychopathology. In this section, we address some hypothesized cognitive and behavioral features that may predispose to panic disorder and discuss what is known about them.

Anxiety Sensitivity

Adults with panic disorder have been observed to misinterpret typical physiological signs of anxiety as catastrophic (130). They tend to respond to physical sensations of arousal with alarm because of the belief that these sensations will have harmful consequences (e.g., interpreting heart palpitations as signals of an impending heart attack) (131). This tendency has been labeled ''anxiety sensitivity'' (132) and is measured in adults using the Anxiety Sensitivity Index (ASI), a 16-item questionnaire that measures fear of sensations of arousal (133). A recent study suggests that the ASI reflects two factors: a primary factor representing fears of somatic sensations of anxiety and a second factor representing fears of loss of mental control (134). Anxiety sensitivity has been shown to be associated with anxiety disorders, including panic disorder (135), agoraphobia (131), and posttraumatic stress disorder (PTSD) (136), as well as with panic attacks (137,138). Anxiety sensitivity predicts relapse and re-emergence in untreated panic patients; it has also been shown to decrease significantly with cognitive-behavioral therapy (139). Studies have shown that anxiety sensitivity is distinct from trait anxiety, the tendency to be anxious across a wide range of situations (140,141).

McNally has proposed that anxiety sensitivity may constitute a cognitive risk factor for the development of panic disorder (131,142). A recent prospective study of a large nonclinical sample supports this view (140). In this study, Army cadets were followed prospectively during military basic training, an intensely stressful 5-week period. The authors found that anxiety sensitivity, measured before the training period, significantly predicted the development of spontaneous panic attacks, the cardinal symptom of panic disorder, even after controlling for history of panic attacks and trait anxiety.

There have been questions as to whether anxiety sensitivity is present during childhood or whether it is a construct that does not begin to emerge and exert its influence until later in life. A children's version of the Anxiety Sensitivity Index (the CASI) has been developed by Silverman and colleagues (143). Like the ASI, this scale has demonstrated the ability to measure a tendency distinct from trait anxiety or fear frequency. However, it has been suggested that anxiety sensitivity in children as measured by the CASI may not emerge as a construct different from general anxiety or fearfulness until the age of 12, the time when most children begin to acquire formal operational (or abstract) thought (144). At this point in development, children become capable of pairing internal sensations of autonomic arousal or anxiety with the potential for future negative consequences or danger, a prerequisite for anxiety sensitivity. Thus, Chorpita and colleagues (144) report that the CASI predicted unique variance in trait anxiety in children with anxiety disorders beyond that accounted for by fear or physical distress in children 12 years and older but not in children age 7 to 11. Kearney and Tillotson (145) confirmed this pattern in a normative sample, finding that the CASI explained variance above that explained by other measures of fear or anxiety in adolescents aged 12 to 15, but less so for children 8 to 12. However, a recent study with a smaller group of elementary-school-age children found that the CASI did uniquely predict state anxiety (148). More work is needed to evaluate the usefulness of the construct of anxiety sensitivity in young children.

Several studies have explored whether anxiety sensitivity differentially characterizes children already affected with anxiety disorders. In one study, anxiety sensitivity scores were found to differentiate children (age 6 to 18) with anxiety diagnoses from children with no diagnoses but not from children with externalizing disorders (e.g., attention-deficit hyperactivity disorder, conduct disorder) (146). However, another study found that anxiety sensitivity scores were able to discriminate between 8- to 17-year-old children with panic disorder and those with anxiety disorders other than panic disorder (147).

It is not yet known whether high anxiety sensitivity in children predicts the later onset of spontaneous panic attacks and/or panic disorder. However, one study has shown that anxiety sensitivity predicts the degree to which elementary-school children become afraid in response to a physiological challenge procedure (148). In this study, children were subjected to a stair-stepping procedure while their heart rates were monitored. Their CASI scores prior to the procedure predicted the increase in their subjectively rated fear, while increase in heart rate alone did not.

In summary, anxiety sensitivity, or the tendency to fear sensations of anxiety, is associated with adult and childhood anxiety disorders, including panic disorder, and seems to predict fear in response to physiological challenge in young children as well as onset of panic attacks in adults under stressful conditions. Prospective studies are needed to assess whether anxiety sensitivity in childhood will predict later onset of panic disorder.

Other Cognitive and Behavioral Patterns

Other cognitive biases have also been observed to be associated with anxiety disorders. Among the types of cognitive distortions observed in adults with anxiety disorders are the tendency to overappraise threat and underestimate resources for coping (149), to interpret ambiguous situations as threatening and to overestimate the likelihood that those events will happen (150), to regard adverse events as being uncontrollable and unpredictable (151,152), and to anticipate adverse outcomes (152). Although we cannot review the evidence for these biases in detail here, they are worth touching upon since they may be hypothesized to mediate coping styles that might trigger or exacerbate panic disorder or associated phobic avoidance.

Prospective studies in children at risk have not been done, but cross-sectional studies of cognitions in anxious children have tended to observe the same sorts of cognitive biases found in adults, at least for children old enough to introspect and report cognitions (generally, children of school age and older). For example, one study found that clinically referred anxious children (ages 7 to 14) were more likely than nonclinic children to interpret ambiguous scenarios as being threatening, and were more likely to formulate avoidant strategies for coping with them (153). Children with anxiety disorders have been found to have lower self-perceived competence (154). Studies of children from both clinical and nonclinical samples have noted an association between external locus of control (the belief that events are controlled by external factors) and higher trait anxiety (155,156) or fearfulness (157,158). Other studies of cognitions associated with anxiety in children have focused on negative attributional style (see Ref. 159 for a review) and on the types of self-statements that individuals use when coping with anxiety-provoking circumstances (160–162). For example, anxious children tend to report or endorse more negative self-statements but *not* fewer positive self-statements (160,162).

With regard to behavioral tendencies, we can hypothesize that limited or unhelpful strategies for coping with anxiety might predispose an individual to develop or respond maladaptively to panic attacks, leading to panic disorder. Thus, individuals who respond to anxiety by retreating from or avoiding the anxiety-inducing situation, or who lack coping strategies that would enable them to feel more control over a situation, might be at higher risk. This might explain in part the link between childhood inhibition or childhood anxiety disorders and later panic disorder. Prospective studies of children at risk are needed in order to examine whether the cognitive and behavioral features discussed in this section predispose to the development of anxiety disorders in general and to panic disorder in particular.

ENVIRONMENTAL INFLUENCES

Individuals may develop heightened risk for panic disorder as a result of exposure to environmental stressors or experiences. When considering such factors, it is important to note that the distinction between individual vulnerability factors and environmental influences is not always clear-cut, but often involves complex interactions. Developmental researchers have long recognized that children act on their environment, just as the environment acts on them. For example, Sameroff has criticized the straightforward "interactional model," which posits that constitution and environment interact to determine an individual's outcome (163,164). By conceptualizing the individual's constitution and environment as being stable and independent of one another, Sameroff argues, the model fails to consider that these factors interact to influence one another. He notes that "the infant is affecting his caretaking environment at the same time that the caretaking environment is affecting the infant." Similarly, Lerner and Lerner (165) regard children as "agents in their own development," who influence their social environments passively, by eliciting particular sets of responses, and actively, by conceptualizing and reacting to the environment in distinctive ways. Caspi and colleagues (166) also emphasize that an individual's style elicits social responses from the environment that reinforce or repeatedly "reinstate" his or her temperamental tendencies. In the section that follows, we discuss influences of parental behavior and of both early and proximal life stressors.

Parental Influences

While some studies link parental behaviors or attitudes to panic disorder—for example, through retrospective reports by adult panic patients—the connections are neither causal nor specific. Thus, there is no evidence that parental behaviors "cause" panic disorder. On the other hand, different parental behaviors or responses are more or less helpful to children who are prone to anxiety. In some cases, the helpfulness of a parental response may depend on the characteristics of the child. Thus, parental behaviors that are unhelpful to an inhibited child (e.g., cueing the child to act cautiously) may be helpful to an impulsive child. On the other hand, some parental behaviors (e.g., negative criticism, abuse, or neglect) are unhelpful in general. In particular, if behavioral inhibition is indeed a risk factor for anxiety disorders, then parental behaviors that increase or maintain behavioral inhibition would be expected to increase risk for anxiety, while behaviors that reduce it might be expected to lower the risk. Similarly, if cognitive and behavioral tendencies such as the ones discussed in the last section increase risk, then parental behaviors that contribute to their development might also put children at higher risk, while behaviors that promote the child's adaptive coping might reduce the child's risk.

With regard to the first point, preliminary evidence suggests that behavioral inhibition can be modified by experience. Kagan has observed that, while most inhibited children from his longitudinal samples maintain their inhibited status, some do not (e.g., 25% from ages 21 months to 7 years) (79). He has hypothesized that the children who change may be those whose parents encourage more outgoing behavior, and he has noted that as children become aware of their own behavioral inhibition at age 4 or 5, they may attempt to control their responses (79,81). Empirical studies of nonhuman primates support the impression of modifiability (104,106,110). Suomi has noted that inhibited-like behavior to novelty (''high-reactivity'') in rhesus monkeys that has a genetic basis can be modified by different rearing experiences (108). Selectively bred high-reactive rhesus infants that were fostered by highly nurturant rhesus mothers (i.e., less physically punishing, more nurturant, and more promoting of independence) showed fewer inhibited-like behaviors than high- or low-reactive infants fostered by normal mothers (109,110). At the other extreme, other investigators found that environmental manipulation of foraging conditions of primate mothers led to sustained long-term inhibited behavior in their infant offspring (167). When primate mothers were periodically and unpredictably required by the experimenters to work several hours per day to obtain full food rations, these investigators created conditions in which mothers were less contingently responsive to their infants. Under these conditions, these primate mothers failed to engage in the usual compensatory behaviors that follow periods of disturbance in the mother–infant connection. Infant primates reared under these conditions exhibited increased timidity, clinging in novel situations, hesitancy to explore, and susceptibility to despair upon separation. They also displayed neurobiological differences, including changes in noradrenergic functioning. This study suggests that in nonhuman primates, inhibited behaviors and associated psychophysiological features may be elicited by environmental adversity and its effect on maternal behavior. Another salient study concerns observation of the early experiences of "high-reactive" (human) infants. As discussed above, high reactivity at age 4 months predicts behavioral inhibition in toddlerhood (86). Arcus conducted naturalistic home observations of a small sample ($N = 12$) of infants classified as "high-reactive" at 4 months in order to explore factors influencing the onset of behavioral inhibition at age 14 months (168). She found that maternal responsivity to fretting or crying (holding the infant proportionately more often when crying or fretting) at ages 5 to 7 months was positively associated with higher inhibition at age 14 months, while limit-setting (issuing firm prohibitions and removing objects) at ages 9 to 13 months was associated negatively with inhibition. She hypothesized that by requiring infants to undergo mild stress, mothers may have facilitated their children's developing strategies for coping with stress. Another possible interpretation is that by setting clear limits about objects unsafe for the infant to hold, the mothers also provide clear information about distinguishing threatening from nonthreatening objects.

With regard to cognitive and behavioral tendencies, we may hypothesize that parent–child experiences that would increase the child's likelihood to develop anxiety would be those that lead children to regard adverse events as uncontrollable and unpredictable, to anticipate adverse outcomes, to have a reduced sense of their own competency, to overappraise threat, to cope via avoidant strategies, and to show coping-skills deficits. Theorists have offered different hypotheses as to what kinds of parent–child experiences might lead to these vulnerabilities. Barlow has proposed that experiences with uncontrollable events might lead to expectancy of not being able to control later events (151). Spence has summarized some hypothesized parental influences, including modeling fearful behavior, influencing children's perceptions of degree of threat and self-efficacy, inhibiting the child's development of coping strategies, encouraging avoidance, and unwittingly reinforcing fearful behavior through attention and social reinforcement (169). In a series of papers, Krohne formulated a model by which parental behaviors influence children's expectancies and generate trait and evaluative anxiety (158,170). He proposes that children's expectancies of negative outcome and their uncertainty about being able to influence these outcomes are influenced by parental punitiveness and inconsistency, respectively. He hypothesizes that children's competencies and expectations of competency are influenced positively by parental support and negatively by parental restrictiveness.

The empirical evidence available by which to evaluate these hypothesized relations, including information about parental behaviors associated with panic disorder and agoraphobia and with their hypothesized childhood precursors (behavioral inhibition, childhood anxiety), derives from retrospective self-reports by adult patients, concurrent self-reports by anxious children or their parents, and observations of parents of anxious children [see also the review by Rapee (171)].

Several studies have examined retrospective reports by adults with panic disorder or agoraphobia about the nature of their parents' behavior during childhood (60,172–175). These studies have used validated questionnaires assessing the two major child-rearing dimensions that have been observed repeatedly in multiple studies and factor analyses (171,175,176), namely, restrictiveness (or control) and nurturance (or affection). The first relates to the parent's tendency to be controlling or make demands on the child's behavior as opposed to the tendency to allow autonomy, and is associated with efforts to protect the child from harm. The second reflects the degree to which the parent is warm and accepting versus critical or rejecting. In tandem, these variables define the construct ''affectionless control,'' or low warmth and high control, which can be a type of parental overprotection (177). Adults with panic disorder without phobic avoidance, compared with controls, reported significantly higher rates of maternal control or protection (60). Although panic patients were more likely than controls to report ''affectionless control'' in their parents (low affection and high control), they were even more likely to report ''affectionate constraint,'' i.e., parenting marked by high control and high affection. Among agoraphobic adults, reports of low affection in parents seems to be the most consistent finding (172-174,178,179). However, these studies suffer from the limitations inherent in retrospective accounts.

To overcome these biases, other investigators have examined the concurrent family environments of children with anxiety disorders or high trait anxiety. These studies are relevant because they provide information on family environments associated with childhood anxiety, which is often a precursor to adult panic disorder with agoraphobia. In studies in which children are the informants, however, findings have tended to be mixed. Some studies have found no associations between children's anxiety or anxiety disorders and parental restrictiveness or rejection (180–182). On the other hand, a few studies have noted associations between anxiety disorders in children and/or low acceptance (183). For example, a study of over 3000 Mexican adolescents from a community sample found negative associations between reported anxiety symptoms and positive aspects of relationships with parents (including parental expressions of affection, friendship, interest, and confidence) (184). Another large study that used reports by 12- to 14-year-old children found a positive association between child anxiety and parental inconsistency with regard to discipline (182). A series of studies by Krohne and colleagues in Germany (reviewed in Ref. 158) found high trait anxiety in 8- to 14-year-old children to be positively associated with child-reported punishment, restrictiveness, and inconsistency. Associations with parental support and positive feedback were insignificant. In these cross-sectional studies, it is unclear whether these parental attitudes are elicited by the child's behavior or contribute to it.

Where parents are assessed directly, the most consistent associations to emerge are those between child anxiety and parental overprotection. Early authors examined this association using case reports and chart reviews, which were limited because they were uncontrolled or relied on information derived from unstandardized interviews by clinicians who themselves may have had hypotheses about the etiology of anxiety (185–187). Nonetheless, such reports did provide preliminary observations linking "timid, dependent, and fearful" behavior in the child with infantilizing or overprotective behavior by the mother (185,188,189). Subsequent studies used nonvalidated questionnaires, but confirmed the association. Thus, studies found that mothers of agoraphobic adults tended to score highly on a measure of overprotectiveness (190) and that mothers of school phobic youngsters preferred their children to be more affectionate and communicative (more emotionally dependent) than mothers of control children, but not more instrumentally dependent (e.g., needing more assistance) (191). Another study found that mothers of school-phobic children were more accepting and more overprotective than mothers of school-refusing children who were not anxious (192). This pattern is consistent with a study by Parker in which retrospective history of school refusal among adult anxiety patients was also associated with ''caring overprotection'' (193). More recently, Rubin and colleagues (194) have reported that withdrawn or anxious behavior in children is associated with the parental belief that more directive teaching strategies (e.g., telling the child how to behave) and coercive ''power-assertive'' (higher control) approaches were appropriate.

Some investigators have instead used a more open-ended interview approach with parents, the 5-minute-speech sample (FMSS) measure of ''expressed emotion,'' in which parental attitudes of criticism, dissatisfaction, or overinvolvement (e.g., self-sacrificing or overprotective behavior) are observed from their narratives about the child, rather than simply queried. In an epidemiological sample, investigators found that the maternal expressed-emotion ''high criticism'' component was associated with disruptive behavior disorders while the ''emotional overinvolvement'' component was associated with anxiety disorders (195). In a small sample of offspring of parents with panic disorder with agoraphobia and psychiatric controls, high emotional overinvolvement on the part of the mother was found to be associated with child separation anxiety disorder (196). In addition, in families in which mothers had a lifetime history of anxiety disorder, child behavioral inhibition was associated with maternal criticism and dissatisfaction (197). Once again, the cross-sectional nature of most of these studies suggests that parents' behavior may well be responses to children's anxiety.

Observational studies of interactions between parents and anxious children have provided support for associations between child anxiety and low parental support or high parental restrictiveness or control. Typically in such studies, parents and children are observed interacting around a laboratory task, and parents are rated for the degree to which they encourage or support the child, express negative affect, or take control from the child. For example, parents of school-age children with high fear of failure who were observed helping their children with difficult problem-solving tasks were observed to respond less to the child's expressed insecurity, to express more irritation, and to withhold more reinforcement after positive solutions (198). Similarly, when 8- to 14-year-olds and their mothers were observed interacting in an unstructured situation in which the child could do homework, the child's self-rated test and state anxiety were associated with maternal aversive behavior (expressions of annoyance, anger, or disappointment about the child's behavior or an implied intention to change the child's behavior in a direct manner against the child's will) (199). In another study using observed discussions of conflictual issues, parents of children with anxiety disorders were rated as being less granting of psychological autonomy than controls (183). Similarly, preliminary data from a study in which clinically anxious children and their parents were observed as the child worked on cognitive puzzles suggest that mothers of anxious children took more control than mothers of non-patient comparison children (200). One microanalytical analysis of 10- to 13-year-olds working on a problem-solving task with their mothers found that associations differed according to the child's gender (201). In this study, mothers of anxious girls were more likely to intervene in their daughter's problem-solving while mothers of anxious boys showed the opposite response. Again, since associations with anxiety are cross-sectional, it is not known whether maternal behaviors contribute to increased anxiety or whether mothers respond differently to anxious children of different genders.

A few studies have begun to test hypotheses about the mechanisms by which parental behaviors influence children's anxiety. Two groups have examined the hypothesis that parental restrictiveness or control increases the child's belief that events are outside his or her control (the child's external locus of control) and increases anxiety. Using structured equational modeling, Chorpita and colleagues found that parental control was positively related to a child's external locus of control, which was associated with children's negative affect and clinical disturbance (202). Similarly, Krohne and colleagues found that external locus of control (which they see as an indication of low competence expectancy) was associated with parental inconsistency, high restriction, and lack of support (158). This group also found that actual competence expectancies measured in an achievement situation were predicted by parental restriction and inconsistency.

Other groups have explored whether parents influence anxious children to use more avoidant coping strategies. One group found that in a laboratory discussion paradigm, parents of children with anxiety disorders were more likely to encourage avoidant responses and to influence their children to adopt more avoidant strategies than parents of nonanxious children (153,203). Another group, which used a similar approach with a very small sample including both clinical and nonclinical children, found limited support for the hypothesis that parents' anxious statements were associated with children's change in their plans for coping (204).

Therefore, a growing body of evidence supports the association between parental behaviors or attitudes—including overprotection, restriction, rejection, and encouragement of avoidance—and children's excessive anxiety. However, with the exception of the experiments done with monkeys, none of the studies addressing this association can discern whether these parental behaviors are responses or contributing factors to children's temperament or anxiety. That children's anxious behavior may *elicit* parental protectiveness is clear. An experiment in which a 10-year-old confederate acted either ''anxious and withdrawn'' or ''conduct-disordered'' with a series of women subjects showed that anxious behavior evoked more helping and rewarding responses (205). Moreover, a prospective study followed children and their families after a brushfire disaster and looked at correlations between parental behaviors and children's symptoms at several points in time (206). The author found that parental overprotection and irritability were as much determined by behavioral and emotional problems in the child as the child's difficulties were determined by parental factors, thus supporting a bidirectional effect. Another retrospective study, which queried young adult women about their concurrent anxiety and depression, their own adolescent behavior problems, and their parents' behavior during adolescence, found that after partialing out effects of the daughters' behavior problems during adolescence, parental behavior predicted little of the variance in daughters' adult anxiety and depression (207). Such studies suggest that the association between parental and child behaviors is complex, and that children's anxious behaviors may influence parental behaviors, just as parental behaviors may influence children's anxiety. Prospective longitudinal studies are needed to clarify these associations. Nonetheless, based on the studies thus far, it does appear that parental behaviors, even when they are in part responses to child behavior, may themselves exacerbate or ameliorate children's anxious tendencies (153,208). This suggests that parents could be taught ways to help children cope with anxiety more adaptively.

Life Stressors and Traumatic Events

Empirical studies of the association between panic disorder and life stressors have focused on two major questions. First, do adverse events early in life contribute to vulnerability for later onset of panic disorder? Second, do proximate adverse life events serve as precipitants of panic disorder, and, if so, what determines whether the disorder will occur?

Studies have relied on retrospective accounts by adults with panic disorder and/or agoraphobia. Authors have tended to probe for associations with separation events, because of theoretical formulations suggesting that events related to separation and mobilization of attachment behaviors (e.g., protesting separation, seeking proximity to an attachment figure) would be associated with panic and agoraphobia (57,209). Laraia and colleagues (179) found that compared to controls with no history of psychiatric disorder, patients with panic disorder and agoraphobia reported a significantly greater incidence of parental separation and were more likely to have household members with a chronic physical illness or with alcohol or substance use problems. Faravelli and colleagues (210) compared life events through age 15 in a small sample of patients with agoraphobia with panic attacks and normal controls. Agoraphobics reported significantly more adverse life events of all kinds, particularly between the ages of 4 and 15. In particular, parental separations (maternal separation and parental divorce) were more prevalent among the agoraphobics. Another study found, without a priori hypotheses, that patients with panic disorder reported more perinatal problems than patients with simple phobia (211). De Loof and colleagues (212) found that panic disorder patients, compared with OCD patients, had significantly more adverse events over the total course of their lives. However, a chart-review study found no differences in rate of parental death between patients with panic disorder, agoraphobia, or simple phobia (213). A few studies have found associations between certain specific traumatic events (e.g., rape, childhood neglect) and panic disorder (214); however, such events are common in the histories of patients with a range of psychopathology (215). Therefore, while there is some suggestion that early adverse events are common among patients with panic disorder, further work needs to be done to clarify this relationship.

Other investigators have examined the association between panic disorder and proximate triggering events. For example, Faravelli (216) found that panic patients had a higher mean number of stressful life events in the 12 months prior to their first panic attack than controls in a comparable period. The events reported included both loss events and threatening events, suggesting that both may play a role in the onset of panic disorder. In another study of life events in the year preceding onset of panic disorder, Faravelli and Pallanti (217) found that panic patients had significantly higher life stress. This association held regardless of the manner in which life stress was assessed (e.g., number of events, weighted normative scores, contextual scores, and number of subjects with major events). The higher number of life events experienced by panic disorder patients was almost entirely attributable to their experiencing more life stress in the month before onset of the disorder. In this study, events beyond the subjects' control were more frequent and more severe among panic disorder patients than among controls, and loss events had the strongest relationship to panic disorder. The authors conclude, however, that even though life events may play a precipitating role in the onset of panic disorder, the degree of association was not large (i.e., only 30–39% of their cases were associated with stressful life events). In a naturalistic study of 223 panic disorder patients, 80% of the subjects reported the occurrence of at least one negative life event in the year prior to the onset of disorder (218).

Perhaps more important than the occurrence of life events is the way those events are viewed by the patient. For example, one group found that while panic disorder patients and controls did not differ in the number of total life events in the year prior to panic onset, patients did experience more events that happened to them personally (as opposed to happening to a member of their family or support system) than controls did (219). Although patients and controls did not differ in the objective degree of life change or stress (i.e., the degree of stress the events could be expected to evoke in an average person), patients rated their experiences as being more subjectively distressing (i.e., uncontrollable, undesirable, and aversive). Similarly, in a study that used both anxiety disorder patients and nonanxious subjects as controls, Rapee, Litwin, and Barlow (220) found that panic disorder patients did not differ significantly from either control group in the number of recent life events reported. However, the panic disorder and anxiety disorder subjects rated the life events that did occur as having a significantly greater negative impact on them than the nonanxious subjects did. This finding suggests that the tendency to experience life events as subjectively distressing may play a precipitating role in panic disorder.

To summarize, the hypothesized association between panic disorder and life events is as yet not conclusive. Studies are limited by the biases of retrospective recall and, with a few exceptions, by failure to control for the degree to which the life events are influenced in some way by a patient's behavior or premorbid tendencies. Therefore, it cannot be determined whether the higher frequency of reported life events in some subjects is a cause or effect of panic disorder or agoraphobia. With regard to precipitating events, it has not been clear whether precipitating events occur more frequently in the lives of those who develop panic disorder, whether they occur at equal frequency (and it is the individual's biological vulnerability to panic disorder that determines onset and level of distress) or whether it is the person's cognitive-emotional response to the event that influences whether the disorder will begin. The apparent influence of the individual's interpretation and responses to the life events suggests that individuals' temperamental tendencies and cognitive and behavioral predispositions may influ-

Table 5 Potential Indicators of Risk for Panic Disorder

Constitutional factors	
Genetic factors	Family history of panic disorder[a,b]
Childhood psychopathology	Childhood anxiety disorders: separation anxiety disorder, social phobia, avoidant disorder, or overanxious disorder[c,d]
Temperamental factors	Behavioral inhibition to the unfamiliar: a tendency to exhibit fear (toddlerhood) and quiet restraint (early childhood) in response to novel situations[c,d]
	Heightened limbic-sympathetic arousal in response to novel situations in some inhibited children[d]
Psychological vulnerability factors	
Cognitive predispositions	Anxiety sensitivity: a tendency to catastrophically misinterpret and fear physiological sensations associated with arousal[e,h,i]
	?Other cognitive biases: tendency to misperceive and magnify threat, tendency to underestimate competency for coping, expectations of unpredictability and uncontrollability of negative events, overestimation of risk of adverse outcome
Behavioral tendencies	Tendency to cope via escape or avoidant strategies[e]
	Negative self-talk in situations that induce anxiety[e]
	?Deficit of skills for coping with anxiety-inducing situations

Table 5 Continued

Environmental factors	
Parental influences	Overprotection[c,e,f]
	Encouragement of avoidant behavior[g]
	Low warmth or high rejection[c,e]
	Parental restrictiveness and control[c,e]
	High criticism[g]
	High punitiveness[e]
	Inconsistency[e]
Life events	Negative life events associated with subjective distress serve as precipitants[c]
	History of adverse or traumatic life events[c]

Nature of supporting evidence: [a]Family studies, [b]twin studies, [c]retrospective accounts by adults with panic disorder with or without agoraphobia, [d]studies of offspring of patients with panic disorder; [e]reports by children with anxiety disorders, [f]reports by parents of patients with anxiety disorders, [g]observations of parent–child interactions in families of anxiety-disordered or high-trait anxious children, [h]prospective study of adults who develop panic attacks, [i]experiment with children.

Question marks indicate factors hypothesized based on associations with panic disorder or other anxiety disorders in adults or children.

ence the onset of panic disorder, similar to the way that attributional style has been shown to influence the onset of affective disorders (221–223).

SUMMARY OF HYPOTHESIZED RISK FACTORS AND TENTATIVE ETIOLOGICAL MODEL

The hypothesized risk factors reviewed in this chapter are summarized in Table 5. While our understanding has not progressed to the point that we can formulate a clear etiological model, several points are worth considering. First, the pathway to panic disorder is most likely multi-factorial. That is, a number of factors can be expected to increase the likelihood of panic disorder, including genetic, temperamental, child-hood, and life stress factors. With regard to debilitating panic, associ-ated with higher phobic avoidance, individuals most at risk would be those who 1) had a family history of panic disorder, 2) evinced early signs of anxious disposition (including inhibited temperament in child-hood and/or childhood anxiety disorders), 3) had a tendency to become fearful in response to physiological signs of anxiety, and 4) had devel-oped some habits of thought and behavior that tend to exacerbate anxi-ety (e.g., deficits in coping skills and a tendency to cope via avoidance). A history of traumatic events or losses early in life or of unhelpful parental attitudes such as excessive restrictiveness or rejection might contribute to the development of these maladaptive habits or tenden-cies. Individuals with some or many of these risk factors would be more likely than most people to respond to adverse events or life stressors by developing panic disorder with agoraphobia.

CLINICAL IMPLICATIONS

Clinicians should be cognizant that children of patients with panic dis-order are at risk to develop anxiety disorders in childhood. Although anxiety disorders are the most prevalent psychiatric disorder of child-hood, affected children are often not referred for treatment because they do not disturb classrooms or family life to the same degree that children with disruptive behavior disorders do. Nonetheless, it is likely that early cognitive-behavioral treatment for mild to moderate anxiety problems may foster strategies for coping with anxiety that might mitigate the severity, or potentially reduce the likelihood, of later difficulties. More-over, although not dealt with in this chapter, childhood anxiety may be associated with difficulties in peer adjustment that might also lead to future difficulties if left untreated (224,225). In addition, difficulties in parent–child interactions (such as a parent's tendency to be more protective or controlling or to offer less support) may prevent the child from developing coping skills that might assist him or her in managing anxiety.

    While clinicians ought to be aware of which individuals are at potential risk, they should also recognize that having many constitutional risk factors does not doom an individual to a future of psychiatric disorder. Intervention early in life—e.g., parental guidance (226), treatment of parents' anxiety disorders, cognitive-behavioral treatment of anxiety disorders of childhood or adolescence (227–229), cognitive-behavioral therapy emphasizing coping actively with life stressors (169), and, in some cases, pharmacological treatment of extant anxiety disorders—may be able to prevent or minimize future dysfunction.

ACKNOWLEDGMENTS

The preparation of this chapter was supported in part by the Brandon Shedd Memorial Fund.

REFERENCES

1. Brown FW. Heredity in the psychoneuroses. Proc R Soc Med 1942; 35:785–790.
2. Cohen ME, Badal DW, Kilpatrcik A, Reed EW, White PD. The high familial prevalence of neurocirculatory asthenia (anxiety neurosis, effort syndrome). Am J Hum Genetics 1951; 3:126–158.
3. Wheeler ED, White PD, Reed EW. Familial incidence of neurocirculatory asthenia (''anxiety neurosis,'' ''effort syndrome''). J Clin Invest 1948; 27:562.
4. Moran C, Andrews G. The familial occurrence of agoraphobia. Br J Psychiatry 1985; 146:262–267.
5. Gruppo Italiano Disturbi d'Ansia GID. Familial analysis of panic disorder and agoraphobia. J Affect Disord 1989; 17:1–8.
6. Hopper JL, Judd FK, Derrick PL, Burrows GD. A family study of panic disorder. Genet Epidemiol 1987; 4:33–41.
7. Kushner MG, Thomas AM, Bartels KM, Beitman BD. Panic disorder history in the families of patients with angiographically normal coronary arteries. Am J Psychiatry 1992; 149:1563–1567.
8. Battaglia M, Bertella S, Politi E, Bernardeschi L, Perna G, Gabriele A, Bellodi L. Age at onset of panic disorder: influence of familial liability to the disease and of childhood separation anxiety disorder. Am J Psychiatry 1995; 152:1362–1364.

9. Crowe RR, Noyes R, Pauls DL, Slymen D. A family study of panic disorder. Arch Gen Psychiatry 1983; 40:1065–1069.
10. Harris EL, Noyes R Jr, Crowe RR, Chaudry DR. Family study of agoraphobia: report of a pilot study. Arch Gen Psychiatry 1983; 40:1061–1064.
11. Noyes R, Crowe RR, Harris EL, Hamra BJ, McChesney CM, Chaudhry DR. Relationship between panic disorder and agoraphobia: a family study. Arch Gen Psychiatry 1986; 43:227–232.
12. Mendlewicz J, Papdimitriou G, Wilmotte J. Family study of panic disorder: comparison with generalized anxiety disorder, major depression and normal subjects. Psychiatr Genetics 1993; 3:73–78.
13. Maier W, Lichtermann D, Minges J, Oehrlein A, Franke P. A controlled family study in panic disorder. J Psychiatr Res 1993; 27:79–87.
14. Maier W, Minges J, Lichtermann D. The familial relationship between panic disorder and unipolar depression. J Psychiatr Res 1995; 29:375–388.
15. Weissman MM, Wickramaratne P, Adams PB, Lish JD, Horwath E, Charney DS, Woods SW, Leeman E, Frosch E. The relationship between panic disorder and major depression: a new family study. Arch Gen Psychiatry 1993; 50:767–780.
16. Goldstein RB, Weissman MM, Adams PB, Horwath E, Lish JD, Charney DS, Woods SW, Sobin C, Wickramaratne PJ. Psychiatric disorders in relatives of probands with panic disorder and/or major depression. Arch Gen Psychiatry 1994; 51:383–394.
17. Mannuzza S, Chapman TF, Klein DF, Fyer AJ. Familial transmission of panic disorder: effect of major depression comorbidity. Anxiety 1994/1995; 1:180–185.
18. Fyer AJ, Mannuzza S, Chapman TF, Martin LY, Kelin DF. Specificity in familial aggregation of phobic disorders. Arch Gen Psychiatry 1995; 52:564–573.
19. Goldstein RB, Wickramaratne PJ, Horwath E, Weissman MM. Familial aggregation and phenomenology of "early" onset (at or before age 20 years) panic disorder. Arch Gen Psychiatry 1997; 54:271–278.
20. Pauls DL, Bucher KD, Crowe RR, Noyes R Jr. A genetic study of panic disorder pedigrees. Am J Hum Genetics 1980; 32:639–644.
21. Vieland JE, Hodge SE, Lish JD, Adams P, Weissman MM. Segregation analysis of panic disorder. Psychiatr Genetics 1993; 3:63–71.
22. Vieland V, Goodman D, Chapman T, Fyer A. New segregation analysis of panic disorder. Am J Med Genetics 1996; 67:147–153.

23. Torgersen S. Genetic factors in anxiety disorders. Arch Gen Psychiatry 1983; 40:1085–1089.
24. Andrews G, Stewart G, Allen R, Henderson AS. The genetics of six neurotic disorders: a twin study. J Affect Disord 1990; 19:23–29.
25. Skre I, Onstad S, Torgersen S, Lygren S, Kringlen E. A twin study of DSM-III-R anxiety disorders. Acta Psychiatr Scand 1993; 88:85–92.
26. Kendler KS, Neale MC, Kessler RC, Heath AC, Eaves LJ. Panic disorder in women: a population-based twin study. Psycholog Med 1993; 23:397–406.
27. Perna G, Caldirola D, Arancio C, Bellodi L. Panic attacks: a twin study. Psychiatry Res 1997; 66:69–71.
28. Lander ES, Schork NJ. Genetic dissection of complex traits. Science 1994; 265:2037–2048.
29. Lander E, Kruglyak L. Genetic dissection of complex traits: guidelines for interpreting and reporting linkage results. Nature Genetics 1995; 11:241–247.
30. Risch N, Merikangas K. The future of genetic studies of complex human diseases. Science 1996; 273:1516–1517.
31. Crowe RR, Noyes R Jr., Wilson AF, Elston RC, Ward LJ. A linkage study of panic disorder. Arch Gen Psychiatry 1987; 44:933–937.
32. Crowe RR. The Iowa linkage study of panic disorder. In: Gershon ES, Cloninger CR, eds. Genetic Approaches to Mental Disorders. Washington, DC: American Psychiatric Association Press, 1994:291–310.
33. Vieland VJ, Knowles JA, Fyer AJ, Stephanovich M, Freimer NF, Lish J, Adams P, Woodley K, Rassnick H, Heiman GA, White P, Das K, Klein DF, Ott J, Weissman MM, Gilliam TC. Linkage study of panic disorder: a preliminary report. In: Gershon ES, Cloninger CR, eds. Genetic Approaches to Mental Disorders. Washington, DC: American Psychiatric Association Press, 1994:345–354.
34. Mutchler K, Crowe RR, Noyes R Jr, Wesner RW. Exclusion of the tyrosine hydroxylase gene in 14 panic disorder pedigrees. Am J Psychiatry 1990; 147:1367–1369.
35. Wang ZW, Crowe RR, Noyes R Jr. Adrenergic receptor genes as candidate genes for panic disorder: a linkage study. Am J Psychiatry 1992; 149:470–474.
36. Crawford F, Hoyne J, Diaz P, Osborne A, Dorotheo J, Sheehan D, Mullan M. Occurrence of the Cys311 DRD2 variant in a pedigree multiply affected with panic disorder. Am J Med Genetics 1995; 60:332–334.

37. Ohara K, Xie D-W, Ishigaki T, Deng Z-L, Nakamura Y, Suzuki Y, Miyasato K, Ohara K. The genes encoding the 5HT1Dα and 5HT1Dβ receptors are unchanged in patients with panic disorder. Biolog Psychiatry 1996; 39:5–10.

38. Kato T, Wang ZW, Zoega T, Crowe RR. Missense mutation of the cholecystokinin B receptor gene: lack of association with panic disorder. Am J Med Genetics 1996; 67:401–405.

39. Crowe RR, Wang Z, Noyes R, Albrecht BE, Darlison MG, Bailey MES, Johnson KJ, Zoega T. Candidate gene study of eight GABA$_A$ receptor subunits in panic disorder. Am J Psychiatry 1997; 154:1096–1100.

40. Steinlein OK, Deckert J, Nothen MM, Franke P, Maier W, Beckmann H, Propping P. Neuronal nicotinic acetylcholine receptor alpha4 subunit (CHRNA4) and panic disorder: an association study. Am J Med Genetics 1997; 74:199–201.

41. Tsuang MT, Faraone SV, Lyons MJ. Identification of the phenotype in psychiatric genetics. Eur Arch Psychiatry Clin Neurosci 1993; 243: 131–142.

42. Noyes R, Clarkson C, Crowe RR, Yates WR, McChesney CM. A family study of generalized anxiety disorder. Am J Psychiatry 1987; 144: 1019–1024.

43. Kendler KS, Walters EE, Truett KR, Heath AC, Neale MC, Martin NG, Eaves LJ. A twin-family study of self-report symptoms of panic-phobia and somatization. Behav Genetics 1995; 25:499–515.

44. Rosenbaum JF, Biederman J, Hirshfeld DR, Faraone SV, Bolduc EA, Kagan J, Snidman N, Reznick JS. Further evidence of an association between behavioral inhibition and anxiety disorders: results from a family study of children from a non-clinical sample. J Psychiatr Res 1991; 25:49–65.

45. Biederman J, Rosenbaum JF, Bolduc EA, Faraone SV, Hirshfeld DR. A high-risk study of young children of parents with panic disorder and agoraphobia with and without major depression. Psychiatr Res 1991; 37:333–348.

46. Coryell W, Endicott J, Andreasen NC, Keller MB, Clayton PJ, Hirschfeld RMA, Scheftner WA, Winokur G. Depression and panic attacks: the significance of overlap as reflected in follow-up and family study data. Am J Psychiatry 1988; 145:293–300.

47. Coryell W, Endicott J, Winokur G. Anxiety syndromes as epiphenomena of primary major depression: outcome and familial psychopathology. Am J Psychiatry 1992; 149:100–107.

48. George DT, Nutt DJ, Dwyer BA, Linnoila M. Alcoholism and panic disorder: is the comorbidity more than coincidence? Acta Psychiatr Scand 1990; 81:97–107.

49. Leckman JF, Weissman MM, Merikangas KR, Pauls DL, Prusoff BA. Panic disorder and major depression: increased risk of depression, alcoholism, panic, and phobic disorders in families of depressed probands with panic disorder. Arch Gen Psychiatry 1983; 40:1055–1060.

50. Skre I, Onstad S, Edwardsen J, Torgersen S, Kringlen E. A family study of anxiety disorders: familial transmission and relationship to mood disorder and psychoactive substance use disorder. Acta Psychiatr Scand 1994; 90:366–274.

51. Last CG, Hersen M, Kazdin AE, Orvaschel H, Perrin S. Anxiety disorders in children and their families. Arch Gen Psychiatry 1991; 48:928–934.

52. Maier W, Minges J, Lichtermann D. Alcoholism and panic disorder: co-occurrence and co-transmission in families. Eur Arch Psychiatry Clin Neurosci 1992; 243:205–211.

53. Munjack DJ, Moss HB. Affective disorder and alcoholism in families of agoraphobics. Arch Gen Psychiatry 1981; 38:869–871.

54. Kendler KS, Walter EE, Neale MC, Kessler RC, Heath AC, Eaves LJ. The structure of the genetic and environmental risk factors for six major psychiatric disorders in women. Arch Gen Psychiatry 1995; 52:374–383.

55. Faraone SV. Personal communication.

56. Klein D. Delineation of two-drug reponsive anxiety syndromes. Psychopharmacologia 1964; 5:397–408.

57. Klein DF. Anxiety reconceptualized. In: Klein DF, Rabkin J, eds. Anxiety: New Research and Concepts. New York: Raven Press, 1981:235–262.

58. Delito J, Perugi G, Maremmani I. The importance of separation anxiety in the differentiation of panic disorder from agoraphobia. Psychiatr Develop 1986; 4:227–236.

59. Lipsitz JD, Martin LY, Mannuzza S, Chapman TF, Liebowitz M, Klein DF, Fyer AJ. Childhood separation anxiety disorder in patients with adult anxiety disorders. Am J Psychiatry 1994; 151:927–929.

60. Silove D, Parker G, Hadzi-Pavlovic D, Manicavasagar V, Blaszczynski A. Parental representations of patients with panic disorder and generalized anxiety disorder. Br J Psychiatry 1991; 159:835–841.

61. Otto M, Pollock M, Rosenbaum JF, Sachs GS, Asher RH. Childhood history of anxiety in adults with panic disorder: association with anxiety

sensitivity and comorbidity. Harvard Rev Psychiatry 1994; 1:288–293.

62. Aronson T, Logue C. On the longitudinal course of panic disorder: developmental history and and predictors of phobic complications. Compr Psychiatry 1987; 28:344–355.

63. Pollack MH, Otto MW, Sabatino S, Majcher D, Worthington JJ, McArdle ET, Rosenbaum JF. Relationship of childhood anxiety to adult panic disorder: correlates and influence on course. Am J Psychiatry 1996; 153:376–381.

64. Lipsitz JD, Mannuzza S, Liebowitz M, Klein DF, Fyer AJ. Childhood separation anxiety disorder and adult anxiety disorders in a non-clinical sample. Presented at ADAA 17th National Conference, New Orleans, 1997.

65. Biederman J, Faraone S, Marrs A, Moore P, Garcia J, Ablon S, Mick E, Gershon J, Kearns M. Panic disorder and agoraphobia in consecutively referred children and adolescents. J Am Acad Child Adolesc Psychiatry 1997; 36:214–223.

66. Weissman MM, Leckman JF, Merikangas KR, Gammon GD, Prusoff BA. Depression and anxiety disorders in parents and children: results from the Yale family study. Arch Gen Psychiatry 1984; 41:845–852.

67. Sylvester CE, Hyde TS, Reichler RJ. The Diagnostic Interview for Children and Personality Inventory for Children in studies of children at risk for anxiety disorders or depression. J Am Acad Child Adolesc Psychiatry 1987; 26:668–675.

68. Warner V, Mufson L, Weissman MM. Offspring at high and low risk for depression and anxiety: mechanisms of psychiatric disorder. J Am Acad Child Adolesc Psychiatry 1995; 34:786–797.

69. Beidel D, Turner S. At risk for anxiety. I. Psychopathology in the offspring of anxious parents. J Am Acad Child Adolesc Psychiatry 1997; 36:918–924.

70. Klein RG, Last CG. Anxiety Disorders in Children. Newbury Park, CA: Sage Publications, 1989.

71. Barlow D, DiNardo P, Vermilyea B, Blanchard E. Comorbidity and depression among anxiety disorders: issues in diagnosis and classification. J Nerv Mental Dis 1986; 174:63–72.

72. Maser J, Cloninger C. Comorbidity of Mood and Anxiety Disorders. Washington, DC: American Psychiatric Association Press, 1990.

73. Brady E, Kendall P. Comorbidity of anxiety and depression in children and adolescents. Psychol Bull 1992; 111:244–255.

74. Kendall PC, Kortlander E, Chansky TE, Brady EU. Comorbidity of anxiety and depression in youth: treatment implications. J Consult Clin Psychol 1992; 60:869–880.

75. Sachs G, Lafer B, Thibault A. Childhood psychopathology in 52 adult bipolar patients. Presented at Annual Meeting of the American Psychiatric Association, Philadelphia, 1994.

76. Garcia-Coll C, Kagan J, Reznick JS. Behavioral inhibition in young children. Child Dev 1984; 55:1005–1019.

77. Kagan J, Reznick JS, Clarke C, Snidman N, Garcia-Coll C. Behavioral inhibition to the unfamiliar. Child Dev 1984; 55:2212–2225.

78. Reznick JS, Kagan J, Snidman N, Gersten M, Baak K, Rosenberg A. Inhibited and uninhibited behavior: a follow-up study. Child Dev 1986; 57:660–680.

79. Kagan J, Reznick JS, Snidman N. The physiology and psychology of behavioral inhibition in children. Child Dev 1987; 58:1459–1473.

80. Kagan J, Reznick JS, Snidman N. Biological bases of childhood shyness. Science 1988; 240:167–171.

81. Kagan J, Reznick JS, Snidman N, Gibbons J, Johnson MO. Childhood derivatives of inhibition and lack of inhibition to the unfamiliar. Child Dev 1988; 59:1580–1589.

82. Kagan J. Temperamental contributions to social behavior. Am Psychol 1989; 44:668–674.

83. Kagan J, Reznick JS, Gibbons J. Inhibited and uninhibited types of children. Child Dev 1989; 60:838–845.

84. Snidman N. Behavioral inhibition and sympathetic influence on the cardiovascular system. In: Reznick J, ed. Perspectives on Behavioral Inhibition. Chicago: University of Chicago Press, 1989:51–70.

85. Gersten M. Behavioral inhibition in the classroom. In: Resnick J, ed. Perspectives on Behavioral Inhibition. Chicago: University of Chicago Press, 1989:71–91.

86. Kagan J, Snidman N. Infant predictors of inhibited and uninhibited profiles. Psycholog Sci 1991; 2:40–44.

87. Kagan J, Snidman N. Temperamental factors in human development. Am Psychol 1991; 46:856–862.

88. Kagan J. Galen's Prophecy: Temperament in Human Nature. New York: Basic Books, 1994.

89. Asendorpf JB. Development of inhibition during childhood: evidence for situational specificity and a two-factor model. Dev Psychol 1990; 26:721–730.

90. Kochanska G, Radke-Yarrow M. Inhibition in toddlerhood and the dy-

namics of the child's interaction with an unfamiliar peer at age five. Child Dev 1992; 63:325–335.

91. Scarpa A, Raine A, Venables P, Mednick S. The stability of inhibited/ uninhibited temperament from ages 3 to 11 years in Mauritian children. J Abnorm Child Psychol 1995; 23:607–618.

92. Matheny AP. Children's behavioral inhibition over age and across situations: genetic similarity for a trait during change. J Pers 1989; 57: 215–235.

93. Robinson JL, Kagan J, Reznick JS, Corley R. The heritability of inhibited and uninhibited behavior: a twin study. Dev Psychol 1992; 28: 1030–1037.

94. DiLalla L, Kagan J, Reznick J. Genetic etiology of behavioral inhibition among 2-year-old children. Infant Behav Development 1994; 17:405– 412.

95. Calkins SD, Fox NA, Marshall TR. Behavioral and physiological antecedents of inhibited and uninhibited behavior. Child Dev 1996; 67: 523–540.

96. Davis M. The role of the amygdala in fear and anxiety. Annu Rev Neurosci 1992; 15:353–375.

97. Kagan J, Reznick J, Snidman N, Johnson M, Gibbons J, Gersten M, Biederman J, Rosenbaum J. Origins of panic disorder. In: Ballenger JC, ed. Clinical Aspects of Panic Disorder. New York: Alan R Liss, 1990:71–87.

98. Davidson R. Emotion and affective style: hemispheric substrates. Psycholog Sci 1992; 3:39–43.

99. Davidson R. Anterior cerebral asymmetry and the nature of emotion. Brain Cognition 1992; 20:125–151.

100. Charney DS, Woods SW, Nagy LM, Southwick SM, Krystal JH, Heninger GR. Noradrenergic function in panic disorder. J Clin Psychiatry 1990; 51:5–11.

101. Krystal J, Deutsch D, Charney D. The biological basis of panic disorder. J Clin Psychiatry 1996; 57:23–31.

102. Goddard A, Charney D. Toward an integrated neurobiology of panic disorder. J Clin Psychiatry 1997; 58:4–11.

103. Adamec R, Stark-Adamec C. Behavioral inhibition and anxiety: dispositional, developmental and neural aspects of the anxious personality of the domestic cat. In: Reznick J, ed. Perspectives on Behavioral Inhibition. Chicago: University of Chicago Press, 1989:93–124.

104. Suomi SJ, Kraemer GW, Baysinger CM, DeLizio RD. Inherited and

experiential factors associated with individual differences in anxious behavior displayed by rhesus monkeys. In: Klein DF, Rabkin J, eds. Anxiety: New Research and Changing Concepts. New York: Raven Press, 1981:179–200.

105. Suomi SJ. The development of affect in rhesus monkeys. In: Fox N, Davidson R, eds. The Psychobiology of Affective Disorders. Hillsdale, NJ: Lawrence Erlbaum Associates, 1984.

106. Suomi SJ. Anxiety-like disorders in young nonhuman primates. In: Gittleman R, eds. Anxiety Disorders of Childhood. New York: Guilford Press, 1986:1–23.

107. Silove D, et al. Is early separation anxiety a risk factor for adult panic disorder?: a critical review. Comprehen Psychiatry 1996; 37:167–179.

108. Suomi S. Genetic and maternal contributions to individual differences in rhesus monkey biobehavioral development. In: Krasnegor NA, Blass EM, Hofer MA, Smotherman WP, eds. Perinatal Development: A Psychobiological Perspective. New York: Academic Press, 1987:397–419.

109. Suomi SJ. Neurobiology of anxiety like syndromes in rhesus monkey juveniles and adolescents. Presented at Annual Meeting of the American Academy of Child and Adolescent Psychiatry, Philadelphia, 1996.

110. Suomi SJ. Early determinants of behaviour: evidence from primate studies. Br Med Bull 1997; 170–184.

111. Berg I, Marks I, McGuire R, Lipsedge M. School phobia and agoraphobia. Psycholog Med 1974; 4:428–434.

112. Caspi A, et al. Behavioral observations at age 3 years predict adult psychiatric disorders: longitudinal evidence from a birth cohort. Arch Gen Psychiatry 1996; 53:1033–1039.

113. Deltito JA, Perugi G, Maremmani I, Mignani V, Cassano GB. The importance of separation anxiety in the differentiation of panic disorder from agoraphobia. Psychiatr Dev 1986; 4:227–236.

114. Rosenbaum JF, Biederman J, Gersten M, Hirshfeld DR, Meminger SR, Herman JB, Kagan J, Reznick JS, Snidman N. Behavioral inhibition in children of parents with panic disorder and agoraphobia: a controlled study. Arch Gen Psychiatry 1988; 45:463–470.

115. Manassis K, Bradley S, Goldberg S, Hood J, Swinson R. Behavioural inhibition, attachment and anxiety in children of mothers with anxiety disorders. Can J Psychiatry 1995; 40:87–92.

116. Battaglia M, Bajo S, Strambi LF, Brambilla F, Castronovo C, Vanni

G, Bellodi L. Physiological and behavioral responses to minor stressors in offspring of patients with panic disorder. J Psychiatr Res 1997; 31: 365–376.

117. Biederman J, Rosenbaum JF, Hirshfeld DR, Faraone SV, Bolduc EA, Gersten M, Meminger SR, Kagan J, Snidman N, Reznick JS. Psychiatric correlates of behavioral inhibition in young children of parents with and without psychiatric disorders. Arch Gen Psychiatry 1990; 47: 21–26.

118. Biederman J, Rosenbaum JF, Bolduc-Murphy EA, Faraone SV, Chaloff J, Hirshfeld DR, Kagan J. A 3-year follow-up of children with and without behavioral inhibition. J Am Acad Child Adolesc Psychiatry 1993; 32:814–821.

119. Hirshfeld DR, Rosenbaum JF, Biederman J, Bolduc EA, Faraone SV, Snidman N, Reznick JS, Kagan J. Stable behavioral inhibition and its association with anxiety disorder. J Am Acad Child Adolesc Psychiatry 1992; 31:103–111.

120. Richman N, Graham P, Stevenson J. Preschool to School: A Behavioral Study. London: Academic Press, 1982.

121. Reznick JS, Hegeman IM, Kaufman E, Woods SW, Jacobs M. Retrospective and concurrent self-report of behavioral inhibition and their relation to adult mental health. Development Psychopathol 1992; 4: 301–321.

122. Angst J, Vollrath M. The natural history of anxiety disorders. Acta Psychiatr Scand 1991; 84:446–452.

123. Kochanska G. Patterns of inhibition to the unfamiliar in children of normal and affectively ill mothers. Child Dev 1991; 62:250–263.

124. Rosenbaum JF, Biederman J, Pollock RA, Hirshfeld DR. The etiology of social phobia. J Clin Psychiatry 1994; 10–16.

125. Hirshfeld DR, Rosenbaum JF, Fredman SJ, Kagan J. Childhood anxiety disorders. In: Charney D, Nestler E, Bunney B, eds. Neurobiological Foundations of Mental Illness. Oxford: Oxford University Press. In press.

126. Reichler RJ, Hyde TS, Sylvester CE. Biological studies of offspring of panic disorder probands. In: Dunner D, Gershon E, Barrett J, eds. Relatives at Risk for Mental Disorder. New York: Raven, 1988:103–125.

127. Grillon C, Dierker L, Merikangas K. Startle modulation in children at risk for anxiety disorders and/or alcoholism. J Am Acad Child Adolesc Psychiatry 1997; 36:925–932.

128. Sallee R, Greenawald J. Neurobiology. In: March J, ed. Anxiety Disorders in Children and Adolescents. New York: Guilford Press, 1995.

129. Turner SM, Beidel DC, Epstein LH. Vulnerability and risk for anxiety disorders. J Anx Dis 1991; 5:151–166.

130. Clark D. A cognitive approach to panic. Behav Res Ther 1986; 24: 461–470.

131. McNally RJ, Lorenz M. Anxiety sensitivity in agoraphobics. J Behav Ther Exper Psychiatry 1987; 18:3–11.

132. Reiss S, McNally R. Expectancy model of fear. In: Reiss S, Bootzin R, eds. Theoretical Issues in Behavior Therapy. San Diego: Academic Press, 1985:107–121.

133. Reiss S, Peterson RA, Gursky M, McNally RJ. Anxiety sensitivity, anxiety frequency, and the prediction of fearfulness. Behav Res Ther 1986; 24:1–8.

134. Blais MA, Otto MW, Zucker BG, McNally RJ, Fava M, Pollack MH. Structure of the Anxiety Sensitivity Index: suggestions for scale refinement based on item and factor analyses. Submitted for publication.

135. Rapee R, Ancis J, Barlow D. Emotional reactions to physiological sensations: panic disorder patients and non-clinical Ss. Behav Res Ther 1988; 26:265–269.

136. McNally RJ, Luedke DL, Besyner JK, Peterson RA, Bohm K, Lips OJ. Sensitivity to stress-relevant stimuli in post-traumatic stress disorder. J Anx Dis 1987; 1:105–116.

137. Donnell C, McNally R. Anxiety sensitivity and panic attacks in a non-clinical population. Behav Res Ther 1990; 28:83.

138. Asmundson GJG, Norton GR. Anxiety sensitivity and its relationship to spontaneous and cued panic attacks in college students. Behav Res Ther 1993; 31:199–201.

139. Otto MW, Reilly-Harrington NA. Impact of treatment on anxiety sensitivity. In: Taylor SA, ed. Anxiety sensitivity: theory, research and treatment of the fear of anxiety. In press.

140. Schmidt NB, Lerew DR, Jackson RJ. The role of anxiety sensitivity in the pathogenesis of panic: prospective evaluation of spontaneous panic attacks during acute stress. J Abnorm Psychol 1997; 106:355–364.

141. McNally RJ. Anxiety sensitivity is distinguishable from trait anxiety. In: Rapee RM, eds. Current Controversies in the Anxiety Disorders. New York: Guilford Press, 1996:214–227.

142. McNally RJ. Psychological approaches to panic disorder: a review. Psychol Bull 1990; 108:403–419.

143. Silverman WK, Fleisig W, Rabian B, Peterson RA. Childhood Anxiety Sensitivity Index. J Clin Child Psychol 1991; 20:162–168.

144. Chorpita BF, Albano AM, Barlow DH. Child Anxiety Sensitivity Index: considerations for children with anxiety disorders. J Clin Child Psychol 1996; 25:77–82.

145. Kearney CA, Tillotson CA. The developmental progression of anxiety sensitivity in youngsters. Presented at Annual Convention of the Associated for the Advancement of Behavior Therapy, Miami, 1997.

146. Rabian B, Peterson RA, Richters J, Jensen PS. Anxiety sensitivity among anxious children. J Clin Child Psychol 1993; 22:441–446.

147. Kearney CA, Albano AM, Eisen AR, Allan WD, Barlow DH. The phenomenology of panic disorder in youngsters: an empirical study of a clinical sample. J Anx Dis 1997; 11:49–62.

148. Rabian B, Embry L, MacIntyre D. Behavioral validation of the CASI in young children. Presented at Annual Convention of the Association for the Advancement of Behavior Therapy, Miami, 1997.

149. Beck AT, Emery G, Greenberg RL. Anxiety Disorders and Phobias: A Cognitive Perspective. New York: Basic Books, 1985.

150. Butler G, Matthews A. Cognitive processes in anxiety. Adv Behav Res Ther 1983; 5:51–62.

151. Barlow D. Anxiety and Its Disorders. New York: Guilford Press, 1988.

152. Alloy LB, Kelly KA, Mineka S, Clements CM. Comorbidity of anxiety and depressive disorders: a helplessness-hopelessness perspective. In: Maser J, Cloninger C, eds. Comorbidity of Mood and Anxiety Disorders. Washington, DC: American Psychiatric Association Press, 1990: 499–544.

153. Barrett PM, Rapee RM, Dadds MM, Ryan SM. Family enhancement of cognitive style in anxious and aggressive children. J Abnorm Child Psychol 1996; 24:187–203.

154. Messer SC, Beidel DC. Psychosocial correlates of childhood anxiety disorders. J Am Acad Child Adolesc Psychiatry 1994; 33:975–983.

155. Finch AJ, Kendall PC, Deardorff PA, Anderson J, Sitarz AM. Reflection-impulsivity, persistence behavior, and locus of control in emotionally disturbed children. J Consult Clin Psychol 1975; 43:748.

156. Nunn G. Concurrent validity between the Nowicki-Strickland Locus of Control Scale and the State-Trait Anxiety Inventory for Children. Educational and Psychological Measurement 1988; 48:435–438.

157. Ollendick TH. Reliability and validity of the revised Fear Survey

Schedule for Children (FSSC-R). Behav Res Ther 1983; 21:685–692.

158. Krohne H. Developmental conditions of anxiety and coping: a two-process model of child-rearing effects. In: Hagtvet K, Johnsen T, eds. Advances in Test Anxiety Research. Vol 7. Amsterdam: Swets & Zeitlinger, 1992:143–155.

159. Bell-Dolan D, Wessler AE. Attributional style of anxious children: extensions from cognitive theory and research on adult anxiety. J Anx Disord 1994; 8:79–96.

160. Treadwell KR, Kendall PC. Self-talk in youth with anxiety disorders: states of mind, content specificity, and treatment outcome. J Consult Clin Psychol 1996; 64:941–950.

161. Zatz S, Chassin L. Cognitions of test-anxious children under naturalistic test-taking conditions. J Consult Clin Psychol 1985; 53:393–401.

162. Prins P. Children's self-speech and self-regulation during a fear-provoking behavioral test. Behav Res Ther 1986; 24:181–191.

163. Sameroff AJ. Early influences on development: fact or fancy? Merril Palmer Quarterly 1975; 21:267–294.

164. Sameroff A. Transactional models in early social relations. Hum Dev 1975; 18:65–79.

165. Lerner RM, Lerner JV. Children in their contexts: a goodness-of-fit model. In: Lancaster J, Altman J, Possi A, Sheri L, eds. Parenting Across the Lifespan. New York: Aldive de Gruyter, 1987:377–403.

166. Caspi A, Bem DJ, Elder GH. Continuities and consequences of interactional styles across the life course. J Pers 1989; 57:375–406.

167. Rosenblum L, Coplan J, Friedman S, Bassoff T, Gorman J, Andrews M. Adverse early experiences affect noradrenergic and serotonergic functioning in adult primates. Biolog Psychiatry 1994; 35:221–227.

168. Arcus DM: The experiential modification of temperamental bias in inhibited and uninhibited children. Doctoral dissertation, Harvard University. Ann Arbor, MI: University Microfilms International, 1991.

169. Spence SH. Preventative strategies. In: Ollendick TH, King NJ, Yule W, eds. International Handbook of Phobic and Anxiety Disorders. New York: Plenum, 1994:453–474.

170. Krohne H. Parental child rearing and anxiety development. In: Hurrelmann K, Losel F, eds. Health Hazards in Adolescence: Prevention and Intervention in Childhood and Adolescence. New York: DeGruyter, 1990:115–130.

171. Rapee R. Potential role of childrearing practices in the development of anxiety and depression. Clin Psychol Rev 1997; 17:47–67.

172. Parker G. Reported parental characteristics of agoraphobics and social phobics. Br J Psychiatry 1979; 135:555–560.

173. Arrindell WA, Emmelkamp PMG, Monsma A, Brilman E. The role of perceived parental rearing practices in the aetiology of phobic disorders: a controlled study. Br J Psychiatry 1983; 143:183–187.

174. Arrindell W, Kwee M, Methorst G, Van der Ende J, Pol E, Moritz B. Perceived parental rearing styles of agoraphobic and socially phobic inpatients. Br J Psychiatry 1989; 155:526–535.

175. Gerlsma C, Emmelkamp P, Arrindell W. Anxiety, depression, and perception of early parenting: a meta-analysis. Clin Psychol Rev 1990; 10: 251–277.

176. Rickel AU, Williams DL, Loigman GA. Predictors of maternal child-rearing practices: implications for intervention. J Comm Psychol 1988; 16:32–40.

177. Parker G. Parental Overprotection: A Risk Factor in Psychosocial Development. New York: Grune and Stratton, 1983.

178. Silove D. Perceived parental characteristics and reports of early parental deprivation in agoraphobic patients. Austr NZ J Psychiatry 1986; 20:365–369.

179. Laraia M, Stuart G, Grye L, Lydiard R, Ballenger J. Childhood environment of women having panic disorder and agoraphobia. J Anx Dis 1994; 8:1–17.

180. Muris P, Bogels S, Meesters C, van der Kamp N, van Oosten A. Parental rearing practices, fearfulness, and problem behavior in clinically referred children. Person Individ Differences 1996; 21:813–818.

181. Johnson DL, Teigen K, Davila R. Anxiety and social restriction: a study of children in Mexico, Norway, and the United States. J Cross Cult Psychol 1983; 14:439–454.

182. Kohlmann CW, Schumacher A, Streit R. Trait anxiety and parental child-rearing behavior: support as a moderator variable? Anx Res 1988; 1:53–64.

183. Siqueland L, Kendall P, Steinberg L. Anxiety in children: perceived family environments and observed family interaction. J Clin Child Psychol 1996; 25:225–237.

184. Hernandez-Guzman L, Sanchez-Sosa J. Parent-child interactions predict anxiety in Mexican adolescents. Adolescence 1996; 31:955–963.

185. Levy DM. Maternal Overprotection. New York: Columbia University Press, 1943.

186. Eisenberg L. School phobia: a study in the communication of anxiety. Am J Psychiatry 1958; 114:712–718.

187. Waldron S, Shrier DK, Stone B, Tobin F. School phobia and other childhood neuroses: a systematic study of the children and their families. Am J Psychiatry 1975; 132:802–808.

188. Rosenthal M, Finkelstein M, Ni E, Robertson R. A study of mother-child relationships in the emotional disorders of children. Genet Psychol Monographs 1959; 60:65–116.

189. Rosenthal M. Inconsistent parenting and anxiety in the child. Anx Res 1990; 3:61–63.

190. Solyom L, Silberfield M, Solyom C. Maternal overprotection in the etiology of agoraphobia. Can Psychiatr Assoc J 1976; 21:109–113.

191. Berg I, McGuire R. Are mothers of school phobic adolescents overprotective? Br J Psychiatry 1974; 124:10–13.

192. Hersov L. Persistent non-attendance at school. J Child Psychol Psychiatry 1960; 1:130–136.

193. Parker G. Parental representations of patients with anxiety neurosis. Acta Psychiatr Scand 1981; 63:33–36.

194. Rubin K, Stewart S, Chen X. Parents of aggressive and withdrawn children. In: Bornstein M, ed. Handbook of Parenting. Vol 1. Children and Parenting. Hillsdale, NJ: Lawrence Erlbaum Associates, 1995:255–283.

195. Stubbe DE, Zahner G, Goldstein MJ, Leckman JF. Diagnostic specificity of a brief measure of expressed emotion: a community study of children. J Child Psychol Psychiatry 1993; 34:139–154.

196. Hirshfeld DR, Biederman J, Brody L, Faraone SV, Rosenbaum JR. Associations between expressed emotion and child behavioral inhibition and psychopathology: a pilot study. J Am Acad Child Adolesc Psychiatry 1997; 36:205–213.

197. Hirshfeld DR, Biederman J, Brody L, Faraone SV, Rosenbaum JF. Expressed emotion toward children with behavioral inhibition: associations with maternal anxiety disorders. J Am Acad Child Adolesc Psychiatry 1997; 36:910–917.

198. Hermans HJM, ter Laak JJF, Maes PCJ. Achievement motivation and fear of failure in family and school. Dev Psychol 1972; 6:520–528.

199. Hock M. Exchange of aversive communicative acts between mother and child as related to perceived child-rearing practices and anxiety of the child. In: Hagtvet K, Johnsen T, eds. Advances in Test Anxiety Research. Vol 7. Amsterdam: Swets & Zeitlinger, 1992:156–174.

200. Hudson J, Rapee R. Parenting factors in child anxiety. Presented at Annual Convention of the Association for the Advancement of Behavior Therapy, Miami, 1997.

201. Krohne H, Hock M. Relationships between restrictive mother-child interactions and anxiety of the child. Anxiety Res 1991; 4:109–124.
202. Chorpita BF, Brown TA, Albano AM, Barlow DH. The influence of parenting style on psychological vulnerability for the development of anxiety disorders. AABT 30th Annual Convention Proceedings New York: Association for the Advancement of Behavior Therapy, 1996.
203. Dadds MR, Barrett PM, Rapee RM, Ryan S. Family process and child anxiety and aggression: an observational analysis. J Abnorm Child Psychol 1996; 24:715–734.
204. Chorpita B, Albano A, Barlow D. Cognitive processing in children: relation to anxiety and family influences. J Clin Child Psychol 1996; 25:170–176.
205. Brunk MA, Henggeler SW. Child influences on adult controls: an experimental investigation. Dev Psychol 1984; 20:1074–1081.
206. MacFarlane AC. The relationship between patterns of family interaction and psychiatric disorder in children. Austr NZ J Psychiatry 1987; 21:383–390.
207. Brown T. Parent-child interactions in adolescence and young adult anxiety and depression. Dissertation Abstracts International 1991; 52:4967.
208. McFarlane AC. The relationship between patterns of family interaction and psychiatric disorder in children. Austr NZ J Psychiatry 1987; 21: 383–390.
209. Bowlby J. Separation: Anxiety and Anger. New York: Basic Books, 1973.
210. Faravelli C, Webb T, Ambonetti A, Fonnesu F, Sessarego A. Prevalence of traumatic early life events in 31 agoraphobic patients with panic attacks. Am J Psychiatry 1985; 142:1493–1494.
211. Thyer BA, Nesse RM, Curtis GC, Cameron OG. Panic disorder: a test of the separation anxiety hypothesis. Behav Res Ther 1986; 24:209–211.
212. De Loof C, Zandbergen J, Lousberg H, Pols H, Griez E. The role of life events in the onset of panic disorder. Behav Res Ther 1989; 27: 461–463.
213. Thyer BA, Himle J, Fischer D. Is parental death a selective precursor to either panic disorder or agoraphobia? A test of the separation anxiety hypothesis. J Anx Disord 1988; 2:333–338.
214. Burnam MA, Stein JA, Golding JM, Siegel JM, Sorenson SB, Forsythe AB, Telles CA. Sexual assault and mental disorders in a community population. J Consult Clin Psychol 1988; 56:843–850.

215. Jacobson A. Physical and sexual assault histories among psychiatric outpatients. Am J Psychiatry 1989; 146:755–758.
216. Faravelli c. Life events preceding the onset of panic disorder. J Affect Disord 1985; 9:103–105.
217. Faravelli C, Pallanti S. Recent life events and panic disorder. Am J Psychiatry 1989; 146:622–626.
218. Manfro GG, Otto MW, McArdle ET, Worthington JJ, Rosenbaum JF, Pollack MH. Relationship of antecedent stressful life events to childhood and family history of anxiety and the course of panic disorder. J Affect Disord 1996; 41:135–139.
219. Roy-Byrne PP, Geraci M, Uhde TW. Life events and the onset of panic disorder. Am J Psychiatry 1986; 143:1424–1427.
220. Rapee RM, Litwin EM, Barlow DH. Impact of life events on subjects with panic disorder and on comparison subjects. Am J Psychiatry 1990; 147:640–644.
221. Seligman M, Kaslow NJ, Alloy LB, Peterson C, Tannenbaum R, Abramson LY. Attributional style and depressive symptoms among children. J Abnorm Psychol 1984; 93:235–238.
222. Nolen-Hoeksema S, Girgus J, Seligman M. Learned helplessness in children: a longitudinal study of depression, achievement, and explanatory style. J Pers Soc Psychol 1986; 51:435–442.
223. Turner JE, Cole DA. Developmental differences in cognitive diatheses for child depression. J Abnorm Child Psychol 1994; 22:15–32.
224. Turner SM, Beidel DC, Costello A. Psychopathology in the offspring of anxiety disorders patients. J Consult Clin Psychol 1987; 55:229–235.
225. Rubin K, Stewart S. Social withdrawal. In: Mash E, Barkley R, eds. Child Psychopathology. New York: Guilford Press, 1996.
226. Cobham V, Dadds M. Treatment of childhood anxiety: the role of parental anxiety. AABT 30th Annual Convention Proceedings. New York: Association for the Advancement of Behavior Therapy, 1996.
227. Kendall PC. Treating anxiety disorders in children: results of a randomized clinical trial. J Consult Clin Psychol 1994; 62:100–110.
228. Kendall PC, Southam-Gerow MA. Long-term follow-up of a cognitive-behavioral therapy for anxiety disordered youth. J Consult Clin Psychol 1996; 64:724–730.
229. Barrett PM, Rapee RM, Dadds MR. Family treatment of childhood anxiety: a controlled trial. J Consult Clin Psychol 1996; 64:333–342.

5

The Pharmacotherapy of Panic Disorder

Jerrold F. Rosenbaum and Mark H. Pollack

Massachusetts General Hospital
and Harvard Medical School
Boston, Massachusetts

Steffany J. Fredman

Massachusetts General Hospital
Boston, Massachusetts

INTRODUCTION

Epidemiological studies have reported lifetime prevalence rates of 1.5–3.5% for panic disorder and 3–15% for panic attacks; an additional 2–5% suffer from agoraphobia with or without panic disorder, and the disorder affects three times as many women as men (1–4). Panic disorder most commonly emerges in early adulthood, although many patients report significant anxiety dating back to childhood in the form of separation anxiety, overanxious disorder, school phobia, excessive shyness, or marked behavioral inhibition in novel circumstances. Panic disorder, with or without agoraphobia, tends to be a chronic and fluctuating disorder associated with considerable morbidity and impairment, but which also responds well to pharmacological and cognitive-behavioral treatments.

Treatment of the panic disorder patient has traditionally focused on blocking panic attacks, diminishing anticipatory or generalized anxiety, and reversing phobic avoidance while recognizing and treating comorbid conditions. The current medical model of panic disorder emphasizes qualitative differences between a panic attack and other types of anxiety. According to this view, panic disorder is seen as reflecting a specific genetically influenced neurochemical dysregulation (5–7). Thus, a rational pharmacological treatment intervention would target the neurobiological pathways associated with maladaptive and overreactive fear and alarm mechanisms (see Chapter 3). Putative sites of this dysregulation have included the locus ceruleus and the noradrenergic system (8,9), the serotonergic system (10,11), and the central GABA-benzodiazepine receptor complex (12). Other studies suggest roles for various other factors in the neurobiology of panic disorder. Among them are cortisol-releasing factor, adenosine (13), and a variety of neuropeptides, including cholecystokinin (14). Support for the neurobiological illness model also stems from experimental panic induction from biological challenges (e.g., CO_2 inhalation, lactate infusion, yohimbine), and the success of treatment with pharmacological agents.

Pharmacotherapy of panic disorder was initially shown to be effective with the monoamine oxidase inhibitors (MAOIs) and tricyclic antidepressants (TCAs), with subsequent studies supporting the efficacy of benzodizepines, selective serotonin-reuptake inhibitors (SSRIs), and other agents. The primary goals of pharmacological treatment are to prevent panic attacks, to address comorbid psychiatric conditions, and to extend treatment effects to achieve remission or recovery (i.e., the absence of impairment and other secondary symptoms). Drug treatment aims at reregulating a dysregulated physiological system, addresses the underlying constitutional vulnerability, treats or facilitates the treatment of the disorder's secondary complications, and reduces severe impairment and distress to the point of remission or to the degree that other therapies become acceptable options for patients (e.g., cognitive-behavioral therapy). A variety of agents have shown primary and adjunctive utility for the treatment of panic disorder (see Table 1).

ANTIDEPRESSANTS

Selective Serotonin-Reuptake Inhibitors

In recent years, dysregulation of the central serotonergic system has been considered to play a key role in the pathogenesis of panic disorder (15–18). The notion has also been proposed that pharmacological agents that act primarily on the serotonergic system—namely, the SSRIs and the tricyclic clomipramine—may also exert their antipanic effects by indirectly modulating an abnormally unstable noradrenergic system, although the precise mechanism of action is not yet clearly understood (19). In clinical practice, the SSRIs are now the "first-line" treatment for panic disorder, combining efficacy for panic disorder with a broad spectrum of efficacy for disorders that are frequently comorbid with panic disorder (e.g., depression, social phobia, obsessive-compulsive disorder), their overall safety and tolerability, their safety in overdose, and (compared to benzodiazepines) their low potential for addiction and withdrawal. Furthermore, their relatively favorable side-effect profile predicts greater tolerability and compliance than with the older TCAs and MAOIs, an important consideration because panic disorder is often of a chronic or recurrent nature, requiring long-term treatment.

Approved in 1996 by the FDA as indicated for panic disorder with or without concomitant agoraphobia, paroxetine was the first antidepressant labeled for treatment of panic disorder and has displayed antipanic efficacy in both short- and long-term studies. In a 12-week, parallel group, double-blind, placebo-controlled study of 367 patients with DSM-III-R-defined panic disorder (20), paroxetine was compared to both clomipramine and placebo. At endpoint, paroxetine (20–60 mg daily) and clomipramine (50–150 mg daily) were equally effective, and both were significantly more effective than placebo. However, paroxetine displayed a more rapid onset of action than clomipramine in reducing the number of panic attacks to zero, and subjects in the par-

Table 1 Drug Treatment of Panic Disorder

Available treatments	Advantages	Disadvantages	Next steps
Antidepressants			
SSRIs (e.g., paroxetine, sertraline, fluvoxamine, fluoxetine)	Favorable side-effect profile Broad spectrum of efficacy for comorbid disorders Low potential for abuse Safety in overdose	Associated with initial "jitteriness," restlessness, and increased anxiety Delayed onset of action (3–6 weeks)	Add HPB Add beta-blocker (e.g., propranolol) to decrease somatic anxiety symptoms Add buspirone Add lithium Add TCA (low-dose) Add anticonvulsant (e.g., valproic acid, gabapentin) Add CBT
TCAs (e.g., imipramine, clomipramine)	Cost of drug less than cost of SSRIs SSRI non-responders may respond	Total cost of care may be more expensive than with SSRIs Adverse side-effect profile Associated with initial jitteriness Delayed onset of action (3–6 weeks) Cardiotoxic in overdose	Switch to SSRI Add HPB Add beta-blocker Add lithium Add anticonvulsant Add CBT
MAOIs (e.g., phenelzine, tranylcypromine)	Often effective for the treatment-refractory patient	Adverse side-effect profile Dietary restrictions Drug interactions Danger in overdose	Washout and switch to SSRI/TCA Add HPB Add lithium Add anticonvulsant Add CBT

Table 1 Continued

Available treatments	Advantages	Disadvantages	Next steps
Benzodiaze-pines			
HPBs: clona-zepam, alpra-zolam LPBs: e.g., diaz-epam, lora-zepam	Highly effica-cious (HPBs block panic at-tacks and anticipatory/ generalized anxiety) Rapid onset of action Favorable side-effect profile	Potential for abuse in abuse-prone individuals Withdrawal syn-drome Initiation of treatment as-sociated with sedation and ataxia Short half-life HPB (alpra-zolam) asso-ciated with in-terdose rebound anxi-ety and with-drawal, risk of difficult dis-continuation, and need for frequent dosing Not effective for depression	Add antidepres-sant Add buspirone Add anticonvul-sant Add CBT

HPB = high-potency benzodiazepine; LPB = lower-potency benzodiazepine; MAOI = monoamine oxidase inhibitor; TCA = tricyclic antidepressant.

oxetine group experienced significantly fewer adverse effects, resulting in fewer patients withdrawing due to side effects than in the clomipramine group. In a 9-month extension of this study (21), 176 patients with DSM-III-R-defined panic disorder who completed the 12-week, double-blind study of paroxetine and clomipramine continued their randomized conditions. As in the short-term study, paroxetine was equal to clomipramine in terms of antipanic efficacy, both were significantly more effective than placebo, and paroxetine was better tolerated than clomipramine. In addition, not only was the efficacy of paroxetine maintained from the previous study, but continued improvement was also observed. Studies of paroxetine's superior antipanic efficacy over placebo were also reported by Oehrberg and colleagues (22) and Steiner and colleagues (23) in controlled studies of 12 and 10 weeks, respectively. In the former study, paroxetine and cognitive-behavioral therapy (CBT) was superior to CBT and placebo. Although patients may respond at lower doses, a double-blind, fixed-dose, placebo-controlled trial of 278 subjects with panic disorder revealed 40 mg of paroxetine to be the most clearly effective dose (24).

Sertraline is also now indicated for the treatment of panic disorder (approved by the FDA in 1997), having shown superior efficacy over placebo in reducing panic attack frequency and anticipatory anxiety in controlled studies (25–28). In a 10-center, double-blind, placebo-controlled study of 176 nondepressed patients with panic disorder with and without agoraphobia, Pollack and colleagues (27) investigated the efficacy of flexible-dose sertraline (50–200 mg/day) for 10 weeks (dose was titrated upward during the first week), following a 2-week single-blind washout period. Sertraline-treated patients experienced significantly greater reductions in panic attack frequency—the primary outcome measure—compared to placebo-treated patients. Additionally, patients receiving sertraline experienced significantly greater improvements over patients receiving placebo as measured by the Clinical Global Impression Improvement and Severity Scales, Multicenter Panic Anxiety Scale (MCPAS) ratings, high end-state function assessment, Patient Global Evaluation rating, and quality-of-life scores. Similar results were reported by DuBoff and colleagues (28), who found that when fixed doses of sertraline (50 mg, 100 mg, and 200 mg daily) were compared to placebo in a 12-week, double-blind, placebo-controlled study of 177 patients with DSM-III-R-defined panic disorder, all sertraline doses significantly reduced the number of panic attacks in comparison to placebo. Overall, sertraline doses of 150 mg appear to be the most effective.

Fluvoxamine has displayed greater antipanic efficacy in double-blind trials than placebo (29–32), maprotiline (33) and ritanserin (34), and comparable efficacy to clomipramine (35) and imipramine (29). Fluvoxamine has also been shown to attenuate panic symptoms in response to challenges with panicogenic agents such as yohimbine (36), CO_2 (37), and CCK-4 (38).

In a 10-week, multicenter, double-blind, placebo-controlled study of panic disorder patients, the SSRI fluoxetine at doses of 10 mg/day or 20 mg/day was significantly better than placebo at reducing panic attack frequency, agoraphobic avoidance, and global distress (39). This finding, in addition to data from open trials (40,41), is consistent with clinical experience suggesting fluoxetine's efficacy for panic disorder. In a study of seven panic patients who showed an inadequate response to open treatment with either fluoxetine or a tricyclic, all seven showed a reduction in panic attacks with combined TCA-fluoxetine treatment (42), consistent with previous reports suggesting the effectiveness of this strategy for treatment-refractory depression (43).

The SSRIs, generally well-tolerated and free of many of the side effects of the TCAs, are now first-line treatments for panic disorder. Although each SSRI heretofore mentioned has demonstrated antipanic efficacy in both double-blind and open trials, there is a lack of direct comparative studies of the various SSRIs in the pharmacotherapy of panic disorder. Nonetheless, nearly all SSRIs (as well as the TCAs) have the potential for restlessness, "jitteriness," and increased anxiety upon initial dosing. Further, panic disorder patients are especially sensitive to bodily sensations of all types (e.g., GI). Thus, starting with low doses (e.g., paroxetine 10 mg/day, sertraline 25 mg/day, fluvoxamine 50 mg/day, and fluoxetine 10 mg/day) is good practice, and then gradually titrating upward to therapeutic levels over the first few weeks often reduces the increased anxiety associated with initiation of these antidepressants. The ultimately optimally effective doses will often be moderate to high (e.g., paroxetine 40 mg/day, sertraline 150 mg/day, fluvoxamine 150 mg/day, or fluoxetine 40 mg/day).

Tricyclic Antidepressants

Imipramine, a TCA, was the first pharmacological agent noted to treat panic disorder (44). In the decades that followed this initial observation, controlled trials have replicated imipramine's anitpanic efficacy (29,45) and have indicated the therapeutic efficacy of other TCAs including, most notably, clomipramine (35,46). Clomipramine's selectivity for serotonergic uptake may be one reason for its superior antipanic efficacy over other TCAs, which are selective for norepinephrine or are less potent at blocking the reuptake of serotonin. In a 12-week, double-blind, placebo-controlled trial comparing clomipramine to imipramine, clomipramine was superior to both imipramine and placebo as measured by reduction in frequency and number of panic attacks as well as decreased scores on the HAM-A (46). Interestingly, maprotiline, a norepinephrine-reuptake inhibitor, failed to show antipanic efficacy (33). Open trials suggest that desipramine (47) and nortriptyline (48) also reduce panic attacks.

Like the SSRIs, the TCAs are associated with jitteriness upon initiation of treatment. Therefore, while typical antidepressant doses of 100–300 mg/day for imipramine may ultimately be used to control the symptoms of panic disorder, it is recommended that treatment be initiated with lower doses (e.g., 10 mg imipramine) and then be titrated upward to minimize exacerbation of anxiety. Once panic symptoms remit, the issue of maintenance treatment becomes central. As in the pharmacotherapy of depression, many clinicians employ full-dose TCA maintenance treatment following a stable response to active treatment for the continued control of panic symptoms. However, in one study (49), TCA maintenance dose was successfully lowered by 50%, although patients had met rigorous criteria for remission before the medication was lowered.

While the antipanic efficacy of the TCAs is well established, their delayed action of onset (usually 4 to 6 weeks) and adverse side-effect profile (e.g., initial jitteriness, anticholinergic effects, orthostatic hypotension, weight gain, sexual dysfunction) may be a barrier to tolerability and compliance in both the short and long term. Noyes and colleagues (50), in a follow-up (mean 2.5 years) assessment of a clinical trial of TCA pharmacotherapy in 107 panic disorder patients, reported that 73 of the 107 patients had discontinued TCA treatment (mean dose 109 mg/day imipramine) for at least a month at follow-up, with 50% citing side effects as the primary reason for terminating pharmacotherapy. Additionally, TCAs are cardiotoxic in overdose, a particular danger in patients with comorbid panic disorder and depression, who are at increased risk for suicide attempts (51).

Monoamine Oxidase Inhibitors

The MAOIs have established efficacy for the treatment of panic disorder as well as a number of other anxiety and affective disorders including atypical depression and social phobia. MAOIs such as phenelzine and tranylcypromine are potent antipanic agents (52). For instance, in a 12-week, placebo-controlled trial of patients with panic disorder, Sheehan and colleagues (52) reported that both phenelzine (45 mg/day) and imipramine (150 mg/day) were significantly better than placebo, with phenelzine more effective than imipramine; however, as many as 40% of patients rated themselves as not improved or only partially improved following phenelzine treatment, consistent with clinical experience that higher doses of the MAOI (e.g., 60–90 mg/day) may be more effective. Similarly, in a 6-month open trial of phenelzine (53), 97% of patients were free from panic symptoms, but 25% required behavior therapy in order to decrease residual phobic avoidance and anxiety.

Optimal doses for phenelzine generally range between 45 and 90 mg/day and for tranylcypromine between 30 and 60 mg/day. Although effective for the reduction of panic symptoms, these agents are typically not used first-line because of adverse effects such as orthostasis, weight gain, insomnia, and sexual dysfunction; moreover, the use of MAOIs necessitates vigilance about lethal drug interactions and dietary restrictions because of the potential for precipitating hypertensive crisis if tyramine-containing foods are ingested. In addition, clinical studies suggest a potential for withdrawal and relapse following treatment with MAOIs (54,55). Consequently, MAOIs are usually reserved for patients who remain symptomatic despite treatment with safer and better-tolerated agents; however, a patient should not be considered truly treatment-refractory to pharmacotherapy until he or she has had an MAOI treatment trial.

BENZODIAZEPINES

Because of their efficacy, rapid onset, and favorable side-effect profile, benzodiazepines are frequently used in the treatment of panic disorder. Common initial side effects of the benzodiazepines are sedation and ataxia, and are usually minimized by initiating treatment with low doses followed by gradual upward dose titration. Treatment with benzodiazepines is generally associated with lower dropout rates (13.1%) than those with TCAs (25.4%) (56,57). Each year, 11–15% of adult Americans use benzodiazepines briefly or occasionally, and 1.65% of the total population take them chronically (i.e., daily for a year or longer) (58). Benzodiazepines may actually be underutilized, however, because of patients' fear of dependence and ambivalence about use of pharmacological treatment for psychological conditions. Clinicians should consider the potential for abuse when prescribing benzodiazepines, although panic patients without a history of alcohol and/or substance abuse or dependence are unlikely to abuse benzodiazepines (59–61). High-potency benzodiazepines (HPBs) are particularly effective in treating panic disorder, both in blocking panic attacks and in reducing anticipatory and phobic anxiety. Alprazolam and clonazepam are two HPBs that have been studied extensively and are often used first-line for treatment of panic disorder when a benzodiazepine is indicated (62). Recently, other benzodiazepines such as diazepam (63) and lorazepam (64) have demonstrated efficacy for the treatment of panic disorder.

Several studies have shown alprazolam, a triazolobenzodiazepine, to be comparably effective and often better tolerated than TCAs, mainly imipramine (65–68). Ballenger and colleagues (65), in the first cross-national collaborative panic study of 481 panic patients, found a mean dose of 5.7 mg/day of alprazolam to be more effective than placebo, with a rapid response that increased in magnitude at each weekly assessment. At endpoint (week 8), 55% of patients in the alprazolam group compared to 32% in the placebo group were panic-free. Schweizer and colleagues (69) later found therapeutic effects of alprazolam and imipramine present at the end of an 8-week trial and at an 8-month follow-up. At long-term follow-up, alprazolam was better tolerated than imipramine. Phase II of the Cross-National Collaborative Panic Study (70), with a study population of 1168 panic patients, also showed alprazolam and imipramine to be effective compared to placebo, with alprazolam having a faster onset of effect.

Alprazolam is given at a starting dose of 0.25–0.5 mg two or three times per day and gradually titrated up to a maintenance dose of 2–10 mg a day (divided into q.i.d. dose). Because alprazolam is a short-half-life HPB, interdose rebound anxiety and withdrawal symptoms on abrupt discontinuation may complicate treatment. Rebound anxiety may limit patients' recovery. Dosing alprazolam four or more times a day may reduce interdose symptoms but foster a cognitive link between anxiolysis and pill-taking that could increase the patient's sense of dependence on the medication. For these reasons, the use of a longer-lasting benzodiazepine, such as clonazepam, may be preferred.

Clinical trials have demonstrated that clonazepam is effective in treating panic disorder and that antipanic benefits are sustained over time without escalation of dosage (71–74). Usually, an initial bedtime dose of 0.25 or 0.5 mg/day is gradually titrated up to the typical effective dose of 1–3 mg/day in morning or bedtime doses. Two recent multicenter, double-blind, placebo-controlled studies, one fixed-dose and the other flexible-dose, have demonstrated clonazepam's efficacy and tolerability for panic disorder patients (75,76). Rosenbaum and colleagues (75) randomly assigned 413 panic patients to receive either placebo or one of five fixed daily doses of clonazepam (0.5 mg, 1.0 mg, 2.0 mg, 3.0 mg, and 4.0 mg). Following 3 weeks of dose escalation, patients received 6 weeks of the fixed dose and were then tapered during a 7-week gradual discontinuation phase. Daily doses of 1.0 mg and higher were equally efficacious in reducing number of panic attacks, and all were well tolerated, although patients in the 1.0- and 2.0-mg-daily dose groups reported fewer adverse symptoms. In addition, although most patients in the clonazepam group worsened during the discontinuation phase (as compared to their functioning at the end of the dose-maintenance phase), they did not revert back to their conditions at baseline, i.e., before initiating clonazepam treatment. Similar results were found by Moroz and Rosenbaum (76), in a study of 438 patients assigned to receive either placebo or flexible doses of clonazepam (daily divided doses of 0.25 to 4.0 mg). At the end of the 6-week therapeutic phase, clonazepam was significantly superior to placebo as demonstrated by number of panic attacks, Clinical Global Impression of Severity of Illness (CGI) scores, patient-impression-of-change scores, and anticipatory anxiety; in addition, adverse effects were reported among those patients taking higher doses of clonazepam. Doses were gradually lowered to cessation during a 7-week discontinuation phase. As in the study by Rosenbaum and colleagues (75), modest clinical deterioration was observed at the end of the discontinuation phase relative to the therapeutic phase, although patients did not deteriorate to their status at baseline. Taken together, these two studies suggest that the optimal dose for clonazepam is approximately 2 mg per day (in divided doses taken in the morning and at night). In a 2-year, open, naturalistic study of 259 panic disorder patients, Worthington and colleagues (77) examined the outcome of patients treated with clonazepam alone or in combination with other treatments compared to those not on clonazepam. Over the 2-year treatment period, patients in all three clonazepam groups tended to improve and maintain their type of treatment. Dosage of clonazepam generally remained constant or decreased from baseline. There were no clinically significant adverse effects associated with clonazepam.

Recently, the antipanic efficacy of other benzodiazepines, such as the lower-potency agent diazepam, has been examined. An 8-week, double-blind, placebo-controlled comparison of diazepam and alprazolam in 241 patients with panic disorder found equal efficacy and tolerability for equivalent doses of diazepam (mean, 43 mg/day) and alprazolam (mean, 4.9 mg/day), and both were superior to placebo (63). This study raises questions as to whether the HPBs are uniquely effective for panic or whether equivalent doses of any benzodiazepine may be efficacious.

Withdrawal symptoms may be associated with benzodiazepine discontinuation and are most intense with shorter-acting agents. In a study by Fyer and colleagues (78), 14 of 17 patients on gradual discontinuation of alprazolam treatment experienced withdrawal symptoms; half of the patients were considered severely symptomatic. Panic attacks recurred or increased for most patients, including 14 of 15 who had been panic-free. In an 8-month follow-up of 48 patients in a placebo-controlled comparison of alprazolam and imipramine treatment for panic disorder (79), nearly all subjects treated with alprazolam had withdrawal during a 4-week gradual taper period, and 33% (mean 5.2

mg/day) were unable to discontinue medication. Clonazepam, as a longer-acting agent, may be a preferable alternative to alprazolam for the maintenance treatment of panic disorder (80,81). Because clonazepam has a longer half-life, it is associated with fewer rebound symptoms and requires less frequent dosing, thus decreasing the patient's sense of dependence on the drug. Of 48 patients receiving alprazolam treatment for panic disorder in a study by Herman and colleagues (82), 41 were able to switch to clonazepam, and 82% of those patients rated clonazepam as "better" treatment because of the need for less frequent administration and a decrease in interdose anxiety.

OTHER AGENTS

The antidepressant venlafaxine has been examined in the treatment of panic disorder, with efficacy suggested by data on 25 patients from one site of a multicenter, randomized, double-blind, placebo-controlled trial (83). A low starting dose of 12.5 mg and gradual upward titration to 255 mg were employed. Preliminary evidence has also suggested usefulness of the 5-HT$_2$ antagonist nefazodone, which may have antipanic efficacy and tolerability at doses between 200 and 600 mg, particularly in those patients with comorbid major depressive disorder or depressive symptoms (84,85). However, trazodone, a compound structurally related to nefazodone, failed to demonstrate antipanic efficacy in a double-blind study by Charney and colleagues (56), and one report suggested that bupropion is relatively ineffective for the treatment of panic disorder (86). The 5-HT$_{1A}$ receptor agonists flesinoxan, buspirone, and ipsapirone, which are effective for generalized anxiety disorder (87), are generally ineffective for panic disorder, although buspirone (in the range of 30–60 mg/day) may be effective as an augmentative strategy in combination with SSRIs or benzodiazepines for patients with refractory panic disorder (88).

Beta-blockers, including propranolol, atenolol, and nadolol, are generally not used as primary treatments for panic disorder since they do not effectively block panic or attenuate the cognitive and emotional experience of fear; however, when used adjunctively with other agents, they may reduce some physical symptoms of autonomic arousal (e.g., tachycardia and tremor) (89). Clonidine, the α_2-receptor agonist, decreases locus ceruleus firing and has been reported to initially—although only transiently—reduce panic attacks in affected patients (90,91). Adjunctive lithium in doses of 300–900 mg/day, in conjunction with antidepressant pharmacotherapy, has been reported to be beneficial in some treatment-refractory panic patients (92). The anticonvulsants valproate (93,94) and gabapentin (95) have apparent efficacy for the treatment of typical, atypical, and treatment-resistant panic patients. See Table 2.

LONG-TERM OUTCOME WITH PHARMACOTHERAPY

It is well established that antidepressants and benzodiazepines are effective for the treatment of panic disorder (96). However, although most patients experience some improvement after treatment is initiated and many actually become panic-free, a substantial number remain symptomatic, requiring long-term treatment to address chronic symptoms and/or recurrent episodes. In addition, it is not uncommon for patients to experience residual anxiety symptoms during pharmacological treatment, and most patients relapse on discontinuation of pharmacotherapy. Approximately 30–75% of patients continue to experience panic attacks and/or other residual symptoms for months to years after initiating treatment (74,97). In a study of 105 panic disorder patients who achieved remission (a Clinical Global Impression-Severity (CGI-S) score of 1 or 2—i.e., not ill or with ''borderline'' illness—for at least 2 months), Pollack and colleagues (61) found that the mean length of remission was 9.2 ± 7.0 months and that 58% of patients experienced a relapse despite continuation treatment.

Enhancing Acute Treatment Response

Not surprisingly, follow-up studies ranging from 8 months to 6 years across several classes of antipanic agents have documented that approximately 50–78% of patients remain on medication following acute treatment trials (50,79,98–101). In light of these findings, it is apparent that the complicated, often chronic nature of panic disorder warrants a long-term approach, the nature of which may vary from patient to

Table 2 Recommended Doses and Administration of Most Commonly Prescribed Antipanic Agents

Drug	Dosage range (mg)	Usual intial dose (mg)	Dosing schedule
SSRIs			
Paroxetine (Paxil)	10–50	10	q.d.
Sertraline (Zoloft)	25–200	25	q.d.
Fluvoxamine (Luvox)	50–300	50	q.d.
Fluoxetine (Prozac)	10–80	10	q.d.
TCAs			
Imipramine (Tofranil)	100–300	10–25	q.d.
Clomipramine (Anafranil)	100–250	12.5–25	q.d.
MAOIs			
Phenelzine (Nardil)	45–90	15	b.i.d.
Tranylcypromine (Parnate)	30–60	10–60	b.i.d.
Benzodiazepines			
Alprazolam (Xanax)	2–10	0.25–0.5	q.i.d.
Clonazepam (Klonipin)	1–5	0.25	b.i.d.
Diazepam (Valium)	5–30	2.5	b.i.d.
Lorazepam (Ativan)	3–16	1.0	t.i.d.–q.i.d.
Atypical antidepressants			
Venlafaxine (Effexor)	75–300	37.5	b.i.d.
Nefazodone (Serzone)	300–500	50	b.i.d.
Azapirones			
Buspirone (Buspar)	15–60	5	t.i.d.
Beta-blockers			
Propranolol (Inderal)	10–160	10–20	b.i.d.
Anticonvulsants			
Valproate (Depakote)	500–2,000	250	b.i.d.
Gabapentin (Neurontin)	300–1,800	100	b.i.d.–t.i.d.

patient. When deciding how best to manage this disorder, it is important to consider the patient's level of response. Since patients who become panic-free at the end of acute treatment may still suffer from residual symptoms or functional impairment, a longer course of treatment to reduce or eliminate symptoms is indicated. Augmentation with combined pharmacotherapy, or the use of CBT to address persistent anxiety sensitivity and maladaptive althoughts or behaviors, may help optimize outcome.

Certain factors may act as a barrier to treatment response, both acutely and over the long term, and they should be addressed. For instance, the presence of comorbid conditions such as depression, anxiety, substance abuse, or personality disorders may increase the levels of distress experienced by patients and predispose to relapse. Although there exists a paucity of empirical data on treatment response in patients with comorbid disorders (due to stringent exclusion criteria in most controlled treatment trials), multiple studies have found that one-half to two-thirds of panic disorder patients suffer from past or present major depression (102,103). The use of agents with a broad spectrum of efficacy such as the SSRIs may help to alleviate comorbid depression and other conditions.

Additionally, medical conditions and the medications used to treat them may interfere with antipanic treatment. For example, hyperthyroidism, hypoglycemia, pheochromocytoma, audiovestibular dysfunctions, and complex partial seizures may cause anxiety symptoms, and the experience of chest pain or cardiac arrhythmias in some panic patients with coronary artery disease may provoke panic. Appropriate management of these medical conditions is critical for maximizing outcome. In addition, medications (e.g., bronchodilators for patients with respiratory disease) and the use of caffeine or such substances as marijuana or cocaine may produce anxiety or panic-like symptoms. The effects of these substances may limit patient compliance and complicate the treatment regimen; therefore, their use should be reduced or eliminated when possible.

Sustaining Treatment Response

Once a patient's panic symptoms and associated impairment have remitted, sustaining the remission becomes paramount. Longer-term maintenance therapy is associated with less relapse in treatment discontinuation (104). However, with relapse rates in excess of 50% during antidepressant discontinuation (49,50) and approximately 60% during discontinuation of benzodiazepines (105), it is clear that many patients require maintenance treatment to remain well. The duration of maintenance treatment typically depends on an individual patient's level of response. If the patient is asymptomatic for a minimum of 1 to 2 years on medication following acute treatment response, then it may be safe to consider medication discontinuation. If, however, the patient only partially responds to treatment (e.g., panic attacks decrease in frequency or intensity but still persist), or the patient continues to experience residual symptoms such as phobic avoidance or anticipatory anxiety, then discontinuation of medication is not recommended.

For patients in whom medication discontinuation is indicated, an extremely gradual taper of pharmacotherapy is crucial (79). This is particularly important when discontinuing treatment with benzodiazepines, discontinuation of which may be accompanied by withdrawal symptoms that mimic anxiety or panic, but it is also pertinent for antidepressant-treated patients (106). The clinical strategy for successful taper requires using the smallest dosing decrements formulated for the agent and communication between patient and physician to monitor patient comfort, return of symptoms, or discontinuation-related new symptoms. CBT during the discontinuation process may reduce discontinuation-related symptomatology; patient and clinician workbooks and manuals are now available to facilitate this process. Otto and colleagues (106) reported that 76% of patients who received CBT while tapering benzodiazepine medication were able to successfully complete the discontinuation process whereas successful discontinuation was achieved by only 25% of those undergoing slow benzodiazepine taper alone. (See Figure 1.)

RATIONALE FOR COMBINATION TREATMENT

As noted earlier, each class of agent used in the pharmacotherapy of panic disorder has both benefits and risks associated with its use. One rationale for coadministering different agents is that the combination

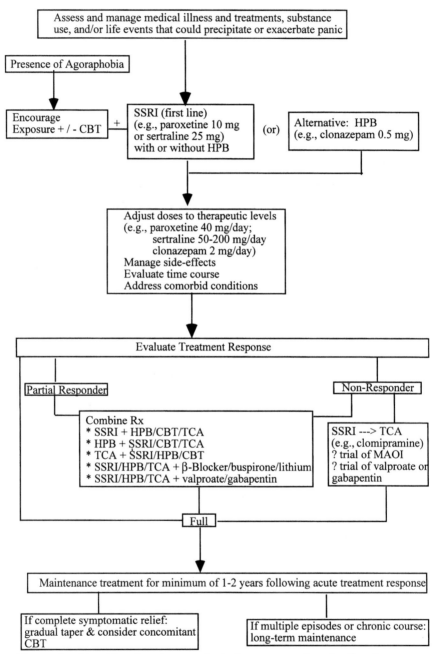

Figure 1   Algorithm for pharmacological treatment of panic disorder.

enables one to capitalize on the positive features of each class of drug while concurrently minimizing negative characteristics or adverse effects. The combination of antidepressants and benzodiazepines provides an illustrative case in point. The benzodiazepines have a rapid onset of action, but are not effective for comorbid depression. In fact, on occasion, depression has been observed to emerge following treatment of panic disorder with benzodiazepines alone. Antidepressants (i.e., TCAs and SSRIs) treat depression yet are associated with initial jitteriness and have a relatively slow onset of action (3–6 weeks). Following the decision to treat a patient with antidepressants, one of the clinician's options is to begin pharmacotherapy concurrently with benzodiazepines to provide early relief of anxiety and minimize antidepressant-associated jitteriness, and then to taper and discontinue the benzodiazepine after a month or two as the patient's condition begins to stabilize. In clinical reality, though, most patients continue on the combination. The long-term combination of benzodiazepines and antidepressants may also exert protective effects compared to treatment with benzodiazepines alone. In a study by Worthington and colleagues (77), patients maintained on a low benzodiazepine dose were more likely to relapse than patients on no medication, patients treated with antidepressants alone, and patients treated with antidepressants and adjunctive benzodiazepines.

As briefly discussed above, the integration of pharmacotherapy and cognitive-behavioral interventions may also maximize treatment gains for certain panic patients, especially those who suffer from agoraphobia and those attempting to discontinue benzodiazepine treatment (107). Adjunctive CBT during acute treatment may improve response to pharmacotherapy (61), block patients' generalized and/or anticipatory anxiety and thereby elevate their panic threshold (108), increase compliance, and decrease the amount of medication required to gain control of symptoms (56,109,110).

ACKNOWLEDGMENT

We thank Maria Bulzacchelli for her assistance in preparing this chapter.

REFERENCES

1. Eaton WW, Kessler RC, Wittchen HU, Magee WJ. Panic and panic disorder in the United States. Am J Psychiatry 1994; 151:413–420.

2. Kessler RC, McGonagle KA, Zhao S, Nelson CB, Hughes M, Eshleman S, Wittchen H, Kendler KS. Lifetime and 12-month prevalence of DSM-III-R Psychiatric Disorders in the United States. Arch Gen Psychiatry 1994; 51:8–19.

3. Myers JK, Weissman MM, Tischler GL, Holzer CE, Leaf PJ, Orvaschel H, Anthony JC, Boyd JH, Burke JD, Kramer M, Stoltzman R. Six-month prevalence of psychiatric disorders in three communities. Arch Gen Psychiatry 1984; 41:959–967.

4. Weissman MM, Merikangas KR. The epidemiology of anxiety and panic disorders: an update. J Clin Psychiatry 1986; 47:11–17.

5. Klein DF. Anxiety reconceptualized. In: Klein DF and Rabkin J, eds. Anxiety: New Research and Concepts. New York: Raven Press, 1981: 235–262.

6. Klein DF, Rabkin JG, Gorman JM. Etiological and pathophysiological inferences from the pharmacological treatment of anxiety. In: Tuma AH, Maser JD, eds. Anxiety and the Anxiety Disorders. Hillsdale, NJ: Erlbaum, 1985:501–532.

7. Sheehan DV. Panic attacks and phobias. N Engl J Med 1982; 307:156–158.

8. Redmond DE, Huang YH, Snyder DR, Maas JW. Behavioral effects of stimulation of the nucleus locus coeruleus in the stump-tailed monkey *Macaca arctoides.* Brain Res 1976; 116:502–510.

9. Gray JA. The Neuropsychology of Anxiety: An Enquiry into the Functions of the Septo-Hippocampal System. New York: Oxford University Press, 1982.

10. Lesch KP, Weismann MM, Hoh A, Muller T, Disselkamp-Tietze J, Osterheider M, Schulte HM. 5-HT1A receptor-effector system responsivity in panic disorder. Psychopharmacology 1992; 106:111–117.

11. Woods SW, Charney DS. Applications of the pharmacologic challenge strategy in panic disorder research. J Anx Dis 1988; 2:31–49.

12. Roy-Byrne PP, Dager SR, Cowley DS, Vitaliano R, Dunner DL. Relapse and rebound following discontinuation of benzodiazepine treatment of panic attacks: alprazolam versus diazepam. Am J Psychiatry 1989; 146:860–865.

13. Uhde TW. Caffeine provocation of panic: a focus on biological mecha-

nisms. In: Ballenger JC, ed. Neurobiology of Panic Disorder. New York: Wiley-Liss, 1990:219–242.

14. Bradwejn J, Koszycki D, Couetoux du Tertre A, Bourin M, Palmour R, Ervin F. The cholecystokinin hypothesis of panic and anxiety disorders: a review. J Psychopharmacol 1992; 6:345–351.

15. Goddard AW, Charney DS. Toward an integrated neurobiology of panic disorder. J Clin Psychiatry 1997; 58:4–11.

16. Krystal JH, Deutsch DN, Charney DS. The biological basis of panic disorder. J Clin Psychiatry 1996; 57(suppl 10):23–31.

17. Westenberg HGM. Developments in the drug treatment of panic disorder: what is the place of the selective serotonin reuptake inhibitors? J Affect Disord 1996; 40:85–93.

18. Westenberg HGM, Den Boer JA. Serotonergic basis of panic disorder. In: Montgomery SA, ed. Psychopharmacology of Panic. Oxford: Oxford University Press, 1993:91–109.

19. Coplan JD, Papp LA, Pine D, Martinez J, Cooper T, Rosenblum LA, Klein DF, Gorman JM. Clinical improvement with fluoxetine therapy and noradrenergic function in patients with panic disorder. Arch Gen Psychiatry 1997; 54:643–648.

20. Lecrubier Y, Bakker A, Dunbar G, Judge R, Collaborative Paroxetine Panic Study Investigators. A comparison of paroxetine, clomipramine and placebo in the treatment of panic disorder. Acta Psychiatr Scand 1997; 95:145–152.

21. Lecrubier Y, Judge R, Collaborative Paroxetine Panic Study Investigators. Long-term evaluation of paroxetine, clomipramine and placebo in panic disorder. Acta Psychiatr Scand 1997; 95:153–160.

22. Oehrberg S, Christiansen PE, Behnke K, Borup AL, Severin B, Soegaard J, Calberg H, Judge R, Ohrstrom JK, Manniche PM. Paroxetine in the treatment of panic disorder: a randomised, double-blind, placebo-controlled study. Br J Psychiatry 1995; 167:374–379.

23. Steiner M, Oakes R, Gergel IP. A fixed-dose study of paroxetine and placebo in the treatment of panic disorder. In: Program and Abstracts on New Research. 148th Annual Meeting of the American Psychiatric Association, Miami, 1995.

24. Ballenger JC, Wheadon DE, Steiner M, Bushnell W, Gergel IP. Double-blind, fixed-dose, placebo-controlled study of paroxetine in the treatment of panic disorder. Am J Psychiatry 1998; 155:36–42.

25. Gorman J, Wolkow R. Sertraline as a treatment for panic disorder. XIXth Collegium International Neuro-psychopharmacologicum Congress, Washington, DC, 1994.

26. Pollack M, Wolkow R, Clary C. Sertraline treatment of panic disorder: combined results from two placebo-controlled trials. 37th Annual Meeting of the NCDEU, Boca Raton, FL, 1997.

27. Pollack MH, Otto MW, Worthington JJ, Wolkow R. Efficacy and safety of sertraline and placebo for the treatment of panic disorder: results from a flexible dose, multicenter trial. Submitted.

28. DuBoff E, Ferguson JM, Londborg PD, Rosenthal MH, Smith W, Wiese C, Wolkow RM. Double-blind comparison of three fixed doses of sertraline and placebo in patients with panic disorder [abstr]. 8th Congress of the European College of Neuropsychopharmacology, Venice, Italy. New York: Elsevier, 1995.

29. Bakish D, Hooper CL, Filteau MJ, Charbonneau Y, Fraser G, West DL, Thibaudeau C, Raine D. A double-blind placebo-controlled trial comparing fluvoxamine and imipramine in the treatment of panic disorder with or without agoraphobia. Psychopharmacol Bull 1996; 32:135–141.

30. Hoehn-Saric R, McLeod DR, Hipsley PA. Effect of fluvoxamine on panic disorder. J Clin Psychopharmacol 1993; 13:321–326.

31. Black DW, Wesner R, Bowers W, Gabel J. A comparison of fluvoxamine, cognitive-therapy, and placebo in the treatment of panic disorder. Arch Gen Psychiatry 1993; 52:44–50.

32. de Beurs E, van Balkom A, Lange A, Koele P, van Dyck R. Treatment of panic disorder with agoraphobia: comparison of fluvoxamine, placebo, and psychological panic management combined with exposure and of exposure in vivo alone. Am J Psychiatry 1995; 152:683–691.

33. den Boer JA, Westenberg HGM. Effects of a serotonin and noradrenaline uptake inhibitor in panic disorder: a double-blind comparative study with fluvoxamine and maprotiline. Int J Clin Psychopharmacol 1988; 3:59–74.

34. den Boer JA, Westenberg HGM. Serotonin function in panic disorder: a double-blind placebo controlled study with fluvoxamine and ritanserin. Psychopharmacology 1990; 102:85–94.

35. den Boer JA, Westenberg HGM, Kamerbeek WDJ, Verhoeven WM, Kahn RS. Effect of serotonin uptake inhibitors in anxiety disorders: a double-blind comparison of clomipramine and fluvoxamine. Int Clin Psychopharmacol 1987; 2:21–32.

36. Goddard AW, Woods SW, Sholomskas DE, Goodman WK, Charney DS, Heninger GR. Effects of the serotonin reuptake inhibitor fluvoxamine on yohimbine-induced anxiety in panic disorder. Psychiatry Res 1993; 48:119–133.

37. Pols JH, Hauzer RC, Meijer JA, Verburg K, Griez EJ. Fluvoxamine attenuates panic induced by 35% CO_2 challenge. J Clin Psychiatry 1996; 57:539–542.

38. van Megen HJGM, Westenberg HGM, den Boer JA, Slaap B, Scheepmaker A. Effect of the selective serotonin reuptake inhibitor fluvoxamine on CCK-4 induced panic attacks. Psychopharmacology 1997; 129:357–364.

39. Lydiard RB, Pollack MH, Judge R, Michelson D, Tamura R. Fluoxetine treatment of panic disorder: a randomized, placebo-controlled, multicenter trial. European College of Neuropharmacology (ECNP) Annual Meeting, Vienna, 1997.

40. Gorman JM, Liebowitz MR, Fyer AJ, Goetz D, Campeas RB, Ryer MR, Davies SO, Klein DF. An open trial of fluoxetine in the treatment of panic attacks. J Clin Psychopharmacol 1987; 7:329–332.

41. Schneier FR, Leibowitz MR, Davies SO, Fairbanks J, Hollander E, Campeas R, Klein DF. Fluoxetine in panic disorder. J Clin Psychopharmacol 1990; 10:119–121.

42. Tiffon L, Coplan JD, Papp LA, Gorman JM. Augmentation strategies with tricyclic or fluoxetine treatment in seven partially responsive panic disorder patients. J Clin Psychiatry 1994; 55:66–69.

43. Weilburg JB, Rosenbaum JF, Biederman J, Sachs GS, Kelly KA. Fluoxetine added to non-MAOI antidepressants converts non-responders to responders: a preliminary report. J Clin Psychiatry 1989; 50:447–449.

44. Klein DF. Delineation of two-drug responsive anxiety syndromes. Psychopharmacologia 1964; 5:397–408.

45. Boyer W. Serotonin reuptake inhibitors are superior to imipramine and alprazolam in alleviating panic attacks: a meta-analysis. Int Clin Psychopharmacol 1995; 10:45–49.

46. Modigh K, Westberg P, Eriksson E. Superiority of clomipramine over imipramine in the treatment of panic disorder: a placebo-controlled trial. J Clin Psychopharmacol 1992; 12:251–261.

47. Lydiard RB. Desipramine in agoraphobia with panic attacks: an open, fixed-dose study. J Clin Psychopharmacol 1987; 7:258–260.

48. Munjack DJ, Usigli R, Zulueta A, Crocker B, Adatia N, Buckwalter JG, Baltazar P, Kurvink W, Inglove H, Kelly R. Nortriptyline in the treatment of panic disorder and agoraphobia with panic attacks. J Clin Psychopharmacol 1988; 8:204–207.

49. Mavissakalian M, Perel JM. Clinical experiments in maintenance and discontinuation of imipramine therapy in panic disorder with agoraphobia. Arch Gen Psychiatry 1992; 49:318–323.

50. Noyes R, Garvey MJ, Cook B. Follow-up study of patients with panic attacks treated with tricyclic antidepressants. J Affect Disord 1989; 16: 249–257.

51. Angst J, Wicki W. The epidemiology of frequent and less frequent panic attacks. In: Montgomery SA, ed. Psychopharmacology of Panic. Oxford: Oxford University Press, 1993:7–24.

52. Sheehan DV, Ballenger JC, Jacobsen G. Treatment of endogenous anxiety with phobic, hysterical, and hypochondriacal symptoms. Arch Gen Psychiatry 1980; 37:51–59.

53. Buiges J, Vallego J. Therapeutic response to phenelzine in patients with panic disorder and agoraphobia with panic attacks. J Clin Psychiatry 1987; 48:55–59.

54. Tyrer P. Clinical effects of abrupt withdrawal from tricyclic antidepressants and monoamine oxidase inhibitors after long-term treatment. J Affect Disord 1984; 6:1–7.

55. Sheehan DV. Tricyclic antidepressants in the treatment of anxiety disorders. 139th Annual Meeting of the American Psychiatric Association, Washington, DC, 1986.

56. Charney DS, Woods SW, Goodman WK, Rifkin B, Kinch MM, Aiken B, Quadrino LM, Heninger GR. Drug treatment of panic disorder: the comparative efficacy of imipramine, alprazolam, and trazodone. J Clin Psychiatry 1986; 47:580–586.

57. Pollack MH, Rosenbaum JF. Benzodiazepines in panic-related disorders. J Anx Dis 1988; 2:95–107.

58. Salzman C. Benzodiazepine treatment of panic and agoraphobic symptoms: use, dependence, toxicity, abuse. J Psychiatr Res 1993; 27:97–110.

59. Clinthorne JK, Cisin IH, Balter MB, Mellinger GD, Uhlenhuth EH. Changes in popular attitudes and beliefs about tranquilizers. Arch Gen Psychiatry 1986; 43:527–532.

60. Mellinger GD, Balter MB, Uhlenhuth EH. Prevalence and correlates of the long-term regular use of anxiolytics. JAMA 1984; 251:375–379.

61. Pollack MH, Otto MW, Worthington JJ, Sabatino S, McArdle ET, Rosenbaum JF. Predictors of time to relapse in a longitudinal study of panic disorder. Annual Meeting of the American College of Neuropharmacology, San Juan, Puerto Rico, 1994.

62. Davidson JRT. Use of benzodiazepines in panic disorder. J Clin Psychiatry 1997; 58:26–28.

63. Noyes R, Burrows GD, Reich JH, Judd FK, Garvey MJ, Norman TR,

Cook BL, Marriott P. Diazepam versus alprazolam for the treatment of panic disorder. J Clin Psychiatry 1996; 57:349–355.

64. Schweizer E, Pohl R, Balon R, Fox I, Rickels K, Yeragni VK. Lorazepam vs. alprazolam in the treatment of panic disorder. Pharmacopsychiatry 1990; 23:90–93.

65. Ballenger JC, Burrows GD, Dupont RJ, Lesser IM, Noyes R Jr, Pecknold JC, Rifkin A, Swinson RP. Alprazolam in panic disorder and agoraphobia: results from a multicenter trial. I. Efficacy in short-term treatment. Arch Gen Psychiatry 1988; 45:413–422.

66. Charney DS, Woods SW. Benzodiazepine treatment of panic disorder: a comparison of alprazolam and lorazepam. J Clin Psychiatry 1989; 50:418–423.

67. Chouinard G, Annable L, Fontaine R, Solyom L. Alprazolam in the treatment of generalized anxiety and panic disorders: a double-blind, placebo-controlled study. Psychopharmacology 1982; 77:229–233.

68. Munjack DJ, Crocker B, Cabe D, Brown R, Usigli R, Zulueta A, McManus M, McDowell D, Palmer R, Leonard M. Alprazolam, propranolol and placebo in the treatment of panic disorder and agoraphobia with panic attacks. J Clin Psychopharmacol 1989; 9:22–27.

69. Schweizer E, Rickels K, Weiss S, Zavodnick S. Maintenance drug treatment of panic disorder. I. Results of a prospective, placebo-controlled comparison of alprazolam and imipramine. Arch Gen Psychiatry 1993; 50:51–60.

70. Cross-National Collaborative Panic Study Second Phase Investigators. Drug treatment of panic disorder: comparative efficacy of alprazolam imipramine, and placebo. Br J Psychiatry 1992; 160:191–202.

71. Beauclair L, Fontaine R, Annable L, Holobow N, Chouinard G. Clonazepam in the treatment of panic disorder: a double-blind, placebo-controlled trial investigating the correlation between clonazepam concentrations in plasma and clinical response. J Clin Psychopharmacol 1994; 14:111–118.

72. Pollack MH, Rosenbaum JF, Tesar GE, Herman JB, Sachs GS. Clonazepam in the treatment of panic disorder and agoraphobia. Psychopharmacol Bull 1987; 23:141–144.

73. Tesar GE, Rosenbaum JF, Pollack MH, Herman JB, Sachs GS, Mahoney EM, Cohen LS, McNamara M, Goldstein S. Clonazepam versus alprazolam in the treatment of panic disorder: interim analysis of data from a prospective, double-blind, placebo-controlled trial. J Clin Psychiatry 1987; 48(suppl 10):16–21.

74. Tesar GE, Rosenbaum JF, Pollack MH, Otto MW, Sachs GS, Herman

JB, Cohen LS, McNamara M, Spier S. Double-blind, placebo controlled comparison of clonazepam and alprazolam for panic disorder. J Clin Psychiatry 1991; 52:69–76.

75. Rosenbaum JF, Moroz G, Bowden CL. Clonazepam in the treatment of panic disorder with or without agoraphobia: a dose-response study of efficacy, safety, and discontinuance. J Clin Psychopharmacol 1997; 17:390–400.

76. Moroz G, Rosenbaum JF. Efficacy, safety, and gradual discontinuation of clonazepam in panic disorder: a placebo-controlled multicenter study using optimized doses. Submitted.

77. Worthington JJ, Pollack MH, Otto MW, Moroz G, Rosenbaum JF. Long-term experience with clonazepam in patients with a primary diagnosis of panic disorder. Psychopharmacol Bull. In press.

78. Fyer A, Leibowitz M, Gorman J, Campeas R, Levin A, Davies S, Goetz D, Klein D. Discontinuation of alprazolam treatment in panic patients. Am J Psychiatry 1987; 144:303–308.

79. Rickels K, Schweizer E, Weiss S, Zavodnick S. Maintenance drug treatment for panic disorder. II. Short- and long-term outcome after drug taper. Arch Gen Psychiatry 1993; 50:61–68.

80. Albeck JH. Withdrawal and detoxification from benzodiazepine dependence: a potential role for clonazepam. J Clin Psychiatry 1987; 48(suppl 10):43–49.

81. Cohen LS, Rosenbaum JF. Clonazepam: new uses and potential problems. J Clin Psychiatry 1987; 48:50–55.

82. Herman JB, Rosenbaum JF, Brotman AW. The alprazolam to clonazepam switch for the treatment of panic disorder. J Clin Psychiatry 1987; 7:175–178.

83. Pollack MH, Worthington JJ, Otto MW, Maki KM, Smoller JW, Manfro GG, Rudolph R, Rosenbaum JF. Venlafaxine for panic disorder: results from a double-blind, placebo-controlled study. Psychopharmacol Bull 1996; 32:667–670.

84. DeMartinis NA, Schweizer E, Rickels K. An open-label trial of nefazodone in high comorbidity panic disorder. J Clin Psychiatry 1996; 57: 245–248.

85. Zajecka JM. The effect of nefazodone on comorbid anxiety symptoms associated with depression: experience in family practice and psychiatric outpatient settings. J Clin Psychiatry 1996; 57:10–14.

86. Sheehan DV, Davidson J, Manschreck T, Van Wyck Fleet J. Lack of efficacy of a new antidepressant (bupropion) in the treatment of panic disorder with phobias. J Clin Psychopharmacol 1983; 3:28–31.

87. van Vliet IM, Westenberg HGM, den Boer JA. Effects of the 5-HT$_{1A}$ receptor agonist flesinoxan in panic disorder. Psychopharmacology 1996; 127:174–180.

88. Gastfriend DR, Rosenbaum JF. Adjunctive buspirone in benzodiazepine treatment of four patients with panic disorder. Am J Psychiatry 1989; 146:914–916.

89. Pollack MH, Smoller JS. Pharmacologic approaches to treatment-resistant panic disorder. In: Pollack MH, Otto MW, Rosenbaum JF, eds. Challenges in Clinical Practice: Pharmacologic and Psychosocial Strategies. New York: Guilford Press, 1996:89–112.

90. Liberthson R, Sheehan DV, King ME, Weyman AE. The prevalence of MVP in patients with panic disorders. Am J Psychiatry 1986; 143: 511–515.

91. Uhde TW, Stein MB, Vittone BJ, Siever LF, Boulenger JP, Klein E, Mellman TA. Behavioral and physiologic effects of short-term and long-term administration of clonidine in panic disorder. Arch Gen Psychiatry 1989; 46:170–7.

92. Feder R. Lithium augmentation of clomipramine. J Clin Psychiatry 1988; 49:458.

93. Woodman CL, Noyes R. Panic disorder: treatment with valproate. J Clin Psychiatry 1994; 55:134–136.

94. Keck PE, Taylor VE, Tugrul KC, McElroy SL, Bennett JA. Valproate treatment of panic disorder and lactate-induced panic attacks. Biolog Psychiatry 1993; 33:542–546.

95. Pollack MH, Matthews J, Scott EL. Gabapentin for refractory anxiety [letter]. Am J Psychiatry. In press.

96. Gould RA, Otto MW, Pollack MH. A meta-analysis of treatment outcome for panic disorder. Clin Psychiatr Rev 1995; 15:819–844.

97. Roy-Byrne PP, Cowley DS. Course and outcome in panic disorder: a review of recent follow-up studies. Anxiety 1995; 1:151–160.

98. Katschnig H, Stolk J, Klerman GL. Long-term follow-up of panic disorder. I. Clinical outcome of a large group of patients participating in an international multicenter clinical drug trial. 27th Annual Meeting of the American College of Neuropsychopharmacology, San Juan, PR, 1989.

99. Nagy LM, Krystal JH, Woods SW, Charney DS. Clinical and medication outcome after short-term alprazolam and behavioral group treatment of panic disorder. Arch Gen Psychiatry 1989; 46:141–151.

100. Nagy LM, Krystal JH, Charney DS, Merikangas KR, Woods SW. Long-term outcome of panic disorder after short-term imipramine and

behavioral group treatment: 2.9 year naturalistic follow-up study. J Clin Psychopharmacol 1993; 13:16–24.

101. Pollack MH, Otto MW, Tesar GE, Cohen LS, Meltzer-Brody S, Rosenbaum JF. Long-term outcome after acute treatment with clonazepam and alprazolam for panic disorder. J Clin Psychopharmacol 1993; 13: 257–263.

102. Ball SG, Otto MW, Pollack MH, Rosenbaum JF. Predicting prospective episodes of depression in patients with panic disorder: a longitudinal study. J Consult Clin Psychol 1994; 62:359–365.

103. Breier A, Charney DS, Heninger GR. Major depression in patients with agoraphobia and panic disorder. Arch Gen Psychiatry 1984; 41:1129–1135.

104. Mavissakalian M, Perel JM. Protective effects of imipramine maintenance treatment in panic disorder with agoraphobia. Am J Psychiatry 1992; 149:1053–1057.

105. Noyes R, Garvey M, Cook B, Suelzer M. Controlled discontinuation of benzodiazepine treatment for patients with panic disorder. Am J Psychiatry 1991; 148:517–523.

106. Otto MW, Pollack MH, Sachs GS, Reiter SR, Meltzer-Brody S, Rosenbaum JF. Discontinuation of benzodiazepine treatment: efficacy of cognitive-behavior therapy for patients with panic disorder. Am J Psychiatry 1993; 150:1485–1490.

107. Spiegel DA, Bruce TJ. Benzodiazepines and exposure-based cognitive behavior therapies for panic disorder: conclusions from combined treatment trials. Am J Psychiatry 1997; 154:773–781.

108. Otto MW, Pollack MH, Meltzer-Brody S. Cognitive-behavioral therapy for benzodiazepine discontinuation in panic disorder patients. Psychopharmacol Bull 1993; 28:123–130.

109. Charney DS, Heninger GR, Breier A. Noradrenergic function in panic anxiety: effects of yohimbine in healthy subjects and patients with agoraphobia and panic disorder. Arch Gen Psychiatry 1984; 41:751–763.

110. Charney DS, Heninger GR. Abnormal regulation of noradrenergic function in panic disorders: effects of clonidine in healthy subjects and patients with agoraphobia and panic disorder. Arch Gen Psychiatry 1986; 43:1042–54.

6

Cognitive-Behavioral Therapy for Panic Disorder

Theory, Strategies, and Outcome

Michael W. Otto and Thilo Deckersbach
Massachusetts General Hospital
and Harvard Medical School
Boston, Massachusetts

Over the past decade, cognitive-behavioral treatments for anxiety disorders have become increasingly specialized, a consequence of an improved understanding of individual disorders and the patterns that maintain them. These considerations are especially fitting for panic disorder, in which greater understanding of the core fears associated with this disorder—fears of anxiety sensations and their consequences—has led to well-targeted treatment interventions.

In this chapter, the phenomenology of panic attacks and panic disorder are discussed from a cognitive-behavioral perspective. Treatment interventions follow logically from this model, and the elements of treatment and outcome findings are summarized and discussed in relation to a longitudinal perspective on the disorder.

NONCLINICAL PANIC, PANIC ATTACKS, AND PANIC DISORDER

Panic attacks are not unique to panic disorder and appear to be more common than previously suspected. Virtually all patients with anxiety disorders report occasional panic attacks (1); likewise, panic attacks in the absence of panic disorder occur with some frequency in the general population (2–4), suggesting that factors other than the occurrence of panic alone are involved in the etiology or maintenance of the disorder.

Comparison of panic attacks experienced by nonclinical panickers with those who meet criteria for panic disorder suggest that both groups experience similar symptoms, but patients with panic disorder have greater fears and concern about their symptoms. Specifically, fears of dying, having a heart attack, and losing control, as well as worry about attacks, discriminate clinical and nonclinical panickers (5,6). Also, attacks experienced by infrequent panickers tend to occur during stressful situations such as public speaking, interpersonal conflicts, and before tests and exams (3), rather than the more spontaneous panic episodes experienced in panic disorder.

Experimental research on information processing indicates that patients with panic disorder tend to interpret ambiguous internal stimuli as being harmful, especially bodily sensations having a sudden onset, e.g., a skipped heartbeat (7,8). Panic patients also exhibit an attentional bias favoring the processing of threat cues (9–12) and exhibit enhanced memory for threatening information (13–16; but see but see Pickles and van den Broek [17] and Rapee [18] for nonsignificant findings). Patients with panic disorder also overestimate the frequency and severity of panic attacks in retrospective accounts (19–21). Moreover, when assessed before exposure to feared agoraphobic situations, patients with panic disorder and agoraphobia tend to overestimate the amount of fear and the probability of panic attacks in these situations (22–24). Such overestimation of fear and panic are potent predictors of avoidance of agoraphobic situations (25–27).

During panic attacks, patients typically engage in "safety" behaviors designed to prevent feared catastrophic consequences (28–30). For example, the fear of having a "heart attack" was shown to be associated with sitting down, keeping still, and asking people for help. Fear of losing control mobilized efforts to keep control, including moving more slowly and looking for an escape route. Consequently, when patients were asked why they had never lost control, many replied that they escaped from the situation "just in time" (28). In short, the use of "safety" or "escape" behaviors appeared to prevent exposure to corrective information: that somatic symptoms such as palpitations, dizziness, or chest pain are not signs of loss of control or impending physical or mental harm.

A COGNITIVE-BEHAVIORAL MODEL OF PANIC DISORDER

Cognitive-behavioral models of panic disorder focus on the role of fears of bodily symptoms, catastrophic cognitions, and avoidance behavior in the genesis and maintenance of panic disorder. Initial panic episodes typically emerge at a time of stress (31), and are viewed as the firing of the fight-or-flight alarm reaction. Such alarm reactions, occurring in the absence of external danger, may become the focus of fear themselves, due in part to catastrophic misinterpretations of the meaning of the somatic sensations of panic. These misinterpretation often evoke fears of death ("Am I having a heart attack?" "Am I having a stroke?"), disability ("Am I going to lose control?" "What if it gets worse?" "What if I faint?"), and social embarrassment ("They will think something is wrong with me"). These catastrophic thoughts initiate a positive-feedback loop that increases anxiety and intensifies bodily sensations, resulting in a spiraling of anxiety into panic (see Figure 1).

A memory bias toward remembering panic attacks of greater severity and overestimation about the likelihood of future attacks serve as significant sources of increased worry and anxiety about future panic attacks. Anxious anticipation and increased physiological arousal provide additional internal stimuli, and an attentional bias ensures that these feared bodily sensations will be readily detected. The tendency to catastrophically interpret these sensations increases the likelihood of increased anxiety and a panic attack. After repeated panic attacks,

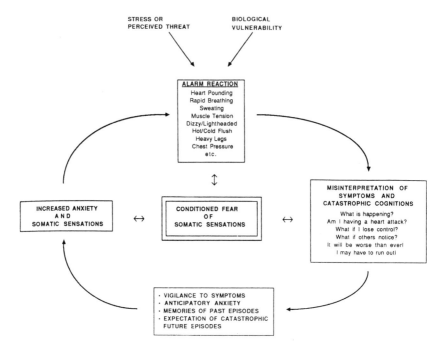

Figure 1 Cognitive-behavioral model of panic disorder. (From Ref. 97.)

phobic responses may become linked directly with somatic sensations of anxiety, such that fearful reactions to somatic sensations may occur without mediation by catastrophic cognitions.

This model of the etiology and maintenance of panic disorder is consistent with data from studies examining the biological provocation of panic attacks in vulnerable individuals. Originally designed as probes to examine panic-related dysfunctions in neurochemical systems, a variety of pharmacological and physiological procedures have been shown to provoke panic attacks in patients with panic disorder but rarely in controls. Procedures such as inhalation of CO_2, infusion of sodium lactate, or hyperventilation share the ability to produce intense bodily sensations that mimic those experienced during panic attacks. According to the cognitive-behavioral model of panic disorder, it is the fear of these provoked symptoms that mediates the emergence of the panic response (32–34). False feedback about an abrupt increased heart rate also appears to increase anxiety and increase physiological arousal in patients with panic disorder but not in control subjects (35).

Manipulations of perceived control and safety cues are also important mediators of anxiogenic responses to provocation procedures. In a 1989 study by Sanderson, Rapee, and Barlow (36), patients who lacked perceived control over the flow of CO_2 reported more catastrophic thoughts and panicked to a higher degree (80%) than those who believed they could exert control (20%). Likewise, panic patients who underwent CO_2 inhalation without being accompanied by a "safe" person showed marked increase in state anxiety and related measures of fear compared to patients who were accompanied by a "safe" person (37). Greater comfort before initiation of provocation also predicts lower intensity of fear and a lower likelihood of panic (38).

Prospective studies have revealed that not all individuals are equally prone to misinterpret bodily sensations as signs of danger, and provide clues about which individuals may be most likely to develop panic disorder after experiencing an initial panic episode. Anxiety sensitivity, defined as the fear of anxiety-related sensations based on beliefs that these sensations have harmful consequences (39,40), is an important concurrent predictor of fearfulness and avoidance in both patients and nonpatients (41–44). Moreover, a number of lines of research suggest that high anxiety sensitivity may identify individuals at risk for panic disorder. Self-reports of panic patients in a study by Fava and associates (45) indicated that worries about bodily feelings and health preceded the first panic attack. Maller and Reiss (46) and Ehlers (47) found that anxiety sensitivity predicted the occurrence of panic attacks in individuals without a history of panic attacks. Further evidence was provided in 1997 by Schmidt, Lerew, and Jackson (48), who examined the emergence of spontaneous panic attacks in a cohort of 1172 cadets at the United Stated Air Force Academy. Anxiety sensitivity emerged as a significant predictor of panic episodes, and remained so when effects of trait anxiety and a history of panic attacks were statistically controlled.

Anxiety sensitivity also predicts the occurrence of panic in biological challenge procedures. Telch and Harrington (49) examined the response to carbon dioxide provocation in college students who had never experienced a panic attack. Subjects with high anxiety sensitivity who experienced unexpected bodily sensations after carbon dioxide inhalation were three times more likely to report a panic attack than subjects informed about the effects of CO_2. Subjects with low anxiety sensitivity were significantly less likely to panic regardless of whether provocation symptoms were expected or unexpected. Likewise, Donnell and McNally (50) found enhanced response to hyperventilation in high-anxiety-sensitivity subjects who did not have a history of panic attacks; subjects low in anxiety sensitivity did not exhibit an anxious response to hyperventilation (50). These studies provide evidence suggesting that anxiety sensitivity, rather than a history of panic attacks, is the critical predictor of future panic attacks.

The similarity between bodily symptoms induced by provocation studies and those experienced during panic attacks also appears to be important in moderating the effects of panic provocation. In a study by Lelliot and Bass (51), only patients who feared cardiovascular and respiratory symptoms during naturally occurring panic attacks responded with increased distress to hyperventilation (51).

TREATMENT CONSIDERATIONS

Given this model of the nature of panic disorder, the challenge of treating panic disorder can be translated into the need to eliminate catastrophic misinterpretations and conditioned fears of body sensations, avoidance, and safety behaviors. To achieve these results, current cognitive-behavioral treatment (CBT) packages commonly include four major components: information about the nature of the disorder, interoceptive and in vivo exposure, cognitive restructuring, and anxiety-management skills. In empirical studies, these interventions are commonly delivered over the course of 12 to 15 sessions (for manuals see Refs 52–54).

CBT for panic disorder is typically initiated with informational interventions that demystify the flood of bodily symptoms experienced during panic attacks and instruct patients about self-perpetuating patterns that maintain the disorder. Emphasis is placed on anxiogenic cognitive and behavioral responses to feared body sensations. Informational interventions can be extended with self-help books (55) or patient manuals that parallel and reinforce protocol-driven treatments (e.g.,

56,57). There is initial evidence that informational interventions combined with supportive treatment alone may have significant treatment effects (58). These interventions, as part of a broader CBT package, also provide the rationale for interventions that follow.

Cognitive restructuring is designed to decatastrophize beliefs about the meaning and the consequences of somatic symptoms and provide patients with corrective information. Using thought records or panic diaries, patients monitor their catastrophic thoughts in panic-provoking situations. Typically, misinterpretations target the meanings of bodily sensations (''This is a heart attack''), distort the degree of catastrophe (''It would be disastrous if I faint''), and/or overestimate the probability of feared outcomes (''I will lose control'') (52). Patients are asked to treat these thoughts as hypotheses, and to evaluate the evidence for or against these and alternative hypotheses. The goal is not to induce falsely positive thinking but to help patients reduce catastrophic interpretations and bring their thoughts in accordance with actual consequences.

Cognitive interventions by themselves have been applied as a treatment (59), but frequently cognitive restructuring interventions are applied in conjunction with exposure interventions. Cognitive-restructuring provides patients with a helpful framework for attempting their initial exposure to feared bodily sensations or feared situations. Exposure itself is perhaps the most central component of CBT of panic disorder. Interoceptive exposure targets fears of somatic sensations of anxiety; situational (in vivo) exposure targets fears of situations in which panic may occur.

Interoceptive exposure is designed to induce bodily sensations that mimic those experienced during panic attacks. For example, running up stairs may be used to produce tachycardia and shortness of breath. Shaking the head from side to side or spinning in a chair produces dizziness and disorientation; breath-holding induces chest tightness and smothering feelings; and hyperventilation frequently induces dizziness, numbness, tingling, and hot flushes (52). During exposure, patients are asked to induce sensations, note what the sensations feel like, and allow the sensations to remain without doing anything to control them (e.g., ''tensing up'' or using safety cues). With repeated exposure to these feared body sensations, patients habituate to the sensations and learn that they do not signal impending harm and need not be feared. In addition, exposure helps solidify cognitive change by providing patients with real-world experiences by which to evaluate their cognitive hypotheses. This latter procedure is formalized in "behavioral experiments." In a behavioral experiment, patients are provided with experience by which to evaluate catastrophic expectations. Patients are first asked to generate hypotheses about the consequences of feared sensations or events (e.g., "If I am in public and feel dizzy, I won't be able to concentrate, people will stare at me, I will get even more dizzy, and then I will faint"). Patients are then provided with the opportunity to examine their hypotheses in a real-world situation (e.g., dizziness may be induced with interoceptive exposure exercises before the patient must interact with others in a store). The patient and therapist then evaluate the actual results of the behavioral test, relative to the catastrophic expectations.

In a number of treatment protocols (54), interoceptive exposure is first rehearsed in therapy sessions (e.g., with hyperventilation), followed by home practice of these procedures. As treatment progresses, interoceptive exposure is then transferred into less "safe" environments (e.g., the patient's office at work). Later in treatment, interoceptive exposure is gradually replaced by natural activities producing critical symptoms (exercise, drinking coffee, etc.). For patients suffering from agoraphobic avoidance, situational (in vivo) exposure is then introduced. Patients are instructed to re-enter avoided situations and, if anxiety sensations are encountered, to react to these initial sensations in a manner similar to their interoceptive exposure practice.

When applying interoceptive and in vivo exposure, clinicians must be aware of subtle avoidance behaviors used by patients to provide themselves with cues for safety (60). For example, patients may brace themselves against the leg of a chair during hyperventilation and may lean against the wall of an elevator during in vivo exposure as an attempt not to "lose control." Completion of exposure in the presence of safety cues or attributing success to the presence of safety cues (e.g., "I would have lost control if I hadn't done that") may prevent exposure to corrective information that such exposure is indeed "safe." Wells and colleagues (61) demonstrated this effect in patients with social phobia who were exposed to feared social situations. Patients allowed to use their usual safety cues reported less benefit from exposure relative to patients encouraged to refrain from their safety cues (61).

The last component of treatment, anxiety-management skills, provide patients with skills for preventing anxiogenic responses to initial anxiety sensations. These skills include diaphragmatic and slow breathing techniques, muscle-relaxation training, and self-instructions (52–54). Relative to other components of CBT, this training might be of less importance and caution should be taken that patients do not utilize these skills to avoid bodily sensations (60).

TREATMENT-OUTCOME FINDINGS

CBT emphasizing informational, exposure, cognitive restructuring, and anxiety-management interventions is associated with some of the strongest treatment-outcome findings in the panic disorder literature, with panic-free rates in the range of 74% to 85% following short-term treatment, and evidence of good maintenance of treatment gains over follow-up periods of 1 to 2 years (62–67).

CBT compares well to pharmacological alternatives. In a recent (1995) meta-analysis, Gould, Otto, and Pollack (68) examined the effect sizes observed in well-controlled trials of cognitive-behavioral interventions and pharmacological treatments (antidepressants and benzodiazepines) published between 1974 and 1994. Both treatment modalities and their combination were effective in the short term, but results were more positive for CBT (see Figure 2). In addition, analysis of follow-up studies revealed that treatment benefits following CBT tended to remained stable, whereas patients treated with medications tended to lose benefits following medication discontinuation (see Figure 3). Moreover, CBT was associated with lower attrition rates (5.6%) than those with pharmacological (19.8%) or combined treatments (22%) (68).

Findings from the meta-analytical review by Gould et al. (68) are consistent with the results of a large, multicenter trial of the relative and combined efficacy of CBT and imipramine. Early reports of the results indicate that CBT offered greater treatment benefit that imipramine. Furthermore, the apparent advantages of adding imipramine to placebo appeared to be accounted for by the nonspecific effects of pill-taking alone (69). However, these studies were largely conducted before the widespread use of selective serotonine-reuptake inhibitors

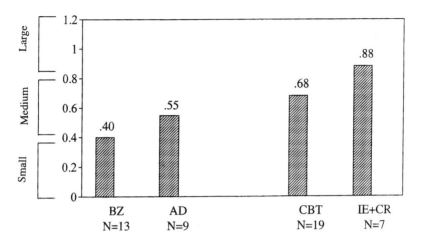

Figure 2 Between-group effect sizes for active treatments compared to waitlist or placebo control groups. BZ = benzodiazepine treatment; AD = antidepressant treatment; CBT = cognitive-behavioral treatment, broadly defined; IE+CR = CBT treatments emphasizing the combination of interoceptive exposure and cognitive-restructuring interventions. Data from a meta-analytic review of 43 studies. (Data from Ref. 68.)

(SSRIs) for panic disorder. Further studies will need to target the relative efficacy of CBT, SSRIs, and their combination.

Attention to panic-free rates in any study design, however, may overestimate the success of the treatment. Patients may achieve periods of freedom from panic attacks, but elevated anxiety sensitivity, anticipatory anxiety, and avoidance may remain and place patients at risk for further panic attacks and relapse. CBT-response rates drop when criteria for high endstate are applied, although the advantage of CBT over pharmacological treatments is preserved in individual studies (64,65). For example, Clark and associates (64) found that 85% of patients who received CBT were panic-free at 15-month follow-up, but only 70% met criteria for a return to normal or near-normal functioning (64). In comparison, only 45% of patients treated with imipramine met criteria for endstate high functioning. Similar, Craske and colleagues (65) reported 81% panic-free patients in the CBT condition at 2-year follow-up, but only 50% additionally fulfilled criteria for high endstate functioning (65). These data suggest that CBT may be offering some

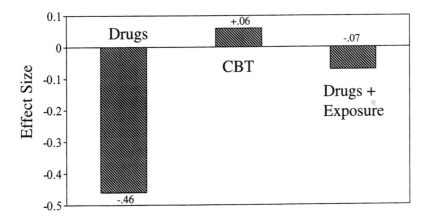

Figure 3 Within-group effect sizes representing the change in treatment efficacy between the end of the acute treatment trial and follow-up assessments. Negative values represent a loss in treatment efficacy. (Data from Ref. 68.)

of the highest outcome findings in the literature, but that additional strategies for success are still required for patients who do not fully respond to short-term treatment (60). For patients who do not respond to exposure therapy alone, it appears that additional exposure homework may offer benefit equal to that of other modalities of treatment (70).

Although the combination of pharmacotherapy and CBT may have some short-term synergistic effects, combination treatments do not appear to be more effective than CBT alone in the long run (71), although these studies have not been completed with SSRIs. Moreover, pharmacotherapy may at times hinder the treatment effects afforded by CBT. It appears that patients receiving combined treatment may be at greater risk for relapse if gains are attributed to medications (68,72). For example, Basoglu and associates (72) found that agoraphobic patients who remitted from their disorder (following a combination of exposure and alprazolam treatment) and attributed gains to medication felt less confident in coping without medication and had greater loss of treatment gains than patients who attributed their gains to their own efforts during treatment. Baseline illness severity, greater age, higher expectations from drug treatment, and alpralozam-related side effects predicted more external attributions but did not independently predict relapse. In addition, Otto, Pollack, and Sabatino (73) found that panic patients who achieved remission with combined CBT and medication (and continued medication—predominantly benzodiazepine—treatment) relapsed sooner than patients who achieved remission with CBT alone. Baseline anxiety severity, chronicity, comorbidity, and avoidance could not account for differences in relapse rates between these treatment groups.

Despite the consistency of findings from both meta-analytical reviews (68,74) and the recent multicenter trial (69), controversy surrounds the apparent success of cognitive-behavioral interventions relative to medications (75–79). Challenges to empirical studies include speculation as to whether patients treated in one modality or another are truly representative of clinic populations, and whether procedures used to ensure high internal validity in studies (e.g., selection of patients with low comorbidity or of those willing to undergo randomization) do not insulate findings from what may be achieved in clinic practice. Otto and colleagues (80) recently addressed some of these issues in a ''services'' research study of the effectiveness of pharmacological and CBT delivered in clinical practice. Pharmacotherapy treatment was not controlled and reflected current practices, and tended to emphasize the application of SSRIs prescribed alone or in combination with high-potency benzodiazepines. CBT was delivered in a program of 12 individual or group sessions. The findings indicated that the symptoms of patients seeking treatment with either modality tended to be of equal severity, and CBT provided patients with benefit at least equal to that provided by pharmacological therapy. In short, this research provided evidence that the experimental treatment literature is accurately representing the relative efficacy of cognitive-behavioral and pharmacological treatments applied in clinical practice. In addition, Otto et al. (80) provided data indicating that CBT is also less costly than pharmacotherapy, especially when longer-term outcome is considered.

PREDICTORS OF RESPONSE AND RELAPSE

In general, predictors of poorer outcome with CBT appear to be the same as those that predict poorer outcome from pharmacotherapy. Although findings are somewhat inconsistent, poorer outcome in CBT has been associated with greater baseline panic and agoraphobic severity, depressed mood, personality psychopathology, and marital dissatisfaction, as well as lower motivation for treatment (81,82). Although greater agoraphobic avoidance is a negative predictor of overall treatment outcome, there is evidence that these patients achieve reductions in severity similar those in less avoidant patients, but remain further from remission at the end of brief treatment (83).

Concerning relapse, a cognitive-behavioral account of panic disorder suggests that reemergence of panic and avoidance would be especially likely when patients continue to fear bodily sensations after treatment. Evidence to support this proposition was provided by Clark et al. (64), who found that posttreatment fears of anxiety sensations predicted outcome at a 15-month follow-up assessment. These fears also predicted relapse at 15-month follow-up in patients who had been panic-free posttreatment, and this association held when the level of catastrophic and agoraphobic cognitions at pretreatment were statistically controlled.

Relapse of patients who have achieved remission during active treatment underscores the importance of including relapse-prevention strategies in current CBT packages. This is particularly important given recent evidence of a waxing and waning course of panic, even in patients who may appear to be panic-free at cross-sectional assessments (84). Also, as noted by Craske and colleagues (65), success of CBT in the treatment of panic attacks should not overshadow the importance of fully treating agoraphobic avoidance to ensure full response. Current CBT packages often include written manuals to provide patients with guidelines on how to continue therapy after active treatment has ended, or offer a limited number of booster sessions (54,64). Ost (85) has shown that such programs aid the maintenance of treatment gains.

APPLICATIONS OF CBT

In addition to the documented efficacy of CBT as an initial strategy for panic disorder, there is also evidence that it can be used to: 1) enhance pharmacological treatment, 2) treat patients who have failed to respond to pharmacotherapy, and 3) aid patients who wish to discontinue pharmacotherapy.

A variety of studies suggest that adding exposure instruction helps extend the treatment gains afforded by medication treatment (71,86–88). In addition, exposure instruction alone was found to be superior to reassurance alone for panic disorder patients presenting to an emergency ward (89). Indeed, if behaviorally trained clinicians are not available in a service area, application of self-help techniques (e.g., self-help books) can be used as an initial strategy, or to extend gains from pharmacotherapy (for a review of the efficacy of self-help strategies, see Gould and Clum [98]).

CBT should also be considered for patients who have failed pharmacological treatment. Pollack and associates (90) examined the role of CBT in patients who were nonresponsive or partially responsive to medication treatment. Short-term CBT was found to offer additional treatment gains, even in the context of medication discontinuation in several patients. In a separate study, Otto and colleagues (80) found that CBT was equally effective for patients who failed to respond to an adequate dose and duration of pharmacotherapy as well as those who failed to respond to lower doses of medication. The latter group of patients—those not treated with adequate levels of medication—appear to be especially common in clinical practice.

CBT has also been found to be effective for patients wishing to discontinue pharmacotherapy for panic disorder. Medication discontinuation is associated with high rates of relapse, in the range of 54% to over 70% (91–93). Discontinuation of benzodiazepine treatment has received particular attention, due not only to high rates of relapse but also to the emergence of discontinuation symptoms that prevent many panic patients from completing a successful medication taper. Short-term CBT, delivered during and after the taper phase, is associated with successful discontinuation and helps patients maintain a medication-free status while controlling symptoms (94–96).

CBT FOR PSYCHOPHARMACOLOGISTS

Several elements of CBT can be easily and routinely added to standard pharmacological care for panic disorder. At treatment outset, patients should be presented with an integrated biopsychosocial model of the disorder. The cognitive-behavioral model discussed earlier not only provides a reasonable rationale for the use of medication (to reduce baseline arousal, the frequency and intensity of panic, and the degree of phobic concern), but it also provides patients with a broad model for understanding the range of phobic concerns inherent in the disorder (including fears of interoceptive symptoms) as well as a ready-made model if the physician or patient elects to pursue more-formal behavior therapy in the future.

Because panic patients are typically anxious during treatment evaluations and initial sessions, and may not fully process spoken material delivered during the session, it is helpful to provide visual as well as auditory information. Figure 1 provides a schematic that can be used as a basis for discussion of panic patterns; likewise, treatment manuals are replete with such materials that can be taken home by patients (52,54,56,57). Moreover, such discussions and materials are especially helpful for preparing patients for the anxiety and catastrophic thoughts that may be experienced during re-entry into avoided situations. As noted, such programmed re-entry, otherwise known as stepwise exposure, has repeatedly been shown to extend treatment gains from pharmacotherapy (71,86–89), and appears to reduce the loss of treatment gains when medication use is discontinued (68). Even if no other element of CBT is integrated into pharmacological care, encouragement of stepwise exposure should be considered an essential element of pharmacotherapy for panic disorder.

Stepwise exposure is initiated with a discussion of the range of situations avoided by the patient, and organization of these situations into a general hierarchy (from least to most feared). Exposure assignments should begin with slight to moderately avoided items, and should always be preceded with a discussion of the patient's concerns about the experience. Patients should be reminded that anticipatory anxiety is a natural part of re-entry into any avoided situation, and encouraged to ''allow'' the natural feelings of arousal during the exposure. These feelings of arousal and anxiety should be differentiated from negative or catastrophic thoughts (detailed earlier in the chapter), and more-adaptive self-talk should be encouraged. Patients should also be encouraged to stay in the avoided situation until anxiety dissipates (e.g., the goal is not to "hurry through" the feared situation). Progress with exposure assignments should be reviewed during subsequent sessions, and, if appropriate, the next item on the hierarchy should be assigned.

Manuals for therapists (52,54) and patients (56,57) are available to aid clinicians in this work. Alternatively, self-help books (e.g., Ref. 55), available at many bookstores, can be assigned and monitored by the clinician to facilitate application of self-help skills in conjunction with medication treatment.

SUMMARY

Cognitive-behavioral therapy for panic disorder appears to be an acceptable and effective treatment that can be offered in an individual or a group format and offers high rates of improvement in acute trials with acceptable longer-term maintenance of treatment gains. Given the success of current treatment packages, additional attention is now being devoted to maximizing longer-term outcome and improving interventions to the patients who do not respond to initial trials. In addition to being a cost-effective first-line treatment for panic disorder, CBT is an excellent strategy for boosting the effects of pharmacological treatment, treating patients who fail to respond fully to pharmacotherapy, and helping patients discontinue their antipanic medication while maintaining clinical benefits.

REFERENCES

1. Barlow DH, Vermilyea J, Blanchard EB, Vermilyea BB, Di Nardo PA, Cerny JA. The phenomenon of panic. J Abnorm Psychol 1985; 94:320–328.
2. Norton GR, Cox BJ, Malan J. Nonclinical panicers: a critical review. Clin Psychol Review 1992; 12:121–139.
3. Norton GR, Dorward J, Cox BJ. Factors associated with panic attacks in nonclinical subjects. Behav Ther 1986:17:239–252.
4. Norton GR, Harrison B, Hauch J, Rhodes L. Characteristics of people with infrequent panic attacks. J Abnorm Psychol 1985; 94:216–221.

5. Telch MJ, Lucas JA, Nelson P. Nonclinical panic in college students: an investigation of prevalence and symptomatology. J Abnorm Psychol 1989; 98:300–306.

6. McNally RJ, Hornig CD, Donnell CD. Clinical cersus nonclinical panic: a test of suffocation false alarm theory. Behav Res Ther 1995; 33:127–131.

7. Harvey JM, Richards JC, Dziadosz T, Swindell A. Misinterpretation of ambiguous stimuli in panic disorder. Cogn Ther Res 1993; 17:235–248.

8. McNally RJ, Foa EB. Cognition and agoraphobia: bias in the interpretation of threat. Cogn Ther Res 1987; 11:567–581.

9. Asmundson GJG, Sandler LS, Wilson KG, Walker JR. Selective attention towards physical threat in patients with panic disorder. J Anxiety Disord 1992; 6:295–303.

10. Burgess IS, Jones LM, Robertson SA, Radcliffe WN, Emerson E. The degree of control exerted by phobic and non-phobic verbal stimuli over recognition behavior of phobic and non-phobic subjects. Behav Res Ther 1981; 19:233–243.

11. Ehlers A, Margraf J, Davies SO, Roth WT. Selective processing of threat cues in subjects with panic attacks. Cognition Emotion 1988; 2:201–219.

12. McNally RJ, Riemann BC, Kim E. Selective processing of threat cues in panic disorder. Behav Res Ther 1990; 28:407–412.

13. Becker E, Rink M, Margraf J. Memory bias in panic disorder. J Abnorm Psychol 1994; 103:396–399.

14. Cloitre M, Liebowitz MR. Memory bias in panic disorder: an investigation of the cognitive avoidance hypothesis. Cogn Ther Res 1991; 15: 371–386.

15. Becker E, Rink M, Margraf J. Memory bias in panic disorder. J Abnorm Psychol 1994; 103:396–399.

16. McNally RJ, Foa EB, Donnel CD. Memory bias for anxiety information in patients with panic disorder. Cognition Emotion 1989; 3:27–44.

17. Pickles AJ, van den Broek MD. Failure to replicate evidence for phobic schemata in agoraphobic patients. Br J Clin Psychol 1988; 27:271–272.

18. Rapee RM. Failure to replicate a memory bias in panic disorder. J Anxiety Disord 1994; 8:291–300.

19. Margraf J, Taylor B, Ehlers A, Roth WT, Agras WS. Panic attacks in the natural environment. J Nerv Mental Dis 1987; 175:558–565.

20. Rapee RM, Craske MG, Barlow DH. Subject-described features of panic attacks using self-monitoring. J Anxiety Disord 1990; 4:171–181.

21. De Beurs E, Lange A, Van Dyck R. Self-monitoring of panic attacks and retrospective estimates of panic: discordant findings. Behav Res Ther 1992; 30:411–413.
22. Rachman S, Lopatka C, Levitt K. Experimental analysis of panic. II. Panic patients. Behav Res Ther 1988; 26:33–40.
23. Schmidt NB, Jacquin K, Telch MJ. The overprediction of fear and panic in panic disorder. Behav Res Ther 1994; 32:701–707.
24. van Hout WJPJ, Emmelkamp PMG. Overprediction of fear in panic disorder with agoraphobia: does the (mis)match model generalize to exposure in vivo therapy? Behav Res Ther 1994; 32:723–734.
25. Craske MG, Rapee RM, Barlow DH. The significance of panic expectancy for individual patterns of avoidance. Behav Therapist 1988; 19: 577–592.
26. Rachman S, Lopatka C. Match and mismatch in the prediction of fear. Behav Res Ther 1986; 24:387–393.
27. Telch MJ, Brouillard M, Telch CF, Agras WS, Taylor CB. Role of cognitive appraisal in panic-related avoidance. Behav Res Ther 1989; 27:373–383.
28. Salkovskis PM, Clark DM, Gelder MG. Cognitive-behavior links in the persistence of panic. Behav Res Ther 1996; 34:453–458.
29. Salkovskis PM. The importance of behavior in the maintenance of anxiety and panic: a cognitive account. Behavioural Psychother 1991; 19: 6–19.
30. Salkovskis PM. Avoidance behavior is motivated by threat beliefs: a possible resolution of the cognitive-behaviour debate. In: Salkovskis PM, ed. Key Trends in Cognitive-Behavior Therapy. New York: Wiley, 1996.
31. Manfro GG, Otto MW, McArdle ET, Worthington JJ, Rosenbaum JF, Pollack MH. Relationship of antecedent stressful life events to childhood and family history of anxiety and the course of panic disorder. J Affect Disord 1996; 41:135–139.
32. Rapee R, Mattick R, Murell E. Cognitive mediation in the affective component of spontaneous panic attacks. J Behav Ther Experimental Psychiatry 1986; 17:245–253.
33. Whittal ML, Goetsch VL. Physiological, subjective and behavioral responses to hyperventilation in clinical and infrequent panic. Behav Res Ther 1995; 33:415–422.
34. Yeragani V, Balon R, Pohl R. Lactate infusions in panic disorder patients and normal controls: autonomic measures and subjective anxiety. Acta Psychiatrica Scandinavica 1989; 79:32–40.

35. Ehlers A, Margraf J, Roth WT, Taylor CB, Birbaumer N. Anxiety induced by false heart rate feedback in patients with panic disorder. Behav Res Ther 1988; 26:1–11.
36. Sanderson WC, Rapee RM, Barlow DH. The influence of percieved control on panic attacks induced via inhalation of 5.5% CO_2 enriched air. Arch Gen Psychiatry 1989; 46:157–162.
37. Carter MM, Hollon SD, Carson, R, Shelton RC. Effects of a safe person on induces distress following a biological challenge in panic disorder with agoraphobia. J Abnorm Psychol 1995; 104:156–163.
38. Rapee RM, Telfer LA, Barlow DH. The role of safety cues in mediating the response to inhalations of CO_2 in agoraphobics. Behav Res Ther 1991; 24:1–8.
39. Reiss S. The expectancy model of fear, anxiety, and panic. Clin Psychol Review 1991; 11:141–153.
40. Reiss S, McNally RJ. The expectancy model of fear. In: Reiss S, Bootzin RR, eds. Theoretical Issues in Behavior Therapy. New York: Academic Press, 1985:107–121.
41. McNally RJ, Lorenz M. Anxiety sensitivity in agoraphobics. J Behav Ther Experimental Psychiatry 1987:18:3–11.
42. Otto MW, Pollack MH, Rosenbaum JF, Sachs GS, Asher RH. Childhood history of anxiety in adults with panic disorder: association with anxiety sensitivity and avoidance. Harvard Rev Psychiatry 1994; 1:288–293.
43. Reiss S, Peterson RA, Gursky DM, McNally RJ. Anxiety sensitivity, anxiety frequency and the prediction of fearfulness. Behav Res Ther 1986; 24:1–8.
44. Taylor S, Rachman S. Fear and avoidance of aversive affective states: dimensions and causal relations. J Anxiety Disord 1992; 3:25–32.
45. Fava GA, Grandi S, Rafenelli C, Canestrari R. Prodromal symptoms in panic disorder with agoraphobia: a replication study. J Affect Disord 1992; 85:85–88.
46. Maller RG, Reiss S. Anxiety sensitivity in 1984 and panic attacks in 1987. J Anxiety Disord 1992; 6:241–247.
47. Ehlers A. A 1-year prospective study of panic attacks: clinical course and factors associated with maintenance. J Abnorm Psychol 1995; 104:164–172.
48. Schmidt NB, Lerew DR, Jackson RJ. The role of anxiety sensitivity in the pathogenesis of panic: prospective evaluation of spontaneous panic attacks during acute stress. J Abnorm Psychol 1997; 106:355–364.
49. Telch MJ, Harrington PJ. Anxiety sensitivity and expectedness of

arousal mediating affective response to 35% carbon dioxide inhalation. Poster presented at the Annual Meeting of the Association for the Advancement of Behavior Therapy, Boston, Nov 1992.

50. Donnell CD, McNally RJ. Anxiety sensitivity and history of panic attacks as predictors of response to hyperventilation. Behav Res Ther 1989; 27:325–332.

51. Lelliot P, Bass C. Symptom specificy in patients with panics. Br J Psychiatry 1990; 157:593–597.

52. Craske MG, Meadows E, Barlow DH. Mastery of Your Anxiety and Panic and Agoraphobia Supplement (Therapist Guide). 2nd ed. San Antonio, TX: Psychological Corporation, 1994.

53. Margraf J, Schneider S. Panik: Angstanfaelle und ihre Behandlung. Berlin: Springer, 1990.

54. Otto MW, Jones JC, Craske MG, Barlow DH. Stopping Anxiety Medication: Panic Control Ther apy for Benzodiazepine Discontinuation (Therapist Guide). San Antonio, TX: Psychological Corporation, 1996.

55. Clum GA. Coping with panic: a drug-free approach to dealing with anxiety attacks. Pacific Grove: Brooks/Cole, 1990.

56. Barlow DH, Craske MG. Mastery of Your Anxiety and Panic (Client Workbook). 2nd ed. San Antonio, TX: Psychological Corporation, 1994.

57. Otto MW, Pollack MH, Barlow DH. Stopping Anxiety Medication: A Workbook for Patients Wanting to Discontinue Benzodiazepine Treatment for Panic Disorder. San Antonio, TX: Psychological Corporation, 1995.

58. Shear KS, Pilkonis PA, Cloitre M, Leon AC. Cognitive-behavioral treatment compared with nonprescriptive treatment of panic disorder. Arch Gen Psychiatry 1994; 51:395–401.

59. Margraf J, Barlow DH, Clark DM, Telch MJ. Psychological treatment of panic: work in progress on outcome, active ingredients and follow-up. Behav Res Ther 1993; 31:1–8.

60. Otto MW, Gould RA. Maximizing treatment-outcome for panic disorder: cognitive-behavioral strategies. In: Pollack MH, Otto MW, Rosenbaum JF, eds. Challenges in Clinical Practice: Pharmacologic and Psychosocial Strategies. New York: Guilford Press, 1996:113–140.

61. Wells A, Clark DM, Salkowskis, PM, Ludgate J, Hackmann A, Gelder M. Social phobia: the role of in-situation safety behaviors in maintaining anxiety and negative beliefs. Behav Ther 1995; 26:153–161.

62. Barlow DH, Craske MG, Cerny JA, Klosko JS. Behavioral treatment of panic disorder. Behav Ther 1989; 20:261–282.

63. Beck AT, Sokol L, Clark DM, Berchick R, Wright F. A crossover study of focused cognitive therapy for panic disorder. Am J Psychiatry 1992; 149:778–789.
64. Clark DM, Salkovskis PM, Hackmann A, Middleton H, Anastasiades P, Gelder M. A comparison of cognitive therapy, applied relaxation and imipramine in the treatment of panic disorder. Br J Psychiatry 1994; 164:759–769.
65. Craske MG, Brown TA, Barlow DH. Behavioral treatment for panic disorder: a two-year follow up. Behav Ther 1991; 22:289–304.
66. Margraf J, Barlow DH, Clark DM, Telch MJ. Psychological treatment of panic: work in progress on outcome, active ingredients and follow-up. Behav Res Ther 1993; 31:1–8.
67. Telch MJ, Lucas JA, Schmidt NB, Hanna HH, LaNae Jaimez T, Lucas RA. Group cognitive-behavioral treatment of panic disorder. Behav Res Ther 1993; 31:279–287.
68. Gould R, Otto MW, Pollack MH. A meta-analysis of treatment outcome for panic disorder. Clin Psychol Rev 1995; 15:819–844.
69. Barlow DH, Gorman JM, Shear MK, et al. Results from the multi-center comparative treatment study of panic disorder: acute and maintenance outcome. Presentation at the 1997 British Association of Behavioural and Cognitive Psychotherapy in Canterbury, England, July 8–12, 1997.
70. Fava GA, Savron G, Zielezny M, Grandi S, Rafanelli C, Conti S. Overcoming resistance to exposure in panic disorder with agoraphobia. Acta Psychiatrica Scandinavica 1997; 95:306–312.
71. Telch MJ, Lucas RA. Combined pharmacological and psychological treatment of panic disorder: current status and future directions. In: Wolfe BE, Maser JD, eds. Treatment of Panic Disorder. Washington, DC: American Psychiatric Association Press, 1994.
72. Basoglu M, Marks IM, Kilic C, Brewin, CR, Swinson RP. Alpralozam and exposure for panic disorder with agoraphobia: attribution of improvement to medication predicts subsequent relapse. Br J Psychiatry 1994; 164:652–659.
73. Otto MW, Pollack MH, Sabatino SA. Maintenance of remission following cognitive-behavior therapy for panic disorder: possible deleterious effects of concurrent medication treatment. Behav Ther 1996; 27:473–482.
74. Clum GA, Clum GA, Surls R. A meta-analysis of treatments for panic disorder. J Consulting Clin Psychol 1993; 61:317–326.
75. Klein DF. Discussion of "methodological controversies in the treatment of panic disorder." Behav Res Ther 1996:34:849–853.

76. Klein DF. Preventing hung juries about therapy studies. J Consulting Clin Psychol 1996:64:81–87.
77. McNally RJ. Methodological controversies in the treatment of panic disorder. J Consulting Clin Psychol 1996:64:88–91.
78. McNally RJ. More controversies about panic disorder: a reply to Klein. Behav Res Ther 1996; 34(11/12):855–858.
79. Otto MW, Pollack MH. Treatment strategies for panic disorder: a debate. Harvard Rev Psychiatry 1994; 2:166–170.
80. Otto MW, Pollack, MH, Maki KM, Penava SJ. Delivering empirically-supported treatments for panic disorder: issues, costs, and benefits. In review.
81. Keijsers GPJ, Hoogduin CAL, Schaap CPDR. Prognostic factors in the behavioral treatment of panic disorder with and without agoraphobia. Behav Ther 1994; 25:689–708.
82. Chambless DL, Gracely EJ. Prediction of outcome following in vivo exposure treatment of agoraphobia. In: Hand I, Wittchen HU, eds. Panic and Phobias 2: Treatment and Variables Affecting Outcome. New York: Springer, 1988:209–220.
83. Jansson L, Ost L-G, Jeramalm A. Prognostic factors in the treatment of agoraphobia. Behav Psychother 1987; 15:31–44.
84. Brown TA, Barlow DH. Long-term outcome in cognitive-behavioral treatment of panic disorder: clinical predictors and alternative strategies for assessment. J Consulting Clin Psychol 1995; 63:754–765.
85. Ost L-G. A maintenance program for behavioral treatment of anxiety disorders. Behav Res Ther 1989; 27:123–139.
86. Mavissakalian M. Sequential combination of imipramine and self-directed exposure in the treatment of panic disorder with agoraphobia. J Clin Psychiatry 1990; 51:184–188.
87. Mavissakalian M, Michelson L. Agoraphobia: relative and combined effectiveness of therapist-assisted in vivo exposure and imipramine. J Clin Psychiatry 1986; 47:117–122.
88. Telch MJ, Agras WS, Taylor CB, Roth WT, Gallen C. Combined pharmacological and behavioral treatment for agoraphobia. Behav Res Ther 1985; 23:325–335.
89. Swinson RP, Soulios C, Cox BJ, Kuch K. Brief treatment of emergency room patients with panic attacks. Am J Psychiatry 1992; 149:944–946.
90. Pollack MH, Otto MW, Kaspi SP, Hammerness PG, Rosenbaum JF. Cognitive-behavior therapy for treatment-refractory panic disorder. J Clin Psychiatry 1994; 55:200–205.
91. Mavissakalian M, Perel JM. Clinical experiments in maintenance and

discontinuation of imipramine therapy in panic disorder with agoraphobia. Arch Gen Psychiatry 1992; 49:318–323.

92. Noyes R, Garvey MJ, Cook BL, Samuelson L. Problems with tricyclic antidepressant use in patients with panic disorder or agoraphobia: results of a naturalistic follow-up study. J Clin Psychiatry 1989; 50:163–169.

93. Noyes R, Garvey MJ, Cook B, Suelzer M. Controlled discontinuation of benzodiazepine treatment for patients with panic disorder. Am J Psychiatry 1991; 148:517–523.

94. Hegel MT, Ravaris CL, Ahles TA. Combined cognitive-behavioral and time-limited alprazolam treatment of panic disorder. Behav Ther 1994; 25:183–195.

95. Otto MW, Pollack MH, Sachs GS, Reiter SR, Meltzer-Brody S, Rosenbaum JF. Discontinuation of benzodiazepine treatment: efficacy of cognitive-behavior therapy for patients with panic disorder. Am J Psychiatry 1993; 150:1485–1490.

96. Spiegel DA, Bruce TJ, Gregg SF, Nuzzarello A. Does cognitive behavior therapy assist slow-taper alprazolam discontinuation in panic disorder? Am J Psychiatry 1994; 151:876–881.

97. Otto MW, Pollack MH, Meltzer-Brody S, Rosenbaum JF. Cognitive-behavioral therapy for benzodiazepine discontinuation in panic disorder patients. Psychopharmacol Bull 1992; 28:123–130.

98. Gould RA, Clum GA. A meta-analysis of self-help treatment approaches. Clin Psycholog Rev 1993; 13:169–186.

7

Clinical Approach to Treatment-Resistant Panic Disorder

Peter Roy-Byrne
University of Washington School of Medicine
and Harborview Medical Center
Seattle, Washington

Deborah S. Cowley
University of Washington School of Medicine
and University of Washington Medical Center
Seattle, Washington

INTRODUCTION

The label "treatment-resistant" is customarily applied to patients who have seen a psychiatrist or other clinician for a period of time, received either a pharmacological or a psychological intervention, and failed to improve. As we emphasize in this chapter, this label is a misnomer. Many patients labeled "treatment-resistant" have actually not received an adequate treatment trial, due to either administration of the wrong treatment, administration of the right treatment in the wrong way, or failure of the patient to tolerate or otherwise comply with the recommended treatment intervention for an adequate period of time. Only if the patient has actually received an adequate treatment trial can the term "treatment resistance" be used. Hence, for the duration of this chapter, we use the term ''treatment-refractory'' to refer to patients who have failed to respond to clinical intervention.

Until quite recently, most of the literature on treatment resistance in nonpsychotic outpatients has focused on major depression. Only recently have there been discussions and reviews of treatment resistance as it applies to panic disorder (1–3). Few, if any, published studies have systematically examined the reasons for treatment nonresponse in this patient population. In this chapter, we review published data that bear on the various reasons for treatment nonresponse. We also report data we have collected on this subject. While of some interest, the retrospective nature of these data limits their generalizability and suggests that prospective studies documenting treatment nonresponse and its causes in panic disorder patients are clearly needed.

DEFINITION AND PREVALENCE

A panic disorder patient can be defined as treatment-refractory if he or she has failed to attain at least a partial response to a known effective antipanic treatment. In the depression literature, a partial response is frequently defined as a 50% improvement (i.e., 50% reduction in symptoms of depression). The case of panic, however, is more complicated than depression because the panic syndrome consists not only of symptoms of anxiety that might be measured, for example, with a Hamilton anxiety scale, but also frequency and intensity of panic attacks and severity of panic attack consequences such as phobic avoidance and hypochondriacal concerns (4). In addition, as with all syndromes, there is an increasing emphasis on degree of work-related and personal-relationship-related disability as well as effects on life satisfaction and quality of life (4).

A number of panic treatment studies have attempted to develop a combined treatment outcome measure that would consider several of these response dimensions. One frequently used measure, particularly in the behavioral literature, is the so-called ''high endstate'' (5), which is usually defined as the absence of panic attacks and reduction in both anxiety and phobic avoidance to minimal levels. A more recently developed scale has attempted to rate a number of these dimensions with the same Likert-like ordinal scale, producing a summary score so that a given cutoff score could more conveniently be used to indicate a high endstate (6).

Despite the above considerations, the majority of published treatment studies use a variety of different response measures and frequently focus on panic attack frequency and phobic avoidance severity as their main measures. In acute (i.e., 8- to 12-week) pharmacotherapy studies, all of which are double-blind and placebo-controlled, approximately 30% of panic patients fail to attain partial response, although the exact figure can vary from study to study (7–9). The majority of longer-term (more than 1 year) studies that provide meaningful data are uncontrolled and naturalistic but suggest that about 20% of patients fail to attain at least partial response in the long run (10,11). It is quite likely that both these figures are underestimates since patients participating in controlled and even naturalistic treatment studies are frequently without significant axis I comorbidity (i.e., co-occurring depression, other phobic disorder, or substance abuse) because of the selection and entry criteria of such studies, and without significant axis II personality pathology because such patients are unlikely to volunteer for research studies or, if they volunteer, are much less likely to stay in the study long-term. In fact, one brief report (12) indicated that certain personality traits such as novelty seeking and impulsivity are associated with premature termination from clinical trials.

DETERMINANTS OF TREATMENT-REFRACTORY PANIC

Because this chapter focuses on approaches to the treatment-refractory panic patient, we assume that an accurate diagnosis has been made and that the patient is indeed suffering from primary panic disorder. This fact should not, however, be taken for granted by any clinician faced with a treatment-refractory patient. There are multiple medical causes of panic that, although they account for an extremely small proportion of panic disorder presentations, are nonetheless vital to identify. Most common is panic secondary to the effect of ingested or other abused substances. While the link may be quite clear when the substance use is obvious, patients may minimize or deliberately obscure evidence of their use in their report to the clinician. These factors, which can also be present as complicating rather than exclusively causal factors, are discussed in more detail later in the chapter. Of other medical conditions, hyperthyroidism and complex partial seizure disorder are two of the more likely candidates that need to be ruled out. The more exotic medical causes of panic such as pheochromocytoma, other endocrinopathy, hypoglycemia, or cardiopulmonary disease—especially pulmonary embolism in young, apparently medically healthy women—also should be considered.

Once the diagnosis can be established with confidence, there are three major reasons for treatment failure in panic disorder patients: inadequate treatment, patient intolerance of treatment, and true treatment resistance, in which the patient fails to respond to adequately administered treatment. We discuss each of these areas in some detail, reviewing critical contributing factors and providing a reasonable clinical approach for each area.

Treatment Adequacy

Four studies (13–16) have examined the proportion of patients with panic disorder in different settings who were prescribed adequate pharmacotherapy. These studies have all focused on patients treated in the 1980s, prior to the introduction of most of the selective serotonin-reuptake inhibitors (SSRIs). Only two of the studies (13,14) also provided information on adequate psychological treatment (i.e., cognitive-behavioral treatment). The proportion of patients receiving adequate pharmacological treatment in these studies ranged from 10 to 45%. The lowest figures (10 and 15%) occurred in two studies (13,14) in which the patients were probably not in a treatment relationship (one sample was recruited by advertisement from the community for a treatment study and the other sample comprised individuals presenting to an emergency room for evaluation of panic attacks). In our recent analysis of 106 panic disorder patients (16), only 43 (41%) received an adequate medication trial, a figure surprisingly close to the 45% figure reported in the most recent report by Yonkers et al. (15). It should be emphasized that both of these studies involved a highly selected group of panic patients who had already seen a number of clinicians and had been in treatment for a period of time with different psychiatrists. Given this fact, it is striking and surprising that over half these patients had not received an adequate treatment trial with medication, despite contact with multiple clinicians. The only comparable figures that we have for behavioral treatment are from the first two studies (13,14), in which only 15% and 11% of individuals had received any behavioral treatment. In a more recently published study (17) that did not focus on panic disorder per se but, rather, examined all the anxiety disorders, a considerably higher incidence of patients had received some kind of cognitive-behavioral or behavior therapy (67%).

It should be noted that in our study (16) we inquired about treatment responsivity in patients even if they had had an inadequate trial, and were surprised to learn that about 60% of patients who had reported inadequate treatment, in either type or dosage, nonetheless described some positive response to this treatment. Although this does not suggest that inadequate treatment is an infrequent problem, it does suggest that it may not invariably be associated with poor response. Nonspecific factors, including the "placebo response," may contribute to a positive response to inadequate treatment.

Ensuring an adequate treatment trial for panic disorder involves consideration of a number of factors. For pharmacotherapy, it is necessary to use the correct type of medication (i.e., one known to be effective), and to administer it in a sufficient dose for a sufficient period of time. Effective antipanic medications include high-potency benzodiazepines, tricyclic antidepressants, SSRIs, and monoamine oxidase inhibitors (MAOIs) (18). In addition, venlafaxine has recently been shown to be effective (19), and emerging evidence suggests that nefazodone may also be effective (20). Bupropion (21), beta-blockers (22), buspirone (23), and carbamazepine (24) were no better than placebo in controlled trials. Trazodone is also known to have variable efficacy (25). Sodium valproate may be effective but has not been tested in a placebo-controlled trial.

Although it is customary to start with low doses in panic patients, a common error is failure to gradually increase the dose until a standard effective level is reached. Because a transient partial response is often evident in the first few weeks, clinicians not providing ongoing monitoring of symptom intensity or panic frequency may overlook the need for further upward dose increments. Patients, often relieved to finally experience some symptomatic improvement, may be reticent to push for more comprehensive efficacy. Although patients may sometimes experience significant relief at lower doses, the effective doses for panic disorder, according to available studies, are generally in the range of 2.0 to 2.5 mg/kg of imipramine or comparable tricyclic (26); at least 2 mg of alprazolam or its equivalent (27); and at least "antidepressant" doses of SSRIs, although studies indicate that a higher than antidepressant dose (40 mg/day) of paroxetine may be required for optimal antipanic efficacy (28).

Knowledge of the time course of response is also important, as it allows the clinician to convey to the patient the expected course of events during treatment. Although some response is usually evident within several weeks (and within 1 week of initiating benzodiazepine therapy) (8), available data suggest that approximately 10% of patients with panic attacks receiving antidepressants may not respond until sometime between the 8th and 12th weeks (9,29). However, even in these patients, some sign of response is usually seen by 5–6 weeks. While no response in a patient by 6 weeks suggests the need for consideration of additional therapeutic intervention, it is still important to continue treatment for another 4–6 weeks, if some, even minimal, response is seen by week 6.

Determining what constitutes an adequate psychotherapy trial for panic disorder is complicated. The two existing standard cognitive-behavioral treatment packages, developed by Barlow and Craske in New York (30) and David Clark in Oxford, England (31), have demonstrated antipanic efficacy in controlled trials. A more interpersonal and psychodynamically oriented treatment with a strong behavioral focus known as emotion-focused psychotherapy has also recently been shown to have some antipanic efficacy (32). Currently, trials are underway to examine the efficacy of more pure forms of both brief dynamic (33) and interpersonal psychotherapies for panic disorder, and these may prove effective as well.

Despite this emerging database demonstrating the efficacy of structured psychotherapies for panic disorder, studies suggest that the most commonly prescribed psychotherapy for anxiety continues to be an open-ended, supportive psychodynamic treatment without clear-cut focus on panic-related symptoms (17). This approach to treatment should probably not be used to the exclusion of other, more empirically supported approaches.

The ability of a patient to obtain effective psychotherapeutic treatment for panic depends on the availability of trained clinicians who possess the knowledge and ability to deliver these treatments, as well as the availability of funds to cover them. Even if both of these are available, the matching of personal patient and therapist characteristics crucial for a "therapeutic alliance" is also vitally important, as problems with treatment alliance have contributed to poor psychotherapy outcomes in multiple studies. Hence, there are probably more logistical obstacles to psychotherapeutic treatment of panic than there are to pharmacotherapy. Although many psychopharmacologists continue to believe that psychotherapeutic treatments for panic are likely to be most effective for individuals with mild to moderate forms of illness, there is no evidence to support this belief. However, if this were true, delays in referring panic patients for psychotherapy might be problematic, since the severity of the patient's syndrome may evolve over time in the absence of treatment, making it more refractory.

Treatment Intolerance

Panic disorder patients are more sensitive to medication side effects and tolerate them less well than do individuals with other diagnoses. A major unresolved issue is the degree to which this intolerance is cognitive or psychologically mediated, as opposed to representing a particular physiological sensitivity to medication. One study (34) sheds some light on this issue, although it does not resolve it. In this study, three diagnostic patient groups—panic disorder, generalized anxiety disorder (GAD), and major depression—participating in double-blind, placebo-controlled phase 2 and 3 clinical medication trials were studied. All these trials included a 1-week single-blind "placebo run-in," during which time the patient received placebo pills daily. All patients were rated before and after this week of placebo administration. These data were carefully examined to determine what proportion of patients in each diagnostic group improved in their symptoms over the course of 1 week of placebo, and what proportion worsened. While only 3% of depressed patients had a symptomatic worsening of their condition, 8% of panic patients deteriorated, with GAD patients occupying an intermediate rate of 5%. However, more striking was the observation that while twice as many patients with depression and an equal number of GAD patients improved as worsened, only one-half as many patients with panic experienced improvement instead of worsening. Hence, panic patients showed a disproportionately greater tendency to have an aggravation as opposed to an improvement in their symptoms while taking a "medication" that was actually inert. This suggests a role for some psychological factor, perhaps an exaggerated concern about medication's effect on the body or attribution of other bodily sensations to medication, in mediating the experience of adverse effects with pharmacotherapy in panic patients.

Despite this study, it is certain that nonpsychological factors also contribute to medication intolerance since only 8% of panic patients in this particular cohort worsened, whereas overstimulation and jitteriness occur early in the course of antidepressant treatment in some 20–30% of panic patients (35). Although this rate of "jitteriness" has in the past been observed mostly in tricyclic antidepressant studies, it occurs even with SSRIs; over 50% of patients in early open studies with fluoxetine stopped their medication because of jitteriness when administered a 20-mg dose (36)—although the use of lower (5-mg) doses reduced this figure several-fold. Jitteriness and intolerance are not the only kinds of adverse side effects that panic patients may experience. Any side effect (e.g., anticholinergic side effects) can interact with a panic patient's apprehension about bodily sensations and create spiraling anxiety.

In the same way that medication side effects can be aggravated by cognitive factors, the role of certain anxiogenic health habits is also important to consider (37). These include the use of caffeinated beverages, which clearly exacerbate panic anxiety; exposure to even small amounts of alcohol, which produces anxiety as the effect wears off; and relative deprivation of sleep. These factors may contribute to medication intolerance, even if they do not appear to aggravate the patient's clinical condition in the absence of medication.

Finally, in our cohort of 106 patients (16), the best predictors of medication intolerance were higher levels of baseline anxiety and lack of a substance abuse history. While the first finding is readily understandable, the second is less intuitive. One interpretation of this finding is that patients intolerant to medication are less likely to initially abuse substances because of either apprehension about their effects or brief prior adverse experiences.

A number of approaches to reduce medication intolerance may be useful to consider. Careful initial education and preparation of the patient are critical. The explanatory model for panic disorder one uses is crucial; a model that emphasizes a brain that is dysregulated, i.e., homeostatically "out of balance," is more likely to be effective and empowering to a patient than a model that emphasizes a brain that is defective or deficient. This latter model may exacerbate a patient's feeling of being out of control and aggravate medication sensitivity. The out-of-balance model can also be used to show patients that medication initiates a gradual, corrective process that takes some time to fully develop and that may involve some initial discomfort. Prior to the prescription of medication, it is also vital to determine the patient's past experience with medications. This may not necessarily involve his or her own personal exposure, but rather that of a loved one or family member who has had an untoward experience with medication. Finally, the time course of response must be carefully described so that the patient knows not to anticipate a "cure" in a short period of time, but rather to expect a slow, gradual improvement in symptoms over a longer period of time, which may plateau at some point without total symptom resolution or cure.

It is worthwhile to prepare patients for their medication trial by obtaining 1 week's worth of daily ratings of anxiety symptoms, including physical symptoms that usually accompany their anxiety. This will generally reveal that some days are accompanied by more severe symptoms than others. Demonstration of this natural waxing and waning of symptoms from day to day will prevent patients from attributing random symptom exacerbation following medication initiation to an adverse medication effect. It is also suggested that close contact by telephone be maintained with patients, talking to them once or twice a week for at least the first few weeks of medication initiation. This helps build and sustain an alliance, gives patients an opportunity to have any question answered, no matter how small, and reinforces their motivation for treatment.

It is important to emphasize that benzodiazepines (BDZs) are far more tolerable than the older tricyclic antidepressants, as shown by short-term treatment studies in which there is greater subject retention overall with BDZs. In our clinic population of 106 panic patients (16), 50% of individuals demonstrated intolerance to antidepressants at at least some point in the course of their illness, whereas only 7% had a similar intolerance to BZDs. Dropout rates from both acute short-term and longer-term treatment studies with SSRIs (9,28) appear to be lower than with tricyclics (7,8) and somewhat comparable to those seen with BZDs (7,8), although the study populations and studies were quite different. This suggests that use of SSRIs may reduce the high rate of medication intolerance experienced by antidepressant-treated patients with panic disorder. Although it is the clinical impression of some investigators that the more sedating quality of paroxetine compared to other SSRIs results in less overstimulation, there are no controlled data that address this issue.

The possible utility of cognitive-behavioral techniques for improving patient tolerance to medication has not been systematically explored but is nonetheless of clinical interest. Several studies have clearly demonstrated that cognitive-behavioral techniques are effective in helping patients overcome the aversive physical symptoms that accompany tapering and discontinuation of BZDs (38,39). If such techniques are useful in getting patients off medication, why would they not be similarly effective in helping patients get on medication? Techniques that all physicians should use when starting pharmacotherapy for panic disorder are the initiation of low doses with very slow titration and the continuous reframing of side effects to reduce catastrophization and other cognitive distortions about the meaning of those effects. The clinician should try to redefine or reinterpret side effects in a manner that increases the patient's self-control. Interestingly, one trial of paroxetine (28) that also included simultaneous cognitive therapy had an extraordinarily low dropout rate, with 92% of patients completing the study. This suggests that cognitive techniques may be helpful in maintaining medication tolerance and adherence.

Treatment Resistance

Assuming that the diagnosis of panic disorder is accurate, that adequate treatment has been administered, and that the patient has tolerated and complied with the prescribed treatment, there are four key groups of factors to be considered with the refractory patient that can complicate the course of treatment and contribute to apparent treatment resistance: exogenous factors, diagnostic comorbidity, failure to use multimodal treatment, and iatrogenic effects.

Role of Exogenous Anxiogenic Factors

Several key types of exogenous factors may contribute to treatment resistance. The first, briefly discussed in the previous section, is the presence of health habits that may promote anxiety. In addition to the use of caffeine and even small amounts of alcohol, panic disorder patients misattributing sensations of breathlessness to ''allergies'' may take a number of over-the-counter cold preparations containing pseudo-ephedrine and phenylpropanolamine, which greatly aggravate anxiety and panic. Studies indicate that a majority of panic disorder patients will have their anxiety state significantly worsened during total sleep deprivation, with a number of them having panic attacks during the next day (40). Although the effects of less than total sleep deprivation (i.e., reduction of normal amounts of sleep) have not been systematically studied, it is the impression of many clinicians that this can be an important factor in certain individuals. Therefore, the possibility of a change in sleep habits should be systematically explored because it may be related to worsening of anxiety or panic.

The effects of ongoing life events and stress are also quite important. In one study (41), responsivity to cognitive-behavioral therapy was substantially reduced in the presence of ongoing life stress, regardless of the nature (e.g., loss, interpersonal stress) of the particular stressor. A related issue involves the potential perturbation in the marital and/or family system that can be introduced when panic patients are successfully treated. For example, an agoraphobic family member who kept close to home, very dependent on others, and relegated to taking care of household chores may gradually abandon this particular role as he or she improves. This may greatly disturb family members and cause them to subtly sabotage treatment, or indirectly create stress that counteracts the beneficial effects of treatment.

Finally, the presence of substance use, even if it does not meet criteria for abuse and dependence, is important to consider (42,43). Marijuana, for instance, is known to have significant anxiogenic affects in some individuals (44). The use of cocaine and other stimulants (45) may be associated with subsequent panic-anxiety, even if initial administrations were devoid of anxiety and associated only with euphoria.

Contributions of Comorbidity

Acute treatment studies as well as longer-term naturalistic studies have clearly demonstrated that the presence of certain comorbid conditions is associated with a relatively poor response to treatment. These include axis I disorders such as major depression (especially recurrent major depression) (46), agoraphobia (47), social phobia (48), blood injury phobia (49), and personality disorders (50). In addition, absolute severity of panic-related symptoms has also been shown to predict poor response (47,48) whether treatment is with a tricyclic, SSRI, or BZD. The presence of substance abuse has also been associated with poor treatment outcome (43), although this may be related, at least in part, to problems with treatment engagement and compliance. In more adherent patients, drug abuse has a greater effect than alcoholism on treatment outcome (43), possibly because the direct neurochemical effects of stimulant drugs are more likely to interfere with antipanic treatment mechanisms.

The Problem of Unimodal Treatment

Treatment resistance is often due to a failure to use more than one treatment modality. Although there are no systematic data, the few studies referred to in the previous section on treatment adequacy (13,14,17) suggest that there is probably more underutilization of cognitive-behavioral therapy than of pharmacotherapy. Although several studies have shown that combined treatment with medication and behavioral treatment is more effective than either treatment alone in panic patients with agoraphobia (52,53), only one report has examined the role of combined treatment in treatment-refractory patients with panic (54). In this case series, eight treatment-intolerant and seven treatment-resistant patients with agoraphobia received cognitive-behavioral therapy in addition to their medication. Six of the 15 patients remitted. Although treatment effects seemed to be greater for the patients who were medication-intolerant as opposed to medication-resistant, some effectiveness was noted even for medication-resistant patients. The specific focus and goals of cognitive-behavioral therapy, its brief time course, and its empirically based efficacy appear to address the major reasons that many panic patients may not want to have ''psychotherapy'' (i.e., that psychotherapy appears too vague, does not appear to be applicable to their problem with panic attacks, costs too much, and does not work).

There is a parallel problem of failure to utilize proper medication in many psychotherapeutically treated panic patients. A recent survey (55) analyzed the use of psychotropic medication for depressed patients by psychiatrists, psychologists, and general medical clinicians. With respect to antidepressants, both the psychiatrists and the general medical clinicians showed the expected increase in rate of prescription for more severely symptomatic patients compared to more moderately symptomatic patients. In contrast, psychologists and other lay therapists reported no difference in the proportion of their patients receiving medications between those who were more and those who were less severely symptomatic. Although these data were gathered on depressed patients, it is likely that it is generalizable to other outpatient groups including panic patients. This suggests that nonphysician psychotherapists may delay referral for pharmacotherapy evaluation until psychotherapy has completely failed. This scenario frequently results in a patient who is biased against psychological treatment and who may refuse indicated additional psychotherapy even after a positive therapeutic response to medication treatment.

The Role of Iatrogenic Anxiety

In addition to overstimulation due to antidepressants and other psychotropic medications, various other medications may exacerbate anxiety, including xanthine bronchodilators, corticosteroids (56), and ovarian steroid hormones, with reports indicating that both estrogen (57) and progesterone (58) may aggravate anxiety. Other medications could also be implicated despite the absence of prior published reports; therefore, all medications should be carefully reviewed and discontinuation of possibly offending candidates considered, if medically feasible.

Chronic BZD use may also have an anxiogenic effect in some patients with panic disorder. This effect is most likely to occur in individuals who have had a significant elevation of their dose over time because of loss of efficacy at lower doses. In these cases, the patient may have become more sensitized to his anxiety rather than tolerant to it. This notion is consistent with one recent four-cell study of fluvoxamine and behavioral therapy treatment that showed that longer-term BZD use was associated with smaller gains with all treatments in panic patients with concomitant phobic avoidance (59). Another study showed that BZDs actually decreased an individual's tolerance to anxiety discomfort as measured by the anxiety sensitivity index (60). These findings are consistent with data indicating that in some animal studies BZDs appear to retard an animal's ability to deal with stress (61). It is estimated that this phenomenon occurs in a small (10%) proportion of BZD-treated patients.

It is interesting that a pattern of dose escalation in BZD-treated patients is often misinterpreted as abuse or addiction. In some cases, substance abuse treatment of this misdiagnosed ''benzodiazepine addiction'' has been inadvertently successful because it provides needed psychotherapy and social support intervention that assists patients in gradually tapering their medication and perhaps better tolerating their anxiety. Patients presenting to physicians with persistent severe panic symptoms despite high doses of BZDs should be considered for taper and discontinuation. In these cases, although taper may result in initial exacerbation of anxiety, after several weeks off these medications, the patient's symptoms may dramatically improve. Anticonvulsants may be used to assist this taper; in particular, valproate may also serve as a partial antipanic treatment during the intervening period (see the following section).

MEDICATION APPROACHES TO TREATMENT RESISTANCE

When standard BZDs, SSRIs, or tricyclic agents fail, MAOIs should be tried. These agents are used less frequently now that numerous effective and safe agents with different mechanisms of action are available. However, earlier studies did suggest that MAOIs may have slight advantages over tricyclics (62), and clinician-experts in the pharmacology of panic maintain that they may have special utility in treatment-resistant patients (63). Doses of at least 60–75 mg of phenelzine and 30–40 mg of tranylcypromine should be used. Although studies also support the efficacy of the newer, reversible MAOIs such as brofaramine (64), these agents are not widely used or available for the treatment of panic.

Few additional single agents are known to be effective for panic disorder. Most importantly, the efficacy of other agents documented in various reports and studies has never been established in treatment-resistant panic patients. As alluded to in the introduction, venlafaxine

Table 1   Medication Approaches to Treatment-Resistant Panic

Single agents
  MAOIs
    Phenelzine 60–75 mg minimum dose
    Ttranylcypromine 30–40 mg minimum dose
  Venlafaxine
  Nefazodone
  Valproate
  Verapamil
  Inositol

Combination treatment
  SSRI plus TCA
  SSRI or TCA plus BZD
  SSRI plus TCA plus BZD (''triple therapy'')
  Li^+ augmentation
  buspirone augmentation
  Valproate plus clonazepam

has now been shown to be effective compared with placebo (19), and there is evidence that nefazodone may also be effective (20). A single study almost a decade ago (65) demonstrated that the calcium channel blocker verapamil was also effective, and a more recent report suggested that nimodipine is effective for panic patients with dizziness associated with decreased basilar artery flow triggered by hyperventilation (66). Despite these reports, the use of calcium channel blockers for panic disorder has generated little enthusiasm or interest (67), and their utility in antipanic treatment is probably limited to individuals with comorbid hypertension or migraine headaches who might benefit from a single agent to treat both the neurological disorder and the panic.

The anticonvulsant valproic acid (i.e., Depakote) is receiving increasing attention as possibly being effective for anxious individuals who have comorbid substance abuse, "mixed affective" symptoms, or other neurologically based "organic" damage due to either heavy substance abuse, head trauma, cerebrovascular disease, or developmental disability. Many anecdotal reports indicate that Depakote has therapeutic effects on anxiety and agitation. In terms of its antipanic efficacy, several open-case series report effectiveness although no placebo-controlled trial has been reported to date (68). One case series reported that 8 weeks of treatment with Depakote blocked lactate-induced panic in a majority of patients, all of whom had a lactate-induced panic attack at baseline prior to treatment (69). Since evidence suggests that placebo cannot block lactate-induced panic, this suggests that Depakote may have exerted a pharmacologically mediated effect. Its antipanic efficacy may be due to its actions in potentiating neurotransmission at the GABA-BZD complex.

A final interesting placebo-controlled study documents the efficacy for panic of the second-messenger precursor inositol (70). This strategy is of some interest because it is mechanistically novel, devoid of significant side effects, and a natural component of the human diet.

A number of combination treatments for refractory panic have been utilized although none has been empirically tested. SSRIs have been combined with tricyclics and in one case series were shown to be effective (71). However, lower tricyclic antidepressant doses and plasma levels are best used since most SSRIs have effects on the hepatic 2D6 microsomal enzyme system and will elevate tricyclic blood levels. Use of BZDs in combination with antidepressants has also been found to be useful in numerous case series although no controlled data exist (72). ''Triple therapy'' with an SSRI, a tricyclic, and a BZD may also be indicated, and many clinicians have used this with some degree of success. One report indicates that lithium augmentation may have some antipanic efficacy (73). Another report focused on the utility of clonazepam added to valproate, a combination that provided therapeutic benefit and a very potent anticonvulsant spectrum of activity (74). Buspirone augmentation of cognitive-behavioral therapy (75) as well as antidepressants may have some degree of antipanic efficacy, although buspirone alone is no more effective than placebo for panic.

CONCLUSIONS

The ideal approach to the treatment-refractory patient begins with determination of the cause of the treatment refractoriness. The general approach involves confirming the diagnosis, examining whether adequate treatment has been provided (the correct type applied appropriately), confirming whether the patient has been compliant with the treatment or whether treatment intolerance exists, and, finally, examining a number of factors that may contribute to treatment resistance. These include anxiogenic factors, comorbid conditions, the use of unimodal treatment, and iatrogenic effects involving prescribed medication.

Once the previous assessment has been completed, the clinical approach involves careful patient education and preparation, utilization of multidimensional symptom ratings, and informed use of combined medication and psychotherapeutic approaches in a manner that will reinforce their mutual efficacy.

REFERENCES

1. Coplan J, Riffon L, Gorman J. Therapeutic strategies for the patient with treatment-resistant anxiety. J Clin Psychiatry 1993; 54:69–74.
2. Hollander E, Cohen L. The assessment and treatment of refractory anxiety. J Clin Psychiatry 1994; 55(suppl 2):27–31.

3. Rosenbaum J. Treatment-resistant panic disorder. J Clin Psychiatry 1997; 58(suppl 2):61–64.
4. Shear MK, Maser JD. Standardized assessment for panic disorder research. Arch Gen Psychiatry 1994; 51:346–354.
5. Brown TA, Barlow DH. Long-term outcome in cognitive-behavioural treatment of panic disorder: clinical predictors and alternative strategies for assessment. J Consulting Clin Psychol 1995; 63(5):754–765.
6. Shear MK, Brown TA, Barlow DH, Money R, Sholomskas DE, Woods SW, Gorman JM, Papp LA. Multicenter Panic Disorder Severity Scale. Am J Psychiatry 1997; 154:1571–1575.
7. Schweizer E, Fox I, Case G, Rickel K. Lorazepam versus alprazolam in the treatment of panic disorder. Psychopharmacol Bull 1988; 24:224–227.
8. Cross National Collaborative Treatment Study. Drug treatment of panic disorder: comparative efficacy of alprazolam, imipramine, and placebo. Br J Psychiatry 1992; 160:191–202.
9. Black DW, Wessner R, Bowers W, Gabel J. A comparison of fluvoxamine, cognitive therapy and placebo in the treatment of panic disorder. Arch Gen Psychiatry 1993; 54(4):44–50.
10. Roy-Byrne P, Cowley D. Course and outcome in panic disorder: a review of recent follow-up studies. Anxiety 1995; 1:151–160.
11. Katschnig H, Amering M, Stolk JM, et al. Long-term follow-up after a drug trial for panic disorder. Br J Psychiatry 1995; 167:487–494.
12. Wingerson D, Sullivan M, Dager S, Flick S, Dunner D, Roy-Byrne P. Personality traits and early discontinuation from clinical trials in anxious patients. J Clin Psychopharmacol 1993; 13(3):194–197.
13. Taylor C, King R, Margaret J, et al. Use of medication and invivo exposure in volunteers for panic disorder research. Am J Psychiatry 1989; 146:1423–1426.
14. Swinson R, Cox B, Woszxzyna C. Use of medical services and treatment for panic disorder with agoraphobia and for social phobia. Canadian Med Assoc J 1992; 147:878–883.
15. Yonkers K, Ellison J, Shera D, et al. Description of antipanic therapy in a perspective longitudinal study. J Clin Psychopharmacol 1996; 16:223–232.
16. Cowley DS, Ha EH, Roy-Byrne PP. Determinants of pharmacologic treatment failure in panic disorder. J Clin Psychiatry 1997; 58:555–561.
17. Goisman RM, Rogers, MP, Steketee, GS, Warshaw, MG, Cuneo, P, Keller, MB. Utilization of behavioral methods in a multicenter anxiety disorders study. J Clin Psychiatry 1993; 54:213–218.

18. Roy-Byrne PP, Cowley D. Assessment and treatment of panic disorder. In: Dunner DL, ed. Current Psychiatric Therapies II. Philadelphia: WB Saunders, 1997:309–316.

19. Pollack MH, Worthington JJ III, Otto MW, Make KM, Smoller JW, Manfro GG, Rudolph R, Rosenbaum JF. Venlafaxine for panic disorder: results from a double-blind, placebo-controlled study. Psychopharmacol Bull 1996; 32(4):667–670.

20. Demartinis NA, Schweizer E, Rickels K. An open-label trial of nefazodone in high comorbidity panic disorder. J Clin Psychiatry 1996; 57(6): 245–248.

21. Sheehan DV, Davidson J, Manschreck T, et al. Lack of efficacy of a new antidepressant (bupropion) in the treatment of panic disorder with phobias. J Clin Psychopharmacol 1983; 3:28–31.

22. Munjack DJ, Crocker B, Cabe D, et al. Alprazolam, propranolol, and placebo in the treatment of panic disorder and agoraphobia with panic attacks. J Clin Psychopharmacol 1989; 9:22–27.

23. Sheehan, DV, Raj AB, Sheehan KH, Soto S. Is buspirone effective for panic disorder? J Clin Psychopharmacol 1990; 10(1):3–11.

24. Uhde TW, Stein MB, Post RM. Lack of efficacy of carbamazepine in the treatment of panic disorder. Am J Psychiatry 1988; 145:1104–1109.

25. Charney DS, Woods SW, Goodman WK, et al. Drug treatment of panic disorder: the comparative efficacy of imipramine, alprazolam and trazodone. J Clin Psychiatry 47:580–586.

26. Mavissakalian M, Perel JM. Imipramine treatment of panic disorder with agoraphobia: dose ranging and plasma level-response relationships. Am J Psychiatry 1995; 152(5):673–682.

27. Lydiard RB, Lesser LM, Bellenger JC, Rubin RT, Laraia M, DuPont R. A fixed-dose study of alprazolam 2 mg, alprazolam 6 mg, and placebo in panic disorder. J Clin Psychopharmacol 1992; 12:96–103.

28. Steiner M, Oakes R, Gergel IP, et al. A fixed dose study of paroxetine and placebo in the treatment of panic disorder [abstr]. In: New Research Program and Abstracts of the 148th Annual Meeting of the American Psychiatric Association, Miami, May 20–25, 1995.

29. Oehrberg S, Christiansen PE, Behnke K, et al. Paroxetine in the treatment of panic disorder, a randomized, double-blind, placebo-controlled study. Br J Psychiatry 1995; 167:374–379.

30. Caske MG, Brown TA, Barlow DH. Behavioral treatment of panic: a two-year follow-up. Behav Ther 1991; 22:289–304.

31. Clark DM, Salkovskis PM, Hackmann A, et al. A comparison of cogni-

tive therapy, applied relaxation and imipramine in the treatment of panic disorder. Br J Psychiatry 1994; 164:759–769.

32. Shear MK, Cloitre M, Heckeman L. Emotion-focused treatment for panic disorder: a brief, dynamically informed therapy. In: Barber JP, Crits-Christoph P, eds. Dynamic Therapies for Psychiatric Disorders (Axis I). New York: Basic Books, 1995:267–293.

33. Milrod, BL, Busch, FN, Cooper, AM, Shapiro, T. Manual of Panic-Focused Psychodynamic Psychotherapy. Washington, DC: American Psychiatric Association Press, 1997.

34. Loebel AD, Hyde TS, Dunner DL. Early placebo response in anxious and depressed patients. J Clin Psychiatry 1986; 47:230–232.

35. Noyes R, Garvey MJ, Cook BL. Problems with tricyclic antidepressant use in patients with panic disorder or agoraphobia: results of a naturalistic follow-up study. J Clin Psychiatry 1989; 50:163–196.

36. Gorman JM, Liebowitz MR, Fyer AJ. An open trial of fluoxetine in the treatment of panic attacks. Am J Psychiatry 1987; 143:303–308.

37. Roy Byrne PP, Uhde TW. Exogenous factors in panic disorder: clinical and research implications. J Clin Psychiatry 1988; 49:56–61.

38. Otto M, Pollack M, Sachs G, et al. Discontinuation of benzodiazepine treatment: efficacy of cognitive-behavior therapy for patients with panic disorder. Am J Psychiatry 1993; 150:1485–1490.

39. Spiegel LDA, Bruce TJ, Gregg SF, et al. Does cognitive behavior therapy assist slow-taper alprazolam discontinuation in panic disorder? Am J Psychiatry 1994; 151:876–881.

40. Roy-Byrne PP, Uhde TW, Post RM. Effects of one night's sleep deprivation on mood and behavior in panic disorder. Arch Gen Psychiatry 1986. 43:895–899.

41. Wade S, Monroe S, Michelson L. Chronic life stress and treatment outcome in agoraphobia with panic attacks. Am J Psychiatry 1993; 150:1491–1495.

42. Goldenberg IM, Mueller T, Fierman EJ, Gordon A, Pratt L, Cox K, Park T, Lavori P, Goisman RM, Keller MB. Specificity of substance use in anxiety-disordered subjects. Comprehen Psychiatry 1995; 36(5):319–328.

43. Worthington J, Pollack MH, Otto MW, Gould RA, McArdle ET, Rosenbaum JF. Effect of lifetime history of alcohol or substance dependence on severity and treatment of panic disorder. Psychopharmacology 1996; 32(3):531.

44. Thomas H. A community survey of adverse effects of cannabis use. Drug Alcohol Dependence 1996; 42(3):201–207.

45. Louie AK, Lannon RA, Rutzick EA, Brown D, Lewis TB, Jones R. Clinical features of cocaine-induced panic. Biolog Psychiatry 1996; 40(9):938–940.
46. Maddock R, Carter C, Blacker K, et al. Relationship of past depressive episodes to symptom severity and treatment response in panic disorder with agoraphobia. J Clin Psychiatry 1993; 54:88–95.
47. Maier W, Roth SM, Argyle N, et al. Avoidance behaviour: a predictor of the efficacy of pharmacotherapy in panic disorder? Dur Arch Psychiatry Clin Neurosci 1991; 241:151–158.
48. Segu'i J, Salvador L, Canet J, Arag'on C, Herrera C. [Comorbidity of panic disorder and social phobia.] Actas Luso-Espanolas de Neurologia, Psiquiatria y Ciencias Afinas 1995; 23(2):43–47.
49. Slaap GR, van Vliet IM, Westenberg HG, et al. Phobic symptoms as predictors of nonresponse to drug therapy panic disorder patients (a preliminary report). J Affect Disord 1995; 33:31–38.
50. Black DW, Wesner RB, Gabel J, et al. Predictors of short-term response in 66 patients with panic disorder. J Affect Disord 1994; 30:233–241.
51. Pollack MH, Otto MW, Sachs GS, et al. Anxiety psychopathology predictive of outcome in patients with panic disorder and depression treated with imipramine, alprazolam and placebo. J Affect Disord 1994: 30: 273–281.
52. Telch MJ, Agras S, Taylor CB, et al. Combined pharmacological and behavioural treatment for agoraphobia. Behav Res Ther 1985; 23:325–335.
53. Telch MJ, Lucas RA. Combined pharmacological and psychological treatment of panic disorder: current status and future directions. In: Wolfe BE, Maser JD, eds. Treatment of Panic Disorder: A Consensus Development Conference. Washington, DC: American Psychiatric Association Press, 1994:177–197.
54. Pollack MH, Otto MW, Kaspi SP, Hammerness PG, Rosenbaum JF. Cognitive behavior therapy for treatment-refractory panic disorder. J Clin Psychiatry 1994; 55(5):200–205.
55. Wells K, Sturm R. Informing the policy process: from efficacy to effectiveness data on pharmacotherapy. J Consulting Clin Psychol 1996; 64(4):638–645.
56. Ismail K, Wessely S. Psychiatric complications of corticosteroid therapy. Br J Hosp Med 1995; 53(10):495–499.
57. Dembert ML, Dinneen MP, Opsahl, MS. Estrogen-induced panic disorder. Am J Psychiatry 1994; 151(8):1246.

58. Wagner KD, Berenson AB. Norplant-associated major depression and panic disorder. J Clin Psychiatry 1994; 55(11):478–480.

59. Van Bolkom AJ, de Beurs, Koele P, et al. Long-term benzodiazepine use is associated with smaller treatment gain in panic disorder with agoraphobia. J Nerv Ment Dis 1996; 184:133–135.

60. Fava GA. Anxiety sensitivity [letter]. Am J Psychiatry 1996; 153:1109.

61. Roy-Byrne PP, Swinson RP: Interactions on benzodiazepines with psychological and behavioral treatment. In: Roy-Byrne PP, Cowley DS, eds. Benzodiazepines in Clinical Practice: Risks and Benefits. Washington, DC: American Psychiatric Association Press, 1991.

62. Sheehan DV, Ballenger J, Jacobsen G. Treatment of endogenous anxiety with phobic, hysterical, and hypochondrical symptoms. Arch Gen Psychiatry 1980; 37:51–59.

63. Lydiard RB, Ballenger JC. Antidepressant in panic disorder and agoraphobia. J Affect Disord 1987; 13(2):153–168.

64. Van-Vliet, IM, Westenberg, HG, Den-Boer, JA. MAO inhibitors in panic disorder: clinical effects of treatment with brofaromine: a double blinded placebo controlled study. Psychopharmacology 1993; 112(4):483–489.

65. Klein E, Uhde TW. Controlled study of verapamil for treatment of panic disorder. Am J Psychiatry 1988; 145:431–434.

66. Gibbs DM. Hyperventilation-induced cerebral ischemia in panic disorder and effect of nimodipine. Am J Psychiatry 1992; 149(11):1589–1591.

67. Balon R, Ramesh C. Calcium channel blockers for anxiety disorders? Ann Clin Psychiatry 1996; 8(4):215–220.

68. Woodman CL, Noyes R Jr. Panic disorder: treatment with valproate. J Clin Psychiatry 1994: 55(4):134–136.

69. Keck PE Jr, Taylor VE, Tugrul KC, McElroy SL, Bennett JA. Valproate treatment of panic disorder and lactate-induced panic attacks. Biolog Psychiatry 1993; 33(7):542–546.

70. Benjamine J, Levine J, Fux M, Aviv A, Levy D, Belmaker RH. Double-blind, placebo-controlled, crossover trial of inositol treatment for panic disorder. Am J Psychiatry 1995; 152(7):1084–1086.

71. Tiffon I, Coplan JD, Papp LA, et al. Augmentation strategies with tricyclic or fluoxetine treatment in seven partially responsive panic disorder patients. J Clin Psychiatry 1994; 55:66–69.

72. Ries RK, Wittkowsky AK. Synergistic action of alprazolam with tranylcypromine in drug-resistant atypical depression with panic attacks. Biolog Psychiatry 1986; 21:522–526.

73. Cournoyer J. Rapid response of a disorder to the addition of lithium carbonate: panic resistant to tricyclic antidepressants. Can J Psychiatry 1986; 31:335–338.

74. Ontiveros A, Fontaine R. Sodium valproate and clonazepam for treatment-resistant panic disorder. J Psychiatry Neurosci 1992; 17(2):78–80.
75. Cottraux J, Note ID, Cungi C, Legeron P, Heim F, Chneiweiss L, Bernard G, Bouvard M. A controlled study of cognitive behavior therapy with buspirone or placebo in panic disorder with agoraphobia. Br J Psychiatry 1995; 167:635–641.

8

Course and Treatment of Panic Disorder During Pregnancy and the Postpartum Period

Ruta Nonacs and Lee S. Cohen
Massachusetts General Hospital
Boston, Massachusetts

Lori L. Altshuler
UCLA Neuropsychiatric Institute
UCLA Brain Research Institute and
VA Medical Center, West Los Angeles
Los Angeles, California

While the postpartum period has been identified as a period of risk for the development of psychiatric illness, pregnancy has previously been described as a time of emotional well-being during which some psychiatric disorders become more quiescent (1–3). More recent studies, however, suggest that some women may not be "protected" from the onset or re-emergence of psychiatric illness during pregnancy (4–6). Although some investigators have focused on the course of mood disorders during pregnancy and the puerperium, comparatively less is known about the impact of pregnancy and the postpartum period on the natural course of anxiety disorders.

Anxiety disorders are highly prevalent in women. Panic disorder affects 2 to 3% of the general population and occurs commonly in women during the childbearing years. Approximately 70% of women with panic disorder describe the onset of symptoms as occurring between the ages of 18 and 35 (7). Many of these women will have significant symptoms and will be treated with antipanic medications, including high-potency benzodiazepines and antidepressants. A clinical dilemma arises when a women maintained on antipanic medications wishes to conceive or inadvertently becomes pregnant. All psychotropic medications diffuse across the placenta, and their impact on the developing fetus must be considered. Although some patients can successfully taper and discontinue antipanic medications, relapse rates are typically very high after discontinuation of both benzodiazepines and antidepressants (8–10). In addition, uncontrolled panic symptoms during pregnancy may confer risk to the fetus (11–13). Clinicians are thus frequently faced with the question of how to advise their patients regarding the treatment of panic disorder during pregnancy and the puerperium.

Clinical decisions regarding the treatment of psychiatrically ill pregnant women typically involve weighing the risks of fetal exposure to psychotropic medications against the potential adverse effects to both mother and fetus of untreated psychiatric illness. The formulation of appropriate guidelines for the treatment of panic disorder during pregnancy derives from an understanding of the impact of pregnancy on the course of panic disorder. However, little systematically derived data are available regarding 1) the prevalence and course of panic disorder during pregnancy and the puerperium and 2) the risk for relapse in women with histories of panic disorder who discontinue antipanic medications either prior to or during pregnancy. This chapter reviews available information on the prevalence and natural history of panic disorder during pregnancy and the postpartum period. Furthermore, treatment guidelines for pregnant and puerperal women who suffer from panic disorder are outlined.

PANIC DISORDER DURING PREGNANCY

Several anecdotal reports and case series have described a reduction in the severity and frequency of panic symptoms during pregnancy

(14–17). For example, in a retrospective study of 20 women with a total of 33 pregnancies, the majority of women reported a marked symptomatic improvement during pregnancy (14). Other authors found that some patients were able to discontinue antipanic medications during pregnancy without relapse of their panic disorder (15,17).

Other studies have proposed a more variable course of panic disorder during pregnancy, suggesting that while some pregnant women with panic disorder are relatively asymptomatic, a subgroup of women exists who may experience persistence or exacerbation of panic symptoms during pregnancy (18,19). In a retrospective study of 49 women with pregravid panic disorder, Cohen and colleagues (19) demonstrated that 20% experienced worsening panic symptoms, 20% showed improvement, and 60% of women noted no change in status during pregnancy. In this study, women with severe pregravid panic disorder typically failed attempts to discontinue antipanic medications. They were more likely to continue antipanic pharmacotherapy during pregnancy than women with milder forms of panic disorder.

In the only prospective study to date (20), no diminution in panic symptoms during pregnancy was noted in a cohort of women with panic disorder. In fact, nine of the 10 patients in this study continued to meet criteria for panic disorder while pregnant. Half of the women experienced worsening of panic symptoms during pregnancy and increased the dosage of antipanic medication relative to pregravid dosage. This study, although small in size, suggests that women are not necessarily "protected" from panic symptoms during pregnancy, and that some women may actually experience symptom exacerbation. These findings are consistent with recent data describing high rates of relapse during pregnancy in women with histories of recurrent major depression who discontinued antidepressant treatment proximate to conception (21,22).

The impact of pregnancy on panic disorder appears to be variable. Apparently, pregnancy has no effect or may even ameliorate panic symptoms in some patients (15–17), affording these women a chance to discontinue medication. Others may note persistence or exacerbation of symptoms and may require antipanic pharmacotherapy (18–20). The factors that precisely delineate these two groups are unclear, and it is difficult at this time to predict which patients will do well during pregnancy compared to those who may experience significant panic symptoms.

REPRODUCTIVE PHYSIOLOGY AND
PANIC DISORDER

Several authors have attempted to explain the course of panic symptoms during pregnancy in the context of various physiological changes
that occur during pregnancy (17,23). Klein (23,24) has suggested that
the hormonal changes associated with pregnancy may have an anxiolytic effect. Others note that progesterone metabolites possess barbiturate-like activity and may thus be anxiolytic (25). Pregnancy has also
been associated with diminished reactivity of the sympathetic nervous
system to a variety of physiological stressors (26,27). The extent to
which these changes may influence the course of panic disorder during
pregnancy is a topic that requires further study.

PANIC DISORDER DURING THE
POSTPARTUM PERIOD

While the course of panic disorder during pregnancy is variable, the
postpartum period appears to be a time of increased vulnerability to
panic symptoms (15,16,18,20,28,29). Several studies describe the first
onset of panic disorder during the puerperium (29–31). In one study
of women with panic disorder, Sholomskas and colleagues (31) reported the first lifetime onset of panic disorder during the postpartum
period in 10.9% of the 64 women studied, a significantly higher rate
than expected for a given 12-week period. This suggests that the emergence of panic disorder in the puerperium is not simply coincidental.

In other retrospective studies of women with pre-existing panic
disorder, postpartum worsening of panic symptoms has been frequently
described (18,19,28,29). A significant increase in the severity or frequency of attacks during the postpartum period appears to be a consistent finding, occurring in 31% (29) to 63% (18) of women with pregravid panic disorder. Postpartum exacerbation occurs commonly even
in those women who were asymptomatic during pregnancy (29). In one
study, those patients who received antipanic pharmacotherapy during
the third trimester were less likely to develop puerperal worsening of
panic symptoms (28).

In one prospective study (20), 90% of women with panic disorder (some of whom had experienced improvement during pregnancy) were actively symptomatic at 1 to 3 months postpartum. The majority of these women increased the intensity of antipanic pharmacological treatment during the puerperium relative to levels of pharmacotherapy used during the pregravid period and pregnancy. These data suggest not only a vulnerability to panic symptoms during the puerperium, but also a worsening of pre-existing panic disorder during the postpartum period.

This increase in postpartum susceptibility to panic symptoms mirrors the vulnerability to affective worsening observed during the postpartum period in women with histories of mood disorder (4,22,32). Like women with pregravid mood disorder, women with panic disorder appear to be at risk for the emergence of psychiatric symptoms during the postpartum period. The extent to which psychosocial and environmental factors, biological vulnerability, and a changing hormonal environment interact with one another during the postpartum period to drive the development of anxiety symptoms is complex and remains to be more clearly explained

Several hypotheses have been put forth to explain postpartum worsening of panic disorder. Some theorize that the sharp postpartum fall in progesterone levels following delivery may increase vulnerability to panic symptoms (17). Elevated progesterone levels during pregnancy stimulate hyperventilation and a subsequent reduction in Pco_2 levels. After delivery, declining progesterone levels stimulate a rise in Pco_2 levels, which may predispose to panic attacks (23).

REPRODUCTIVE SAFETY OF ANTIPANIC MEDICATIONS

Information regarding the risks associated with prenatal exposure to psychotropic medications is incomplete. While data are available on risks for congenital malformation and neonatal toxicity, much less is known about the extent to which fetal exposure to psychotropic agents may be associated with more subtle neurobehavioral sequelae. There is a natural tendency to discontinue or limit pharmacotherapy in pregnant women; however, some women may experience persistent and severe symptoms and may elect to continue pharmacological treatment during pregnancy and the puerperium. While no medication can be deemed completely without risk, a range of psychotropic medications may be used during pregnancy. When prescribing medications to a pregnant patient, the clinician must first consider several different types of risk associated with prenatal exposure to psychotropic medications: risk of organ malformation, risk of neonatal toxicity, and potential for longer-term neurobehavioral effects.

The consequences of prenatal exposure to benzodiazepines have been debated for over 20 years. Three prospective studies support the absence of increased risk of organ malformation following first-trimester exposure to benzodiazepines (33–35). More controversial has been the issue of whether first-trimester exposure to benzodiazepines increases risk for specific malformations, such as cleft lip or cleft palate. While several studies do not support this association (36,37), a recent meta-analysis (38) calculates a 0.7% risk of oral cleft associated with first-trimester exposure to benzodiazepines. This is an approximately 10-fold increase in risk for oral cleft over that observed in the general population (6 in 10,000, or 0.06%). The limitations of risk estimates derived from this type of meta-analysis have previously been noted (39). Methodological difficulties emerge when several studies are pooled that include exposure to different benzodiazepines at varying dosage and duration in populations ascertained in a noncontrolled fashion. Nonetheless, the likelihood that a woman exposed to benzodiazepines during the first-trimester will give birth to a child with this congenital anomaly, although significantly increased, remains less than 1%. This risk must be discussed with the patient and weighed against the likelihood of relapse after benzodiazepine discontinuation.

Neonatal toxicity, as well as symptoms characteristic of withdrawal, have been described following benzodiazepine exposure at or near the time of delivery (41–43). Case reports have described impaired temperature regulation, apnea, depressed APGAR scores, muscular hypotonia, and failure to feed. Systematically derived data on the long-term neurobehavioral effects of benzodiazepine exposure are sparse. Several studies have reported motor and developmental delays (44,45), although these studies have been criticized for having significant ascertainment biases (34). Other studies have revealed no association between benzodiazepine exposure and developmental delay (33).

While data are available regarding prenatal exposure to benzodiazepines such as diazepam and alprazolam, there is comparatively little information on clonazepam exposure. In one prospective study (40), 38 pregnant women with panic disorder received clonazepam only (0.5 mg to 3.5 mg per day). No evidence of congenital malformation was noted, although this sample was obviously small. Of note, however, is that APGAR scores were uniformly high, and no children showed signs of neonatal withdrawal syndromes or other perinatal difficulties.

Tricyclic antidepressants (TCAs) represent an effective, nonbenzodiazepine alternative for the treatment of panic disorder. To date, three prospective studies and over 10 retrospective studies have investigated the risk for organ malformation following first-trimester exposure to TCAs (38,39,51,52,71,72). Over 400 cases of first-trimester exposure to TCAs have been documented in the literature. When evaluated on an individual basis and when pooled, these studies fail to indicate a significant association between fetal exposure to TCAs and high rates of congenital malformation.

Various case reports describe neonatal toxicity in infants exposed to TCAs. These have included TCA withdrawal syndromes, with characteristic symptoms of jitteriness, irritability, and seizures following exposure to these agents during labor and delivery (46–48). Symptoms attributed to the anticholinergic effect of TCAs, such as functional bowel obstruction and urinary retention, have also been reported (49,50). No systematically derived data are available regarding long-term neurobehavioral sequelae of TCA exposure in humans.

Data regarding the reproductive safety of fluoxetine derives in part from the manufacturer's postmarketing surveillance register (Eli Lilly and Company, personal communication). Data from the manufacturer's register and several prospective studies (51–54) include a total of 1100 fluoxetine-exposed children. No increased risk of organ malformation has been noted in children exposed to fluoxetine, as compared to baseline risk in the general population.

The extent to which prenatal exposure to fluoxetine increases risk of neonatal toxicity or long-term neurobehavioral consequences is still unclear. Data regarding risk for neonatal toxicity have been inconsistent, with at least one study (53) describing higher rates of perinatal complications and two others that did not note perinatal distress in infants exposed to fluoxetine (55,70). In one of the first efforts to systematically study long-term neurobehavioral effects of prenatal exposure to fluoxetine, Nulman and colleagues (56) noted no difference between children exposed to fluoxetine and nonexposed controls.

Information regarding the reproductive safety of other SSRIs (i.e., paroxetine, sertraline, fluvoxamine) is limited to one series of 63 infants with prenatal exposure to paroxetine (57) and anecdotal data obtained from the manufacturer of sertraline (Pfizer Inc., personal communication, 1996). These reports do not reveal incresed rates of congenital malformation or perinatal complications; however, prospectively derived data in larger numbers of women is needed to more adequadely assess the reproductive safety of SSRIs other than fluoxetine. Similarly, scant information is available regarding the reproductive safety of monoamine oxidase inhibitors (MAOIs). One study described an increase in congenital malformations following prenatal exposure to tranylcypromine and phenelzine (58).

TREATMENT GUIDELINES FOR PANIC DISORDER

In making decisions regarding the treatment of women with panic disorder who are pregnant or planning to conceive, the clinician must discuss not only the risks associated with prenatal exposure to various psychotropic agents but also the consequences of untreated panic disorder during pregnancy. Untreated anxiety symptoms may cause significant morbidity in the mother and may also have an effect on fetal outcome.

Panic attacks during pregnancy are not necessarily benign. Panic attacks are associated with increased plasma catecholamine and cortisol levels. Although the impact of these neuroendocrine changes on fetal well-being has not been well studied, the effect of hypercortisolemia on the developing brain is of concern. Data from animal studies suggest that elevated cortisol levels in utero can lead to neuronal death and abnormal development of neural structures in the fetal brain (59–61).

There are also data to suggest that anxiety during pregnancy is associated with poor fetal outcome, including preterm labor, low birth weight, and other obstetrical complications (12,13,62). Cohen and colleagues (11) reported a case of placental abruption related to uncontrolled panic attacks. In addition, preliminary data suggest that postpartum anxiety disorders, like maternal mood disorders, may be associated with adverse effects on child development and maternal–infant emotional regulation (63).

Cognitive-behavioral therapy (CBT) is a highly effective, nonpharmacological option for the treatment of panic disorder and may be especially useful in the treatment of panic disorder during pregnancy (64). CBT may obviate the need for pharmacotherapy altogether or may allow a reduction in the dosage of antipanic medication. While this modality has proven to be very effective in nonpregnant cohorts with panic disorder, further studies are required to evaluate the efficacy of CBT in the treatment of panic disorder during pregnancy and the postpartum period.

Patients with panic disorder who are maintained on antipanic medications and who wish to discontinue pharmacotherapy prior to attempts to conceive should be advised to taper medications slowly. Some patients may inadvertently conceive on antipanic drugs and may present for emergent consultation. Abrupt discontinuation of antipanic medication is not recommended, as it is frequently associated with increased anxiety and rebound panic symptoms (8–10) and, in some cases, potentially dangerous benzodiazepine withdrawal. Adjunctive CBT may be helpful in limiting anxiety symptoms during attempts to discontinue medication and may increase time to relapse (64,65).

Women who are unable to taper their antipanic medications prior to pregnancy or those who develop panic symptoms during pregnancy may elect to take antipanic medications during pregnancy. Pharmacotherapy is an appropriate treatment option when the risks associated with untreated panic disorder outweigh the risks related to fetal exposure to a particular psychotropic agent. While no medication taken during pregnancy is completely without risk, certain drugs (i.e., benzodiazepines, TCAs, and fluoxetine) may be used during pregnancy for the treatment of panic disorder.

Given the first-trimester risk of oral cleft associated with benzodiazepine use, fluoxetine and the TCAs are attractive nonbenzodiazepine alternatives for the treatment of panic disorder during pregnancy, with the SSRI a probable first choice given its more favorable side-effect profile. TCAs are also commonly used during pregnancy, although orthostatic hypotension is sometimes a problem, particularly with the tertiary amines (i.e., imipramine, amitryptyline). Because treatment with either fluoxetine or a TCA is frequently insufficient for the control of panic symptoms, benzodiazepines remain a reasonable alternative. In all cases, use of the lowest possible effective dose for treatment is recommended.

While the choice of an appropriate antipanic agent during pregnancy is based in part on prior treatment response, it is also determined by information regarding the reproductive safety of these medications. In a woman who has been previously treated with fluoxetine or a TCA, one would resume treatment with the agent that was previously effective. However, a clinical dilemma arises when a women stabilized on an MAOI or an SSRI other than fluoxetine becomes or plans to become pregnant. Given the limited information available on the reproductive safety of these agents, they should be avoided during pregnancy. One should therefore make an effort to switch from these agents to fluoxetine or to a TCA (possibly with an adjunctive benzodiazepine) if pharmacotherapy is required during pregnancy. For those patients who have a history of nonresponse to fluoxetine but who have responded to an alternative SSRI such as sertraline or paroxetine, the use of these latter drugs is not absolutely contraindicated. However, the clinician is obliged in this clinical situation to share the absence of reproductive safety data regarding these two compounds.

As the postpartum period appears to be a period of increased vulnerability to panic symptoms, many women with panic disorder may elect to use antipanic medications after delivery. While nonlactating women may be treated according to standard treatment guidelines, women who plan to breastfeed must be warned that all psychotropic medications are secreted into the breast milk. Concentrations of these medications in breast milk vary widely, and the effect of these agents on the neonate vary as well (66,67). The frequency of severe complications, as reported in the literature, appears to be low (68); however, the long-term effects of exposure to even trace amounts of these medications has not been studied.

Clearly breastfeeding has many benefits for both mother and infant, and the use of psychotropic medications should not preclude breastfeeding. There are no data to suggest that any particular medication is safer than another in women who breastfeed while taking psychotropic agents (68,69). It is most reasonable to choose those medications that have been effective in the past and those that have a favorable side-effect profile. If a woman chooses to take psychotropic agents while breastfeeding, the infant should be monitored closely for signs of toxicity. Given the possibility that premature infants may exhibit immature hepatic metabolism and may therefore be unable to effectively clear psychotropic agents present in the breastmilk, breastfeeding in this setting should be deferred or pursued with considerable caution.

The infant's plasma may be assayed for the presence of drug 1 to 2 weeks after initiating therapy or if signs of neonatal toxicity emerge. Sesitivities of the tests used to detect antidepressants and their metabolites vary among laboratories. In the absence of neonatal toxicity, there is no absolute cutoff above which breastfeeding should be avoided or discontinued. While higher levels are more likely to be associated with toxicity in the infant, the impact of even trace amounts of drug on the developing brain are not known. Decisions regarding the use of psychotropic medications while breastfeeding must be made on a case-by-case basis.

CONCLUSION

Although data are limited, the current literature consistently describes the postpartum period as a time of heightened vulnerability for women with panic disorder. In addition, it is frequently associated with the new onset of panic disorder. However, the impact of pregnancy on panic disorder is less clear. For some women, pregnancy does not appear to exacerbate panic symptoms; however, a subgroup of women appears to experience worsening of panic attacks during pregnancy. It is not clear which women are at greatest risk for relapse during pregnancy or the puerperium, although some data suggest that women with more severe pregravid panic disorder may be more likely to have recurrent symptoms (20).

Untreated panic disorder in the mother has been associated with poor fetal outcome. If panic symptoms during pregnancy are severe or unremitting, treatment with benzodiazepines, TCAs, or fluoxetine may be considered. Cognitive-behavioral therapy may be a useful adjunct, both for facilitating medication discontinuation and for reducing panic symptoms.

In order to design thoughtful strategies for the treatment of panic disorder in women during the childbearing years, the course of this disorder during pregnancy and the puerperium demands further investigation. Data derived from prospective studies will enhance our ability to predict the course of panic disorder during pregnancy. This will allow for the implementation of effective interventions in women who are vulnerable to worsening of panic symptoms during pregnancy and will also provide an opportunity to limit exposure to psychotropic medications in women who are likely to experience improvement in panic symptoms during pregnancy.

REFERENCES

1. Zajicek E. Psychiatric problems during pregnancy. In: Wolkind S, Zajicek E, eds. Pregnancy: A Psychological and Social Study. London: Academic Press, 1981:57–73.
2. Kendell RE, Chalmers JC, Platz C. Epidemiology of puerperal psychosis. Br J Psychiatry 1987; 150:662–673.
3. McGrath E, Keita GP, Strickland BR, Russo NF. Women and Depression: Risk factors and Treatment Issues. Washington, DC: American Psychological Association, 1990.
4. O'Hara MW. Social support, life events, and depression during pregnancy and the pueperium. Arch Gen Psychiatry 1986; 43:569–573.
5. Viguera AC, Nonacs R, Baldessarini RJ, Murray A, Cohen LS. Relapse following discontinuation of lithium maintenance in pregnant women with bipolar disorder. Annual meeting of the American Psychiatric Association, San Diego, 1997.

6. Bottolph ML, Holland A. Obsessive-compulsive disorders in pregnancy and childbirth. In: Jenicke M, Baer L, Minicello WE, eds. Obsessive-Compulsive Disorders: Theory and Management. Chicago: Yearbook Medical Publishers, 1990.

7. Robins LN, Helzer JE, Weissman MM, et al. Lifetime prevalence of specific psychiatric disorders in three sites. Arch Gen Psychiatry 1984; 41:949–958.

8. Noyes R, Garvey M, Cook B, et al. Benzodiazepine withdrawal: a review of the evidence. J Clin Psychiatry 1988; 40:382–389.

9. Noyes R, Garvey M, Cook B, et al. Problems with tricyclic antidepressant use in patients with panic disorder or agoraphobia. J Clin Psychiatry 1989; 50:163–169.

10. Pollack MH, Smoller JW. The longitudinal course and outcome of panic disorder. Psychiatr Clin North Am 1995; 18:785–801.

11. Cohen LS, Rosenbaum JF, Heller VL. Panic attack-associated placental abruption: a case report. J Clin Psychiatry 1989; 50:266–267.

12. Istvan J. Stress, anxiety, and birth outcome: a critical review of the evidence. Psychol Bull 1986; 100:331–348.

13. Lobel M. Conceptualizations, measurement, and effects of prenatal maternal stress on birth outcomes. J Behav Med 1994; 17:225–272.

14. Klein DF, Skrobala AM, Garfinkel RS. Preliminary look at the effects of pregnancy on the course of panic disorder. Anxiety 1994/1995; 1: 227–232.

15. George DT, Ladenheim JA, Nutt DJ. Effect of pregnancy on panic attacks. Am J Psychiatry 1987; 144:1078–1079.

16. Cowley DS, Roy-Byrne PP. Panic disorder during pregnancy. J Psychosom Obstet Gynaecol 1989; 10:193–210.

17. Villeponteaux VA, Lydiard RB, Laraia MT, Stuart GW, Ballenger JC. The effects of pregnancy on pre-existing panic disorder. J Clin Psychiatry 1992; 53:201–203.

18. Northcott CJ, Stein MB. Panic disorder in pregnancy. J Clin Psychiatry 1994; 55:539–42.

19. Cohen LS, Sichel DA, Dimmock JA, Rosenbaum JF. Impact of pregnancy on panic disorder: a case series. J Clin Psychiatry 1994; 55:284–288.

20. Cohen LS, Sichel DA, Faraone SV, Robertson LM, Dimmock JA, Rosenbaum JF. Course of panic disorder during pregnancy and the puerperium: a preliminary study. Biolog Psychiatry 1996; 39:950–954

21. Cohen L, Robertson L, Sichel D, Birnbaum C, Grush L, Weinstock L.

Impact of pregnancy on risk for relapse of major depressive disorder. Annual meeting of the American Psychiatric Association, New York, 1996.

22. O'Hara MW, Schlechte JA, Lewis DA, et al. Controlled prospective study of postpartum mood disorders: psychological, environmental, and hormonal factors. J Abnorm Psychol 1991; 100.

23. Klein DF. False suffocation alarms, spontaneous panics, and related conditions. Arch Gen Psychiatry 1993; 50:306–317.

24. Klein DF. Pregnancy and panic disorder. J Clin Psychiatry 1994; 55: 293–294.

25. Majewski MD, Harrison NL, Schwartz RD, et al. Steroid hormone metabolites are barbiturate-like modulators of the GABA receptor. Science 1986; 232:1004–1007

26. Barron WM, Mujais SK, Zinaman M, et al. Plasma catecholamine responses to physiologic stimuli in normal human pregnancy. Am J Obstet Gynecol 1986; 154:80–84

27. Nissel H, Hjemdahl P, Linde B, et al. Sympathoadrenal and cardiovascular reactivity in pregnancy-induced hypertension. II. Responses to tilting. Am J Obstet Gynecol 1985; 152:554–560.

28. Cohen LS, Sichel DA, Dimmock JA, Rosenbaum JF. Postpartum course in women with preexisting panic disorder. J Clin Psychiatry 1994; 55: 289–292.

29. Wisner KL, Peindl K, Hanusa BH. Effect of child-bearing on the natural history of panic disorder with comorbid mood disorder. J Affect Disord 1996; 41:173–180.

30. Metz A, Sichel DA, Goff DC. Postpartum panic disorder. J Clin Psychiatry 1988; 49:278–279.

31. Sholomskas DE, Wickamaratne PJ, Dogolo L, et al. Postpartum onset of panic disorder: a coincidental event? J Clin Psychiatry 1993; 54:476–480.

32. O'Hara MW, Neunaber DJ, Zekoski EM. A prospective study of postpartum depression: prevalence, course, and predictive factors. J Abnorm Psychol 1984; 93:158.

33. Hartz SC, Heinonen O, Shapiro S, Siskind V, Slone D. Antenatal exposure to meprobamate and chlordiazepoxide in relation to malformations, mental development, and childhood mortality. N Engl J Med 1975; 292: 726–728.

34. Milkovich L, van den Berg BJ. Effects of prenatal meprobamate and chlordiazepoxide hydrochloride on human embryonic and fetal development. N Engl J Med 1974; 291:1268–1271.

35. St. Clair SM, Schirmer RG. First-trimester exposure to alprazolam. Obstet Gynecol 1992; 80:843–846.
36. Rosenberg L, Mitchell AA, Parsells JL, et al. Lack of relation of oral clefts to diazepam use during pregnancy. N Engl J Med 1983; 309:1282–1285.
37. Shiono PH, Mills IL. Oral clefts and diazepam use during pregnancy [letter]. N Engl J Med 1984; 311:919–920.
38. Altshuler LL, Cohen LS, Szuba MP, Burt VK, Gitlin M, Mintz J. Pharmacologic management of psychiatric illness in pregnancy: dilemmas and guidelines. Am J Psychiatry 1996; 153:592–606.
39. Cohen LS, Altshuler LL. Pharmacologic management of psychiatric illness during pregnancy and the postpartum period. Paychiatr Clin North Am 1997; 4:522–542.
40. Weinstock L. Clonazepam use during pregnancy. Presented at the annual meeting of the American Psychiatric Association, New York, 1996.
41. Rementaria JL, Blatt K. Withdrawal symptoms in neonates from intrauterine exposure to diazepam. J Pediatr 1977; 90:123–126.
42. Speight A. Floppy infant syndrome and maternal diazepam and/or nitrazepam [letter]. Lancet 1977; ii:878.
43. Fisher JB, Edgren BE, Mammel M. Neonatal apnea associated with maternal clonazepam therapy: a case report. Obstet Gynecol 1985; 66(Sept suppl):34–35.
44. Laegreid L, Olegard R, Conradi N, Hagberg G, Wahlstrom J, Abrahamsson L. Congenital malformations and maternal consumption of benzodiazepines: a case control study. Dev Med Child Neurol 1990; 32: 432–441.
45. Viggedal G, Hagberg BS, Laegreid L, Aronsson M. Mental development in late infancy after prenatal exposure to benzodiazepines: a prospective study. J Child Psychol Psychiatry 1993; 34:295–305.
46. Webster PAC. Withdrawal symptoms in neonates associated with maternal antidepressant therapy. Lancet 1973; ii:318–319.
47. Eggermont E. Withdrawal symptoms in neonates associated with maternal imipramine therapy. Lancet 1973; ii:680.
48. Cowe L, Lloyd DJ, Dawling S. Neonatal convulsions caused by withdrawal from maternal clomipramine. Br Med J 1982; 284:1837–1838.
49. Shearer WT, Schreiner RL, Marshall RE. Urinary retention in a neonate secondary to maternal ingestion of nortriptyline. J Pediatr 1972; 81:570–572.
50. Falterman LG, Richardson DJ. Small left colon syndrome associated

with maternal ingestion of psychotropic drugs. J Pediatr 1980; 97:300–310.

51. Pastuszak A, Schick-Boschetto B, Zuber C, et al. Pregnancy outcome following first-trimester exposure to fluoxetine (Prozac). JAMA 1993; 269:2246–2248.

52. McElhatton PR, Garbis HM, Elefant E, et al. The outcome of pregnancy in 689 women exposed to theraputic doses of antidepressants: a collaborative study of the European Network of Teratology Information Services (ENTIS). Reprod Toxicology 1996; 10:285–294.

53. Chambers CD, Johnson KA, Dick LM, Felix RJ, Jones KL. Birth outcomes in pregnant women taking fluoxetine. N Engl J Med 1996; 335:1010–1015.

54. Goldstein DJ, Corbin LA, Sundell KL. Effects of first-trimester fluoxetine exposure on the newborn. Obstet Gynecol 1997; 89:713–718.

55. Goldstein DJ. Effects of third trimester fluoxetine exposure on the newborn. J Clin Psychopharmacol 1995; 15:417–420.

56. Nulman I, Rovet G, Stewart DE, et al. Neurodevelopment of children exposed in utero to antidepressant drugs. N Engl J Med 1997; 336:258–262.

57. Inman W, Kobotu K, Pearce G, et al. Prescription event monitoring of paroxetine. Prescription Events Monitoring Reports 1993; PXL 1206:1–44.

58. Heinonen O, Sloan D, Shapiro S. Birth Defects and Drugs in Pregnancy. Littleton, MA: Publishing Services Group, 1977.

59. Alves SE, Akbari HM, Anderson GM, Azmitia EC, McEwen BC, Strand FL. Neonatal ACTH administration elicits long-term changes in forebrain monoamine innervation: subsequent disruptions in hypothalamic-pituitary-adrenal and gonadal function. Ann NY Acad Sci 1997; 814:226–251.

60. Uno H, Eisele S, Sakai A, Shelton S, Baker E, DeJesus O, Holden J. Neurotoxicity of glucocorticoids in the primate brain. Horm Behav 1994; 28:336–348.

61. Peters DAV. Maternal stress increases fetal stress and neonatal cortex 5-hydroxytryptophan synthesis in rats: a possible mechanism by which stress influences brain development. Pharmacol Biochem Behav 1990; 35:943–947.

62. Bhagwanani SG, Seagraves K, Dierker LJ, Lax M. Relationship between prenatal anxiety and perinatal outcome in nulliparous women: a prospective study. J Natl Med Assoc 1997; 89:93–98.

63. Weinberg MK. Impact of maternal psychiatric illness on infants. Pre-

sented at the annual meeting of the American Psychiatric Association, New York, 1996.

64. Robinson L, Walker JR, Anderson D. Cognitive-behavioural treatment of panic disorder during pregnancy and lactation. Can J Psychiatry 1992; 37:623–626.

65. Otto MW, Pollack MH, Sachs GS, et al. Discontinuation of benzodiazepine treatment: efficacy of cognitive-behavioral therapy for patients with panic disorder. Am J Psychiatry 1993; 150:1485–1490.

66. Riordah J. Drugs and breastfeeding. In: Riordan J, Auerbach KG, eds. Breastfeeding and Lactation. Boston: Bartlett and Jones, 1993:135–152.

67. Buist A, Norman TR, Dennerstein L. Breastfeeding and the use of psychotropic medication: a review. J Affect Disord 1990; 19:197–206.

68. Wisner K, Perel J, Findling R. Antidepressant treatment during brestfeeding. Am J Psychiatry 1996; 153:1132–1137.

69. American Academy of Pediatrics Committee on Drugs. The transfer of drugs and other chemicals into human milk. Pediatrics 1994; 93:137–149.

70. Cohen LS, Heller VL, Bailey J, Grush L, Rosenbaum JF. Birth outcomes following prenatal exposure to fluoxetine. Presented at the annual meeting of the American Psychiatric Association, San Diego, 1997.

71. Misri S, Sivertz k. Tricyclic drugs in pregnancy and lactation: a preliminary report. Int J Psychiatry Med 1991; 21:157–171.

72. Loebstein R, Koren G. Pregnancy outcome and neurodevelopment of children exposed in utero to psychoactive drugs: the Motherisk experience. J Psychiatry Neurosci 1997; 22:192–196.

9

Panic Disorder

Alcohol and Substance Abuse

James W. Jefferson and John H. Greist

Dean Foundation for Health, Research and Education
Middleton
and University of Wisconsin Medical School
Madison, Wisconsin

INTRODUCTION

Issues abound regarding the relationship between panic disorder and alcohol and other substance use disorders. Are they merely common disorders whose coexistence is explainable by chance alone? Is there an underlying diathesis that predisposes certain individuals toward both conditions? Do the anticipatory anxiety, panic attacks, and avoidance behaviors of panic disorder lead patients to ill-fated attempts at relief through self-medication with alcohol? After all, who can doubt Hippocrates, who said, ''Wine drunk with an equal quantity of water puts away anxiety and terrors'' (quoted in Ref. 1). Do the anxiety-promoting effects of alcohol use and withdrawal serve as catalysts for the subsequent emergence of panic disorder?

Fortunately, there has been no lack of interest in this topic in recent years (1–12). Unfortunately, despite valiant efforts by researchers and reviewers, many of these questions remain unanswered.

In this review, we 1) summarize the prevalence studies of panic disorder, alcohol, and other substance use disorders, and the comorbidity of these conditions, 2) explore reasons for the coexistence of these disorders, 3) present an overview of treatment approaches to dealing with comorbidity, and 4) make recommendations regarding future epidemiological, etiological, and therapeutic studies.

Before preceding, several points should be made. First, although the title of the chapter is "Panic Disorder: Alcohol and Substance Abuse," the vast majority of studies have focused on alcohol alone rather than other substances. In addition, in studies of substance use disorders (including alcohol), distinction is seldom made between abuse and dependence. Next, many studies are not panic-disorder-specific but rather address entities such as "anxiety," "anxiety disorders," "panic-related anxiety," "panic attacks," "panic states," and "agoraphobia." Furthermore, even when the diagnostic entity is the same across studies, the diagnostic methodologies used may differ and hence produce patient populations with the same names but different contents.

Not only is there great variation in diagnostic terminology but comparisons across studies are also difficult for reasons such as subject sources (general population surveys versus patient samples from inpatient or outpatient settings that focus on either anxiety disorders or substance use disorders, but less commonly on both). The phenomenon of "DSM drift" is a further complicating factor because diagnostic criteria change and the concept of diagnostic hierarchies is handled differently across editions of the *Diagnostic and Statistical Manual of Mental Disorders.* For example, DSM-III (1980) lacked a section on substance-induced anxiety disorders. DSM-III-R (1987) contained an Organic Anxiety Syndrome that included panic attacks and generalized anxiety under the category of Organic Mental Syndromes and Disorders. DSM-IV (1994) both separated Substance-Induced Disorders from Mental Disorders Due to a General Medical Condition and moved Substance-Induced Anxiety Disorder to the Anxiety Disorders section (where it now includes panic attacks, generalized anxiety, obsessive-compulsive symptoms, and phobic symptoms as specifers). Well before the successions of DSMs (and perhaps in anticipation of them), Chauncy Leake (13) made a prescient observation: "Let us remember always that whatever truth we may get by scientific study about ourselves and our environment is always relative, tentative, subject to change and correction, and that there are no final answers."

Additional problems with research design include reliance on memory to obtain retrospective information, interrater unreliability, small sample sizes that do not allow generalization, failure to control for additional comorbidities (e.g., depression), and lack of prospective design.

DOES A RELATIONSHIP EXIST?

Let us begin with two sentinel population surveys: the Epidemiologic Catchment Area (ECA) study (14) and the National Comorbidity Survey (NCS) (6,15–16). The ECA study examined the comorbidity of DSM-III mental disorders (including panic disorder and panic disorder with agoraphobia) and substance use disorders (particularly alcohol) in 20,291 individuals in community and institutional populations using a structured interview, the Diagnostic Interview Schedule (DIS) (14,17). Lifetime prevalence rates were 13.5% for alcohol abuse/dependence, 6.1% for other drug abuse/dependence, 5.2% for agoraphobia, 1.6% for panic disorder, and 0.5% for panic disorder with agoraphobia. In patients with a diagnosis of panic disorder, the odds ratio for a diagnosis of alcohol abuse/dependence was 2.6; for other drug abuse/dependence it was 3.2; and for any substance abuse/dependence it was 2.9. Prevalence rates for specific anxiety disorders were not given in those with a diagnosis of alcohol abuse/dependence, but the odds ratio for the presence of any anxiety disorder in this group was 1.5 (14). While comorbidity was common, it was far from universal. For example, DuPont (18) observed that in the ECA study almost three-quarters of people with anxiety disorders never had a substance use disorder diagnosed, and 80% of those with alcohol abuse/dependence and 72% of those with other drug abuse/dependence never had an anxiety disorder diagnosed.

A more detailed evaluation of the community ECA data included people with various anxiety disorder diagnoses who also had a lifetime history of alcohol abuse or dependence (17). The lifetime prevalence of alcohol abuse/dependence was 12.3% in those with agoraphobia without panic, 20.4% in those with panic disorder, and 31.5% in those with agoraphobia with panic attacks. The lower prevalence in those with agoraphobia without panic was attributed to an "oddity in the DIS" that may have miscategorized many individuals with simple phobia as having agoraphobia.

The NCS involved interviews with 8098 noninstitutionalized people (aged 15–54 years) in 48 states using a modification of the Composite International Diagnostic Interview (CIDI) to arrive at DSM-III-R diagnoses (16). Lifetime and 12-month prevalence figures for alcohol abuse and dependence are listed in Table 1. Overall, the lifetime prevalence of alcohol abuse without dependence was 9.4% and that of alcohol dependence was 14.1%. In individuals with a lifetime diagnosis of alcohol abuse or alcohol dependence, the lifetime comorbidities of panic disorder and agoraphobia are shown in Table 2. Overall, the comorbidity figures are higher for alcohol dependence than for alcohol abuse and for women than for men.

Other perspectives of the lifetime prevalence data from the NCS are provided in Tables 3 and 4 (6). These tables must be evaluated against the following overall NCS lifetime prevalence data (16):

Panic disorder	3.5%
Agoraphobia without panic disorder	5.3%
Alcohol abuse without dependence	9.4%
Alcohol dependence	14.1%
Drug abuse without dependence	4.4%
Drug dependence	7.5%
Any substance abuse/dependence	26.6%

With this in mind, the excessive comorbidity between panic disorder and substance abuse disorder is most apparent for alcohol dependence and for other drug dependence.

In summary, while the ECA and NCS comorbidity figures are not identical, both studies found a higher comorbidity than would be expected by chance between panic disorder and substance use disorders.

Table 1 Lifetime and 12-Month Prevalences of National Comorbidity Survey/DMS-III-R Alcohol Abuse and Dependence by Sex

Disorder	Lifetime prevalence				12-month prevalence			
	%	SE	No.	No.$_w$	%	SE	No.	No.$_w$
Alcohol abuse								
Men	12.5	0.8	482	503	3.4	0.4	141	138
Women	6.4	0.6	299	261	1.6	0.2	67	65
Total	9.4	0.5	**781**	**764**	2.5	0.2	**208**	**204**
Alcohol dependence								
Men	20.1	1.0	838	806	6.5	0.7	272	265
Women	8.2	0.7	374	336	2.2	0.3	91	91
Total	14.1	0.7	**1212**	**1142**	4.4	0.4	**363**	**356**

No. = unweighted number of respondents in the numerators of the prevalence estimates (the prevalence estimates, in comparison, are based on weighted data); No.$_w$ = weighted number of respondents in the numerators of the prevalence estimates.
Source: Ref. 15.

Table 2 Lifetime Prevalence of Panic Disorder and Agoraphobia in Men and Women with Alcohol Abuse or Alcohol Dependence Based on Data from the National Comorbidity Survey

	Diagnosis (% of subjects)			
	Alcohol abuse		Alcohol dependence	
	Panic disorder	Agoraphobia	Panic disorder	Agoraphobia
Men	1.6	5.1	3.6	6.5
Women	7.3	9.3	12.0	18.5

Source: Adapted from Ref. 15.

In a community survey of 3258 individuals in Edmonton, Canada, using the DIS to obtain DSM-III diagnoses, the lifetime prevalence of panic disorder was 1.2% (0.8% in men and 1.7% in women) (19). In the panic disorder population, the lifetime prevalence of alcohol abuse/dependence was 54.2% compared to 17.5% in the non-panic-disorder subjects. In addition, the panic disorder subjects were 6.7 times more likely to have a history of drug abuse/dependence (43% vs. 6.7%).

High comorbidity rates were also found in studies of patient populations (e.g., the prevalence of panic disorder in patients with substance use disorders and the prevalence of substance use disorders in patients with panic disorder). One might expect prevalence rates in studies of identified patients to be higher than in the general population because comorbid patients tend to be sicker and, therefore, more likely to seek medical attention.

PANIC DISORDER IN ALCOHOLICS

Schuckit and Hesselbrock (5) summarized the literature on anxiety disorders and alcoholism. They acknowledged potential problems in interpreting the data, including lack of diagnostic consistency, variable periods of abstinence prior to evaluation (early in the course of withdrawal, abstinence symptoms often include marked anxiety), failure to control for additional comorbidity, and reliance on patient recall as the only source of information. With this in mind, across 10 studies of

Table 3 Lifetime Prevalence of Panic Disorder and Agoraphobia in Individuals with Substance Use Disorders Based on Data from the National Comorbidity Survey

| | Diagnosis (% of subjects) | | | | |
	Alcohol abuse without dependence	Alcohol dependence	Other drug abuse without dependence	Other drug dependence	Any substance abuse without dependence
Panic disorder	3.7	6.2	5.4	10.5	5.5
Agoraphobia	6.7	10.3	6.4	15.5	9.3

Source: Adapted from Ref. 6.

Table 4 Lifetime Prevalence of Substance Use Disorders in Individuals with Panic Disorder or Agoraphobia Based on Data from the National Comorbidity Survey

	Diagnosis (% of subjects)	
	Panic disorder	Agoraphobia
Alcohol abuse without dependence	9.6	9.2
Alcohol dependence	24.4	21.4
Other drug abuse without dependence	6.6	4.2
Other drug dependence	22.5	17.5
Any substance abuse/dependence	41.2	36.5

Source: Adapted from Ref. 6.

alcoholics, they found a mean gross adjusted rate for panic disorder of 6% and for agoraphobia of 9%. While these percentages are higher than the prevalence of these disorders in the general population, they are not strikingly higher.

Cox et al. (7) also concluded from a summary of studies of "panic-related anxiety in alcoholics" that the prevalence is higher than in the general population. The studies reviewed were published between 1979 and 1990 (a range that spans DSM-II, -III, and -III-R) and included anxiety conditions such as panic attacks, panic disorder, phobias, agoraphobia, social phobia, and any anxiety disorder. Despite problems with diagnostic heterogeneity, the consensus of reviewers and investigators supports the conclusion that panic disorder is more common in individuals with alcohol abuse/dependence than would be expected based on the prevalence of these two conditions in the general population.

SUBSTANCE USE DISORDERS IN PATIENTS WITH PANIC DISORDER

Studies addressing the issue of comorbidity from the perspective of substance abuse/dependence in patients with anxiety disorders also suffer from diagnostic heterogeneity. Disorders listed by Kushner et al. in their review (4) include anxiety neurosis, social phobia, generalized anxiety disorder, agoraphobia, agoraphobia with panic attacks, and panic disorder. Based on these studies, they concluded that alcohol problems were more common in those diagnosed with agoraphobia or social phobia, but not in those with panic disorder, generalized anxiety disorder, or simple phobia.

Since then, additional studies have found a higher prevalence of alcohol abuse/dependence in panic disorder patients. In a naturalistic study of 100 patients being treated for panic disorder, Otto et al. (20) found a 24% lifetime prevalence of alcohol dependence, although only one patient was actively alcoholic. When the rates of alcohol dependence were compared with those found in the ECA study, they were elevated in women but not men. Finally, the investigators found no association between the presence or absence of agoraphobia and alcohol dependence. A French study of 100 outpatients with panic disorder found a 31% lifetime prevalence of alcohol or other substance abuse (37.8% in men and 27% in women) (21).

All in all, the weight of evidence suggests a higher comorbidity of alcohol and other substance abuse/dependence in panic disorder patients than expected by chance alone, although there is not universal agreement about this conclusion. For example, Schuckit and Hesselbrock (5) state that ''most of the studies do not convincingly demonstrate higher rates of alcoholism [defined differently in different studies] among patients with anxiety disorders, even among those with panic disorder.''

WHICH CAME FIRST AND WHY

When two conditions coexist, the order of onset suggests the possibility that the first may cause the second. This would be especially true if the order differed from the usual age of onset of each disorder when it occurs independently. According to DSM-IV (22), the age of onset of alcohol dependence peaks in the 20s to mid-30s whereas the age of onset of panic disorder is quite similar—''most typically between late adolescence and the mid-30s.''

Most studies that have explored the temporal relationship between panic disorder and substance use disorders relied on the memories of those interviewed to assign a date to the onset of their illnesses. In addition to the unreliability of memory, date of onset is further clouded by differences in time between onset of symptoms and onset of a formal diagnostic entity (6). If one adds to these problems the abovementioned difficulties with diagnostic heterogeneity, it appears that clear resolution of the question of which came first may not be possible. Kushner et al. (4) concluded: ''Panic disorder and obsessive-compulsive disorder, according to the studies reviewed, may typically begin before, after, or at the same time as alcohol problems.'' Schuckit and Hesselbrock (5) refer initially to several studies in which the anxiety disorder predated the alcohol disorder in 40–60% of subjects, but later state that if ''more rigorous'' studies are considered, ''it is the alcohol-related syndromes that appeared first.''

In their study of 100 panic disorder patients, Otto et al. (20) found that the average age of onset was 23.7 years for alcohol dependence and 29.8 years for panic disorder, and that in 83.3% of their patients alcohol dependence came first. Other observations that require further substantiation include an earlier age of onset of panic disorder in patients with preexisting alcohol/drug abuse (23), an increased rate of panic disorder in early-onset alcoholics (24), and an earlier age of onset of substance use disorder when anxiety disorders occur before age 21 (25).

Now that most readers are thoroughly confused, let us summarize this section on epidemiology.

1. Do panic disorder and substance use disorders (particularly alcohol) coexist to an extent greater than expected by chance? *Answer:* yes.

2. Is the prevalence of panic disorder greater in individuals with substance use disorders (particularly alcohol) than in the general population? *Answer:* yes.

3. Is the prevalence of substance use disorders (particularly alcohol) greater in individuals with panic disorder than in the general population? *Answer:* possibly.

4. When comorbidity exists between panic disorder and substance use disorders (particularly alcohol), is there a clear consensus about which disorder occurs first? *Answer:* no.

WHY IS COMORBIDITY INCREASED?

Theories abound that attempt to explain the increased comorbidity of panic disorder and substance use disorders. As do most theories in psychiatry, they incorporate psychological and biological conjectures without providing definitive answers.

The Self-Medication Hypothesis

The self-medication hypothesis posits that anxious people drink because alcohol makes them feel less anxious. Marks (26) refers to Westphal's observation in 1871 that "the use of beer or wine allowed the [agoraphobic] patient to pass through the feared locality with comfort." In a more recent study of agoraphobics, Bibb and Chambless (27) reported that many of their patients drank to control anxiety and that they were motivated to drink because it made them feel more normal.

While this theory makes intuitive sense, attempts to confirm it have produced equivocal results. Schuckit and Hesselbrock (5) point out that even in individuals who report that their anxiety condition preceded the alcohol disorder, careful confirmational studies have shown in up to two-thirds of them that the reverse was actually the case. Wilson, in an invited essay (28), addressed the broad topic of anxiety and alcohol. He points out that studies have variously shown alcohol to increase, decrease, and have no effect on anxiety. Confounding variables included alcohol dose, environmental setting, and individual differences. One individual difference, of course, is whether an anxiety disorder is present and, if so, which anxiety disorder. He speculates that alcohol may be most effective in reducing anxiety characterized by a strong cognitive component such as the anticipatory anxiety of agoraphobia.

Studies in both animals and humans have generally found that alcohol had an acute anxiety/tension-reducing effect (28). When patients with panic disorder were given either alcohol or placebo under single-blind conditions (they were told they were getting alcohol on both occasions) and challenged with carbon dioxide inhalation, they had less anxiety and fewer panic attacks after ingesting alcohol. Nonetheless, the authors acknowledge that "a confluence of factors acts to either promote or inhibit drinking among those with panic" (28).

The potential benefit of alcohol as an anxiety reducer must be weighed against evidence that alcohol can also be an anxiety inducer. Kushner et al. (4) summarized support for this observation pointing out that prolonged alcohol consumption, high doses of alcohol, and alcohol withdrawal have all been linked to increased anxiety. Obviously, the misuse of alcohol can lead to conflicts with society that in turn can exacerbate stress and anxiety.

All in all, the self-medication hypothesis may explain why some anxiety disorder patients use and misuse alcohol, but it is far from a universal answer. As summarized by Wilson (28), "The really important conclusion from the wealth of experimentation the anxiety reducing theory has generated is the absence of an automatic and constant effect of alcohol on anxiety. Rather, alcohol's effects on anxiety . . . including subsequent drinking by non-abusing and abusing drinkers, are conditional on a wide range of biological, psychological, and social influences."

The Alcohol-Causes-Panic Hypothesis

This possibility can be addressed from several perspectives. As mentioned above, alcohol misuse/overuse may cause or worsen anxiety symptoms (4). More specifically, it has been suggested that a succession of alcohol withdrawals may have a kindling-like effect on the central nervous system so that anxiety or panic symptoms occur with greater and greater ease until they eventually develop a life of their own (3). A similar possibility was suggested in a report of three patients whose panic attacks, while initially cocaine-induced, continued spontaneously after drug discontinuation (29). George et al. (3) further propose that conditioned tolerance, a process by which the sedative effects of alcohol may be adapted to by a state of hyperarousal, might contribute to the panicogenic effects of alcoholic kindling. These processes could be invoked to explain the observation in 54 patients that panic disorder tended to have an earlier age of onset in those with a prior history of alcohol or other substance abuse (23).

Whether the panic disorder of alcoholics differs in some intrinsic fashion from the panic disorder of nonalcoholics is unclear. While George et al. (30) found fewer lactate infusion-induced panic attacks in the former group, Cowley et al. (31) found no such difference.

Other Observations of Etiopathological Interest

Cerebrospinal fluid (CSF) was examined in alcoholics with panic disorder, alcoholics without panic disorder, and controls (but not in nonalcoholics with panic disorder) (32). No differences were found with the exception of increased β-endorphin levels in the panic group after correction for the effects of weight, height, and age. This observation led the authors to speculate that "alcoholic patients with panic disorder may have a dysregulation in the interaction between adrenergic and β-endorphin systems."

Another study investigated behavioral and neuroendocrine responses to intravenous clomipramine in a small number of patients with alcohol dependence alone, with panic disorder alone, and with both conditions, as well as in normal controls (33). No neuroendocrine differences were noted across groups, but both groups with panic disorder had more dysphoria and anxiety from clomipramine (perhaps suggesting that panic disorder is panic disorder whether or not alcohol is involved).

As might be expected, both norepinephrine (NE) and gamma-aminobutyric acid (GABA) have been implicated in the panic/anxiety/alcohol intermix, but no firm conclusions have been reached (1,3,34).

IS THERE A GENETIC LINK?

Do family studies show an increased risk for substance use disorders in relatives of probands with panic disorder? Is there an increased risk of panic disorder in relatives of probands with substance use disorders? The answer to both questions is "maybe."

Before discussing data, it would be wise to point out methodological problems in some studies (5). For example, family history information obtained only from the proband is likely to be quite unreliable. Directly interviewing all biological relatives is a much more productive approach, yet it is more time-consuming and expensive. Also, there may be great variability in the methods used to obtain diagnoses. Next, some relatives who are destined to develop a particular condition may be interviewed before the onset of the disorder. Finally, failure to control for comorbidity in the proband may distort interpretation of results.

With these considerations in mind, Schuckit and Hesselbrock (5) conclude that "a review of the literature does not indicate a consistent family crossover between alcoholism and anxiety disorders once morbidity in the proband is controlled for and appropriate assessment methods and criteria are used." They leave the door open, however, to the possibility that "a modest level of crossover might be seen in some pedigrees." In their study involving direct structured interviews of 591 first-degree relatives of alcohol-dependent individuals, they found a lifetime risk for panic disorder of only 3.4% and for agoraphobia of only 1.4% (35).

From the opposite perspective, face-to-face interviews of 78% of first-degree relatives of 40 patients with noncomorbid panic disorder uncovered a greater risk of alcoholism compared to relatives of healthy controls (17.5% versus 7.8%). The difference was more pronounced when the proband had panic disorder with agoraphobia (25%) than panic disorder alone (11.9%) (36). In a similar study, however, the apparent aggregation of alcohol abuse/dependence in relatives of probands with panic disorder appears to have been accounted for by comorbidity in the probands (37).

All in all, while there may be a genetic link between panic disorder and alcohol abuse/dependence, such a link has not yet been forged to a high degree of certainty.

WHAT ABOUT NON-ALCOHOLIC SUBSTANCE ABUSE/ DEPENDENCE AND PANIC DISORDER?

While alcohol has been the major focus of panic disorder/substance use disorder studies, a small body of literature exists on other drugs. As summarized by Cox et al. (7), the onset of "panic-related anxiety" has been associated with the use of cocaine, amphetamines, hallucinogens, inhalants, oxymetazoline nasal spray, and marijuana. A study using brain-electrical activity mapping (BEAM) found an increased use of stimulants in patients with panic disorder and prior drug abuse compared to prior drug abuse patients without panic disorder (38). In a subsample of the ECA study subjects, there was an increased risk of panic attacks in cocaine users compared to nonusers (39).

The Harvard-Brown Anxiety Disorders Project (HARP) explored the lifetime history of substance abuse/dependence in groups that included patients with uncomplicated panic, panic with agoraphobia, and agoraphobia without panic. Small sample sizes within specific anxiety groups and within specific substance use groups limited conclusions. Overall, however, a tendency to avoid CNS stimulants was noted in those with anxiety disorders (40).

In general, the stimulant-type drugs are not favored by individuals with panic disorder, probably because such drugs worsen the condition. Whether stimulants play an etiological role in the genesis of panic disorder is unclear (see above).

The self-medication hypothesis with regard to alcohol use in panic disorder patients has been difficult to prove, and confirming a similar hypothesis involving sedative/hypnotic abuse has been even more difficult. In HARP (40), the odds ratio for a lifetime co-occurence of sedative use disorder was 0.7 in uncomplicated panic, 1.4 in panic with agoraphobia, and 1.6 in agoraphobia without panic. The authors concluded that these figures were not particularly persuasive in terms of establishing a relationship. The issue of whether treatment of panic disorder with benzodiazepines increases the risk of an anxiolytic use disorder is discussed below.

TREATMENT

After all is said and done, it matters little to a clinician faced with a patient with substance abuse/dependence and panic disorder whether the two conditions coexist to a degree greater than expected by chance or whether there are plausible hypotheses to explain the comorbidity. Rather, the clinician is most concerned about how to treat the patient effectively and safely. If the clinician searches for data-oriented studies to guide such treatment, none will be found. The investigational trials that bring antipanic drugs to market invariably exclude patients with a current or recent history of substance abuse/dependence. This has also been the case in most studies of cognitive-behavioral approaches to the treatment of panic disorder. Fortunately, both common sense and the recommendations of experienced clinicians can do much to offer guidance (8,12,18,41,42).

Despite early optimistic observations, admittedly tentative, that imipramine treatment of a "phobic anxiety syndrome" would also resolve coexisting sedative or alcohol dependency (43), most experts agree that a two-pronged approach to treatment is necessary. Obviously, such an approach requires identification of both conditions. While it is likely that the probability of getting treatment is increased in the presence of a dual diagnosis (6), it is not always the case that both diagnoses are readily revealed. Hence, clinicians must be always alert to the possibility that the presenting diagnosis is not the only diagnosis and that one or more additional conditions may lurk beneath the surface. Especially considering the strong use of denial by many substance abusers, involvement of significant others becomes diagnostically (and therapeutically) important. In addition, the use of computer-administered screening interviews utilizing either desktop computers or touch-tone telephones and interactive voice response (IVR) technology should add substantially to the diagnostic yield (44).

DuPont (41) suggests not getting overly involved in developing treatment strategies based on which disorder came first; rather, he states, "The clinician's goal is to identify both disorders and to provide fully effective treatments for both conditions." There is general agreement, however, that treatment of active substance abuse/dependence should take priority, in part because resolution of anxiety/panic symptoms often occurs after withdrawal is complete and a period of sobriety has been achieved. One must also bear in mind that the risk of suicide attempts in panic disorder patients is increased in the presence of a history of substance abuse and/or major depression (21). Appropriate safety precautions should be taken.

If panic attacks persist during sobriety and the diagnosis of panic disorder is confirmed, the standard pharmacological and nonpharmacological approaches to treatment can be pursued. Failure to treat panic disorder effectively can certainly sabotage a substance abuse program both because of the high level of distress caused by the disorder and because agoraphobic avoidance can compromise the ability to attend group meetings such as Alcoholics or Narcotics Anonymous.

The pharmacological approach to panic disorder may require modification in the presence of a substance use disorder. Most experts advise against using benzodiazepines in abuse-prone individuals

(12,41,42), especially if there has not been a long intervening period of sobriety. Nonetheless, when Caraulo et al. (45) reviewed the abuse liability of benzodiazepines in alcoholics, their conclusion was not that cut-and-dried. While they agreed that alcoholics were at greater risk for benzodiazepine abuse, they felt that ''benzodiazepines are relatively safe drugs with many uses in the treatment of alcoholics when prescribed rationally.'' Rational prescription, incidently, is what you always do with your patients, but what your colleagues invariably fail to do with theirs. If benzodiazepines are to be used, those with slower onsets of action (lower lipid solubility) are preferred because they are less abusable (for example, clonazepam or oxazepam rather than alprazolam or diazepam) (45,46). Abuse issues aside, the mixing of benzodiazepines and alcohol is likely to produce serious impairment of judgment, cognition, coordination, and reaction time.

The antidepressant antipanic drugs—selective serotonin-reuptake inhibitors (SSRIs), tricyclics, and monoamine oxidase inhibitors (MAOIs)—have little in the way of abuse potential (there is, however, a small body of literature on tranylcypromine abuse), but there are some potential concerns about their use in patients with substance abuse/dependence. Alcohol-related liver disease may impair metabolism of many of these drugs, and hypoproteinemia may reduce protein binding (the same is true of some benzodiazepines). Unlike the tricyclics, the SSRIs have the advantage of not increasing the adverse mental and motoric effects of alcohol. The MAOIs present the potential for life-threatening interactions with a number of abusable substances such as stimulants, certain opiates, and high tyramine-containing alcoholic beverages.

In the real world, clinicians may be faced with the need to initiate therapy for panic disorder in patients who have not achieved full abstinence from their alcohol or other substance use habits. In such cases, one must tread cautiously, and it would be wise to work preferentially with the antipanic drugs (e.g., SSRIs) that are least likely to interact adversely with substances of abuse. Whether certain anticonvulsants could play a useful role in such situations is unclear. Both valproate and gabapentin have shown some promise as antipanic drugs (the substantiation of which remains to be established). While it may be wise to avoid using valproate in the presence of alcohol-induced hepatic dysfunction, gabapentin (no hepatic metabolism) should be safe under such circumstances (whether it would be effective is another question).

In general, substance use disorders complicate the treatment of panic disorder, but they do not necessarily present overwhelming obstacles to determined clinicians. Despite early expectations to the contrary, successfully treating one condition is unlikely to automatically result in the secondary resolution of the other. Unless a clinician is particularly adept at the comprehensive treatment of both panic disorder and substance use disorders, a multidisciplinary approach is more likely to be effective (although possibly more difficult to implement in a managed-care environment).

RECOMMENDATIONS

Epidemiological studies examining the comorbidity between panic disorder and substance use disorders are likely to continue, but they are unlikely to produce major advances in the field. The next DSM edition may introduce changes in diagnostic criteria that would result in the next generation of epidemiological studies having little similarity to those that came before. On the other hand, advances in the areas of molecular genetics, neuroimaging, and neurochemistry may well promote greater understanding of the complex relationships between these two conditions.

There is a clear need for clinical research that specifically addresses the treatment of patients with panic disorder and substance use disorders. It has been unfortunate, thus far, that what is a relatively common "real-life" problem has generated so little attention from funding sources and from qualified clinical investigators. A recent study that found benefit from fluoxetine in the treatment of depressed alcoholics (both depressive symptoms and alcohol consumption decreased on fluoxetine compared to placebo) is an encouraging step in the right direction (47). Similar results were noted when imipramine was compared with placebo under double-blind conditions in 69 depressed, actively drinking alcoholics (48). Depression improved, there were no serious adverse events, and mood improvement was linked to reduced alcohol consumption. The outcomes of these studies are grounds for cautious optimism and should serve as a stimulus for further research in this area that might examine the treatment of panic disorder in active substance abusers.

REFERENCES

1. Cowley DS. Alcohol abuse, substance abuse, and panic disorder. Am J Med 1992; 92(suppl 1A):1A-41S–1A-48S.
2. Marshall JR. Alcohol and substance abuse in panic disorder. J Clin Psychiatry 1997; 58(suppl 2):46–50.
3. George DT, Nutt DJ, Dwyer BA, Linnoila M. Alcoholism and panic disorder: is the comorbidity more than coincidence? Acta Psychiatr Scand 1990; 81:97–107.
4. Kushner MG, Sher KJ, Beitman BD. The relation between alcohol problems and the anxiety disorders. Am J Psychiatry 1990; 147:685–695.
5. Schuckit MA, Hesselbrock V. Alcohol dependence and anxiety disorders: what is the relationship? Am J Psychiatry 1994; 151:1723–1734.
6. Kessler RC, Nelson CB, McGonagle KA, Edlund MJ, Frank RG, Leaf PJ. The epidemiology of co-occurring addictive and mental disorders: implications for prevention and service utilization. Am J Orthopsychiatry 1996; 66:17–31.
7. Cox BJ, Norton GR, Swinson RP, Endler NS. Substance abuse and panic-related anxiety: a critical review. Behav Res Ther 1990; 28:385–393.
8. Brown TA, Barlow DH. Comorbidity among anxiety disorders: implications for treatment and DSM-IV. J Consult Clin Psychol 1992; 60:835–844.
9. Kushner MG, Mackenzie TB, Fiszdon J, Valentiner DP, Foa E, Anderson N, Wangensteen D. The effects of alcohol comsumption on laboratory-induced panic and state anxiety. Arch Gen Psychiatry 1996; 53:264–270.
10. Cox BJ, Norton GR, Dorward J, Fergusson PA. The relationship between panic attacks and chemical dependencies. Addict Behav 1989; 14:53–60.
11. Maier W, Minges J, Lichtermann D. Alcoholism and panic disorder: co-occurrence and co-transmission in families. Eur Arch Psychiatry Clin Neurosci 1993; 243:205–211.
12. John S, Miller NS. Anxiety disorders and addictions. In: Miller NS, ed.

The Principles and Practice of Addictions in Psychiatry. Philadelphia: Saunders, 1997; 249–254.

13. Leake CD. Unity and communication in science and the health professions. NY State J Med 1960; 60:1496–1500.

14. Regier DA, Farmer ME, Rae DS, Locke BZ, Keith SJ, Judd LL, Goodwin FK. Comorbidity of mental disorders with alcohol and other drug abuse. JAMA 1990; 264:2511–2518.

15. Kessler RC, Crum RM, Warner LA, Nelson CB, Schulenberg J, Anthony JC. Lifetime co-occurrence of DSM-III-R alcohol abuse and dependence with other psychiatric disorders in the National Comorbidity Survey. Arch Gen Psychiatry 1997; 54:313–321.

16. Kessler RC, McGonagle KA, Zhao S, Nelson CB, Hughes M, Eshleman S, Wittchen HU, Kendler KS. Lifetime and 12-month prevalence of DSM-III-R psychiatric disorders in the United States. Arch Gen Psychiatry 1994; 51:8–19.

17. Himle JA, Hill EM. Alcohol abuse and the anxiety disorders: evidence from the Epidemiologic Catchment Area Survey. J Anx Dis 1991; 5: 237–245.

18. DuPont RL. Anxiety and addiction: a clinical perspective on comorbidity. Bull Menninger Clin 1995; 59(suppl A):A53–A72.

19. Dick CL, Bland RC, Newman SC. Panic disorder. Acta Psychiatr Scan 1994:376(suppl):45–53.

20. Otto MW, Pollack MH, Sachs GS, O'Neil CA, Rosenbaum JF. Alcohol dependence in panic disorder patients. J Psychiatr Res 1992; 26:29–38.

21. Lepine JP, Chignon JM, Teherani M. Suicide attempts in patients with panic disorder. Arch Gen Psychiatry 1993; 50:144–149.

22. Diagnostic and Statistical Manual of Mental Disorders. 4th ed. Washington, DC: American Psychiatric Association Press, 1994.

23. Starcevic V, Uhlenhuth EH, Kellner R, Pathak D. Comorbidity in panic disorder. II. Chronology of appearance and pathogenic comorbidity. Psychiatry Res 1993; 46:285–293.

24. Roy A, DeJong J, Lamparski D, Adinoff B, George T, Moore V, Garnett D, Kerich M, Linnoila M. Mental disorders among alcoholics. Arch Gen Psychiatry 1991; 48:423–427.

25. Burke JD, Burke KC, Rae DS. Increased rates of drug abuse and dependence after onset of mood or anxiety disorders in adolescence. Hosp Commun Psychiatry 1994; 45:451–455.

26. Marks IM. Fears, Phobias, and Rituals. New York: Oxford University Press, 1987.

27. Bibb JL, Chambless DL. Alcohol use and abuse among diagnosed agoraphobics. Behav Res Ther 1986; 24:49–58.
28. Wilson GT. Alcohol and anxiety. Behav Res Ther 1988; 26:369–381.
29. Aronson TA, Craig TJ. Cocaine precipitation of panic disorder. Am J Psychiatry 1986; 143:643–645.
30. George DT, Nutt DJ, Waxman RP, Linnoila M. Panic response to lactate administration in alcoholic and nonalcoholic patients with panic disorder. Am J Psychiatry 1989; 146:1161–1165.
31. Cowley DS, Jensen CF, Johannessen D, Parker L, Dager SR, Walker RD. Response to sodium lactate infusion in alcoholics with panic attacks. Am J Psychiatry 1989; 146:1479–1483.
32. George DT, Adinoff B, Ravitz B, Nutt DJ, DeJong J, Berrettini W, Mefford IN, Costa E, Linnoila M. A cerbrospinal fluid study of the pathophysiology of panic disorder associated with alcoholism. Acta Psychiatr Scand 1990; 82:1–7.
33. George DT, Nutt DF, Rawlings RR, Phillips MJM, Eckardt MJ, Potter WZ, Linnoila M. Biol Psychiatry 1995; 37:112–119.
34. Linnoila MI. Anxiety and alcoholism. J Clin Psychiatry 1989; 50(suppl): 26–29.
35. Schuckit MA, Hesselbrock VM, Tipp J, Nurnberger JI, Anthenelli RM, Crowe RR. The prevalence of major anxiety disorders in relatives of alcohol dependent men and women. J Stud Alcohol 1995; 56:309–317.
36. Maier W, Lichtermann D, Minges J, Oehrlein, Franke P. A controlled family study in panic disorder. J Psychiatr Res 1993; 27:79–87.
37. Goldstein RB, Weissman MM, Adams PB, Horwath E, Lish JD, Charney D, Woods SW, Sobin C, Wickramaratne PJ. Psychiatric disorders in relatives of probands with panic disorder and/or major depression. Arch Gen Psychiatry 1994; 51:383–394.
38. Abraham HD, Duffy FH. Computed EEG abnormalities in panic disorder with and without premorbid drug abuse. Biolog Psychiatry 1991; 29: 687–690.
39. Anthony JC, Tien AY, Petronis KR. Epidemiologic evidence on cocaine use and panic attacks. Am J Epidemiol 1989; 129:543–549.
40. Goldenberg IM, Mueller T, Fierman EJ, Gordon A, Pratt L, Cox K, Park T, Lavori P, Goisman RM, Keller MB. Compr Psychiatry 1995; 36:319–328.
41. DuPont RL. Panic disorder and addiction: the clinical issues of comorbidity. Bull Menninger Clinic 1997; 61(suppl A):A54–A65.
42. Frances RJ, Borg L. The treatment of anxiety in patients with alcoholism. J Clin Psychiatry 1993; 54(suppl):37–43.

43. Quitkin FM, Rifkin A, Kaplan J, Klein DF. Phobic anxiety syndrome complciated by drug dependence and addiction. Arch Gen Psychiatry 1972; 27:159–162.
44. Kobak KA, Taylor LvH, Dottl SL, Greist JH, Jefferson JW, Burroughs D, Katzelnick DJ, Mandell M. Computerized screening of psychiatric disorders in an outpatient community mental health clinic. Psychiatr Serv 1997; 48:1048–1057.
45. Ciraulo DA, Sands BF, Shader RI. Critical review of liability for benzodiazepine abuse among alcoholics. Am J Psychiatry 1988; 145:1502–1506.
46. Baron DH, Sands BF, Ciraulo DA, Shader RI. The diagnosis and treatment of panic disorder in alcoholics: three cases. Am J Drug Alcohol Abuse 1990; 16:287–295.
47. Cornelius JR, Salloum IM, Ehler JG, Jarrett PJ, Cornelius MD, Perel JM, Thase ME, Black A. Fluoxetine in depressed alcoholics. Arch Gen Psychiatry 1997; 54:700–705.
48. McGrath PJ, Nunes EV, Steward JW, Goldman D, Agosti V, Ocepek-Welikson K, Quitkin FM. Imipramine treatment of alcoholics with primary depression. Arch Gen Psychiatry 1996; 53:232–240.

10

Panic Disorder, Quality of Life, and Managed Care

Cost-Effectiveness and Treatment Choices

Kathryn M. Connor and Jonathan R. T. Davidson
Duke University
Durham, North Carolina

INTRODUCTION

Panic disorder has been associated with the highest rates of utilization of general medical, emergency, and mental health services when compared to patients with other psychiatric diagnoses. Patients with panic disorder frequently present to nonpsychiatric care providers with multiple medical symptoms that often, after extensive work-up, defy medical explanation and further frustrate patients and their care providers. These evaluations are costly to both the patient and the health care system. In economic terms, unnecessary expenses are incurred by elaborate work-ups and a delay in diagnosis. The social costs impact directly on the patient's quality of life, including domains of personal happiness, role fulfillment, and health status, and indirectly increase the economic burden through lost productivity. Panic disorder is amenable to treatment, however, and treated patients report improved functioning and reduced health care utilization. With early recognition and treatment of patients with panic disorder, social and economic savings could be passed not only to the patient but also to society through a reduction in managed health care expenditures and improved productivity.

In this chapter, we examine quality-of-life (QOL) issues and associated cost factors in patients with panic disorder in the era of managed health care. QOL measures are described and their importance in assessing treatment outcomes discussed. The magnitude of panic disorder in the community and in specific treatment-seeking medical and mental health populations is reviewed. Studies of the QOL in patients with panic disorder are then examined. The cost-effectiveness of treatment is assessed and available therapeutic options are presented. Finally, the role of managed care in identifying panic patients and facilitating treatment to reduce the social and economic costs of panic disorder is discussed.

QUALITY-OF-LIFE MEASURES

QOL may be conceptualized holistically, with an emphasis on the positive aspects of health, rather than on pathology or problems, and on subjective perspectives of the individual. Measures of QOL generally include domains of personal happiness, role fulfillment, and health status. Personal happiness is assessed through reports of the following variables: satisfactory and/or supportive relationships; adequacy of social network; satisfaction in religious and spiritual beliefs; freedom from despair, ideas of suicide, and attempted suicide; and freedom from use of alcohol or illicit drugs. The second domain, role fulfillment, encompasses areas of work adjustment, family functioning, and leisure. Work adjustment may be characterized by employment status, work attendance, productivity, and days of sick leave. Family functioning describes one's ability to carry out expected roles within the family unit, such as homemaking, parenting, fiscal duties, and spousal obligations. Leisure is a more loosely defined concept, but may include time spent on hobbies and social activities and with friends and/or relatives and number of available friends. The third domain, health status, is composed of measures of both general and mental health. Of these three domains, health status has received the most attention, including studies of the following variables: number of medical or psychiatric visits, number of visits to other health care providers or counselors, number of emergency room and hospital visits, use of laboratory tests, use of medication, general physical and psychological health status, number of days in bed, and limitations on physical or mental functioning. Another measure often included in health status is that of vitality, as a measure of perceived energy or fatigue.

Together, these domains of QOL characterize or describe what the patient has experienced as the result of medical care. Measures of QOL may thus serve as useful and important adjuncts to more traditional measures of health status (i.e, physiological, biological, behavioral). However, unlike these more traditional measures of health status, there are currently no standard measures of QOL.

The most widely implemented measure of QOL is the Short-form Health Survey (SF-36) (1), a 36-item questionnaire, originally developed for use in medical outcome studies, that has been psychometrically validated (2,3). The SF-36 is a self-rated scale composed of physical and mental component scales, each of which is divided into four subscales. The Physical Component Scale (PCS) includes items assessing physical functioning, physical health role limits, body pain, and general health perceptions. In contrast, the Mental Component Scale (MCS) consists of questions about social functioning, emotionally related health limitations, vitality, and general mental health subscales.

Several other instruments are currently in use in medical outcome studies or are under development. For example, the Work Productivity Impairment (WPI) questionnaire measures the effects of health status and symptom severity on work productivity (4). To date, this instrument has been validated in one sample of physically ill subjects. Another instrument, the Diagnostic Interview Schedule (DIS), was designed for use in the National Institute of Mental Health (NIMH)-sponsored Epidemiologic Catchment Area (ECA) study conducted in the early 1980s (5). Although not designed as an instrument to specifically assess QOL, the DIS contains items designed to evaluate QOL, general medical and psychological health status, and health service utilization. In recent years, the World Health Organization has also undertaken the development of an instrument to assess quality of life measures (6). Initially planned to complement the tenth edition of the International Classification of Diseases (ICD-10), this instrument remains under development.

In summary, studies examining the relationship between symptoms and dimensions of functioning recognize that the demonstrated variations in functioning cannot be fully explained by biological and physiological variables alone. QOL measures characterize distinct aspects of health status and can assist in identifying important differences not otherwise detected by more traditional clinical variables.

THE PREVALENCE OF PANIC DISORDER

Prevalence estimates for panic disorder vary greatly depending on the population studied: community vs. specialty clinic, age, gender, treatment-seeking individuals vs. non-treatment-seeking. Findings from the ECA study revealed that the prevalence of panic disorder among adults in the community was between 1.2% for current panic disorder and 3.6% for lifetime panic disorder (7). These estimates may actually be low, however, in that—based on criteria defined by the third edition of the *Diagnostic and Statistical Manual for Mental Disorder* (DSM-III)—subjects who reported panic symptoms but concomitantly met criteria for major depression were not diagnosed with panic disorder (8). In a study of inner-city working-class and single mothers in the United Kingdom, the prevalence of panic disorder was estimated at 3.34% and was highly associated with adversity in childhood (9). Other international data support a lifetime prevalence of panic disorder of at least 1% (10,11).

Panic disorder is more common in treatment-seeking samples. Given the wide range of potential somatic experiences in panic disorder, these individuals often present to primary care providers or specialists (e.g., cardiologists, gastroenterologists, pulmonologists) for initial treatment. In a study of outpatients in a cardiology practice, Goldberg and colleagues (12) reported a prevalence of current panic disorder of 9.2%, considerably higher than community estimates of 1 to 3%. In a study of cardiology outpatients with chest pain without objective evidence of coronary artery disease (CAD), 33% had panic disorder and 24% simple panic, while 59% of subjects with atypical or nonanginal chest pain and normal coronary arteries met criteria for panic disorder (13). In another study of cardiac outpatients, 47% of CAD-negative subjects evidenced panic disorder in contrast to 6% of subjects with documented CAD. In a subsample of 26 subjects with panic disorder, 88.5% were without evidence of CAD (14).

The prevalence of panic disorder in primary care settings varies as well. Among distressed, high utilizers of health care services in an HMO primary care practice, Katon et al. (15) reported a prevalence of 11.8% for panic disorder in the last year and 30.2% for a lifetime history of panic disorder.

Elevated rates of panic disorder are also observed in mental health samples, due in part to increased sensitivity for making a diagnosis of panic disorder and in part because patients with recognized panic disorder may be referred to a mental health setting for treatment.

QUALITY OF LIFE IN PANIC DISORDER
IN THE COMMUNITY

Data concerning the QOL in subjects with panic disorder in the community are limited to the findings from the ECA study. Using the DIS, information pertaining to QOL issues was collected and, for the first time in an epidemiological sample, associations with mental illnesses were explored. The findings of these studies are summarized in Table 1, and a brief review of these data follows.

In the ECA study, panic disorder was associated with a variety of adverse social and health consequences. Markowitz et al. (16) reported that these consequences were similar to or greater than those observed in major depression, including significantly higher rates of poor physical health, poor emotional health, alcohol and drug abuse, and attempted suicide. Impairment in role fulfillment was demonstrated through marital dysfunction (e.g., not getting along with partner, seldomly or never confiding in or telling worries to partner) and financial dependency, with 27% of subjects with panic disorder receiving welfare or disability assistance at the time of the interview. Subjects with

Table 1 The Prevalence of Panic Disorder: Community Studies

Author	Population	Diagnostic instrument	Findings
Markowitz et al., 1989 (15)	ECA study: sample from 5 U.S. communities (N > 18,000)	DIS	A diagnosis of panic disorder was associated with pervasive social and health consequences (i.e., subjective feelings of poor physical and emotional health, alcohol and other drug abuse, increased likelihood of suicide attempts, impaired social and marital functioning, financial dependency, and increased use of psychoactive medications, health services, and hospital emergency department for emotional problems) similar to or greater than those associated with major depression. These findings were not explained by comorbid mental illness.
Klerman et al., 1991 (7)	ECA study: sample from 5 U.S. communities (N > 18,000)	DIS	The lifetime community prevalence of panic attacks not meeting full diagnostic criteria for panic disorder was 3.6% of the adult population. These individuals had impairment in perceived physical and emotional health, in occupational and financial functioning, increased use of health care facilities, emergency departments, and psychoactive drugs. Persons with panic attacks were intermediate in severity between those with panic disorder and those with other psychiatric disorders. These findings were not explained by comorbid mental illness.

Brown and Harris, 1993 (9)	Inner-city working-class and single mothers (N = 404)	DSM-III-R	Depression arises much more frequently in ongoing anxiety disorders (excluding mild agoraphobia and simple phobia) than anxiety disorders arise in ongoing depression. In particular, rates of panic disorder were 3.34 per 100 women over the previous year, compared to 1.22 in the ECA. Anxiety conditions were highly related to adversity in childhood (parental indifference, physical abuse, sexual abuse), with panic disorder having the greatest association.
Leon et al., 1995 (17)	ECA study: sample from 5 U.S. communities (N > 18,000)	DIS	The 6-month prevalence of panic disorder was 0.5% for men and 1.0% for women, while the rate for panic attacks not meeting diagnostic criteria for panic disorder was 0.6% in men and 1.1% in women. Of those with panic disorder, 20% of men and 30% of women had comorbid major depression. Approximately 30% of those with panic disorder had used the general medical system for emotional, alcohol, or drug-related problems in the previous 6 months. Along with phobias and obsessive-compulsive disorder, men with panic disorder were more likely to have chronic unemployment and receive disability or welfare in the previous 6 months.

DIS = Diagnostic Interview Schedule.

panic disorder also reported greater use of health services, with increased utilization of general medical, psychiatric, or combined services, and of emergency room services. Psychoactive medications were widely prescribed, with 42% of panic subjects reporting use of minor tranquilizers, 15% of sleeping pills, and 8% of antidepressants within the previous 6 months.

Similar results were reported in ECA subjects with panic attacks not meeting full diagnostic criteria for panic disorder. Klerman et al. (7) concluded that panic attacks have clinical significance, demonstrating social morbidity intermediate in severity between that noted in panic disorder and that in other psychiatric disorders.

In a more recent study, Leon and colleagues (17) examined the social costs of anxiety disorders incurred over the previous 6 months in subjects in the ECA study. The authors found substantial social morbidity associated with anxiety disorders in general (i.e., panic disorder, obsessive-compulsive disorder, and phobia) and panic disorder in particular. In contrast to subjects with other anxiety disorders or no psychiatric diagnosis, subjects with panic disorder were associated with the highest rates of current unemployment (60% in men, 69% in women). When compared to patients with panic attacks (i.e., subclinical panic disorder) or panic disorder and major depression, subjects with panic disorder without major depression demonstrated the greatest rates of current unemployment (65% for men, 70% for women), further underscoring the substantial impairment associated with panic disorder. Similar trends were observed for financial dependence, with 37% of men and 42% of women with panic disorder receiving some type of financial assistance. Substance abuse/dependence rates showed the greatest elevation for both panic disorder and panic attacks, while rates of help-seeking for emotional, drug, or alcohol problems were highest in those with panic disorder, regardless of the presence of comorbid major depression.

QUALITY OF LIFE IN PANIC DISORDER: STUDIES IN TREATMENT-SEEKING, NONPSYCHIATRIC POPULATIONS

Patients with undiagnosed panic disorder often present to nonpsychiatric caregivers for treatment of a variety of panic-related somatic complaints. In the past, for example, patients with complaints of chest pain and dyspnea may have presented to the emergency room or to cardiologists, only to discover after extensive and often invasive work-ups that their symptoms were of noncardiac origin. More recently, with the growth of managed health care, these patients' complaints are often brought first to the attention of primary care physicians rather than to specialists, and these physicians may then commence similar evaluations. Recognizing the substantial physical impairment in these samples, a number of studies have been undertaken to explore the quality of life and social impairment in these individuals with untreated panic disorder (Table 2).

Studies in Samples Under Evaluation for Cardiac Symptoms

Functional impairment has been observed in patients with subjective reports of chest pain but lacking objective evidence of cardiac disease. In an open study of 20 patients with panic disorder and chest pain without significant evidence of CAD, subjects were treated with alprazolam for a minimum of 3 weeks. In addition to measures of anxiety and depression, patients reported work and social functioning over the last week at each visit. Significant differences were observed in all of these measures after the first week of treatment, including: fewer panic attacks; lower scores on physician-rated measures of anxiety, depression, and global functioning; and improvement in work and social functioning based on patient reports, while a marginally significant reduction in chest pain episodes was demonstrated. These changes were sustained throughout the duration of the trial. The authors concluded that other, noncardiac pharmacotherapeutic interventions may be useful in treating these patients (13).

Panic disorder, however, may also be comorbid with cardiac pathology. There is evidence to suggest that untreated panic disorder, with greater frequency of chest pain, may result in physiological worsening of CAD. For example, in subjects with CAD, panic attacks may provoke ischemic pain by increasing cardiac work with increased heart rate, blood pressure, and possibly resistance in collateral coronary vessels (40). Ischemic chest pain can also provoke increased anxiety, resulting in panic attacks (41). These events may result in a vicious circle of panic symptoms → cardiac chest pain → panic symptoms. As anti-

Table 2 The Panic Disorder and Quality of Life: Studies in Primary Care and Nonpsychiatric Specialties

Author	Population	Diagnostic instrument(s)	Findings
Katon et al., 1986 (18)	Patients in a primary care practice (N = 195)	DIS	13% of patients met criteria for panic disorder, while an additional 8.7% had panic attacks consistent with simple panic. When compared to nonpanic controls, these patients had a significantly greater lifetime risk of major depression, multiple phobias, and avoidance behavior. Higher scores were also demonstrated on psychological distress and somatization indices.
Kahn et al., 1987 (19)	Patients under evaluation for clinical cardiac transplantation (N = 60)	Interview	Of 35 patients with idiopathic cardiomyopathy (mean age 38.2 years), 83% had definite or probable panic disorder, in contrast to 16% of 25 patients with postinfarction cardiac failure, rheumatic heart disease, or congenital heart disease.

| Beitman et al., 1988 (13) | Patients seen by cardiologists in a university hospital | SCID-UP | In 33 patients with chest pain and angiographically normal coronary arteries, 33% had panic disorder and 24% simple panic. 43/74 (59%) of outpatients with atypical or nonanginal chest pain and no CAD had panic disorder. After an 8-week trial of alprazolam, 0.5 mg/day, in a group of outpatients with atypical or nonanginal chest pain without evidence of CAD and inpatients with chest pain and angiographically normal coronary arteries, all meeting criteria for panic disorder, patients reported significant improvement in their work and social functioning by the end of week 1 and throughout the 8-week trial. |
| Cormier et al., 1988 (14) | Outpatients with chest pain but no prior history of organic cardiac disease referred for evaluation by cardiologists ($N = 98$) | DIS | 47% of the CAD-negative patients had panic disorder compared to 6% of patients with CAD. Of 26 patients with panic disorder, 88.5% had no evidence of CAD. In a logistic-regression model, knowledge of panic disorder significantly increased the ability to predict a negative cardiac test result, even after adjusting for age, gender, type of pain, and method of testing. |

Table 2 Continued

Author	Population	Diagnostic instrument(s)	Findings
Wuslin et al., 1988 (20)	Patients seen in emergency room (N = 49)	PDRS, CES-D	Of patients presenting with complaints of chest pain, 16% had panic disorder and 43% panic attacks.
Brown FW et al., 1990 (21)	Primary care patients referred for evaluation of unexplained somatic complaints (N = 196)	DIS	119 (60.7%) of patients met criteria for somatoform disorder. Panic disorder was the fourth most common comorbid psychiatric disorder (26.6%), behind major depression, GAD, and phobic disorders. Compared to general population data from the ECA, however, these patients were 16.25 times more likely to have panic disorder than patients without somatoform disorder.
Goldberg et al., 1990 (12)	Ambulatory patients in a cardiology practice (N = 414)	SCID-UP	Of 414 patients in the practice, panic disorder was suspected in 104 of 310 respondents. Interviews with 52 of 104 patients substantiated diagnoses of panic disorder, for a prevalence of 9.2%. 44% of the 52 patients used psychotropic medications. In examining duration of panic disorder, longer-duration panic disorder developed before age 30 and followed a chronic course, while shorter-duration panic disorder had a later onset following the development of cardiac disease.

Katon et al., 1990 (15)	Outpatients in HMO primary care clinics (N = 119)	DIS	In a chart review of distressed high utilizers of health services, 11.8% met criteria for current panic disorder, while 30.2% met criteria for lifetime panic disorder.
Chignon et al., 1993 (22)	Patients referred for ambulatory ECG recordings (N = 197)	HADS, SADS-LA	Of 50 anxious patients identified with the HADS, 62% met criteria for panic disorder. The prevalence of panic disorder was similar in patients with and without ECG abnormalities, indicating that in anxious patients the presence of panic disorder does not rule out organic cardiac disease.
Sullivan et al., 1993 (23)	Patients referred for otological evaluation of dizziness	DIS, HAM-A, HAM-D, HSC	Of 71 patients evaluated, 33 (46%) had no evidence of vestibular dysfunction. These patients also had significantly greater rates of lifetime psychiatric illness, particularly panic disorder, depression, and somatization disorder. These patients also reported more current and lifetime unexplained medical symptoms, as well as more frequent and severe anxiety, depression, and somatic systems.

Table 2 Continued

Author	Population	Diagnostic instrument(s)	Findings
Ormel et al., 1994 (11)	A multinational sample of patients in primary care clinics (N = 25,916)	GHQ, CIDI	After controlling for physical disease severity, psychopathology was consistently associated with increased disability, as measured by patient-reported physical disability, number of disability days, and interviewer-rated occupational role functioning. Disability was most prominent among patients with major depression, panic disorder, GAD, and neurasthenia.
Cohen et al., 1994 (24)	Pregnant females with a pregravid history of panic disorder (N = 49)	Chart review, DSM-III-R criteria	In following 45 patients through three trimesters of pregnancy, 78% had insignificant change in status or improvement, while 20% demonstrated more severe panic symptoms. Pregnancy did not increase the likelihood of successful discontinuation from antipanic medication.

Cohen et al., 1994 (25)	Postpartum females with a pregravid history of panic disorder (N = 40)	Chart review, DSM-III-R criteria	Between the third trimester and postpartum week 12, 65% of patients maintained or improved their clinical status, while 35% had puerperal worsening. Patients who received pharmacotherapy in the third trimester were significantly less likely to experience puerperal worsening than those who did not receive medication prior to the puerperium.
Hollifield et al., 1994 (26)	Outpatients in a primary care clinic in Lesotho, Africa (N = 126)	DIS	Prevalence estimates for panic disorder (24%), major depression (23%), and GAD (29%) are reported. Patients with panic disorder or major depression presented with significantly more physical symptoms, notable for a greater percentage of pain or autonomic symptoms.
Lyiard et al., 1994 (27)	Community sample (ECA) (N = 13,537)	DIS	Individuals with panic disorder had a significantly higher rate of reporting GI symptoms, including those associated with IBS, than individuals with other or without psychiatric diagnoses.

Table 2 Continued

Author	Population	Diagnostic instrument(s)	Findings
Simpson et al., 1994 (28)	Outpatients in general practices with panic disorder ($N = 100$) and controls ($N = 100$)	Chart review	Compared to controls, patients with panic disorder had significantly higher rates of general consultation over the 10-year period prior to the diagnosis of panic disorder. Panic disorder patients were also prescribed more psychiatric and nonpsychiatric medications, received more secondary referrals, and reported higher rates of minor illnesses and somatic complaints (e.g., cardiac, GI, and CNS).
Klein et al., 1995 (29)	Patients admitted to the general emergency service of an urban medical center in Israel ($N = 517$)	SCID	Patients were in one of four groups: patients presenting with somatic complaints without a physical disorder ($N = 100$), patients with somatic complaints and found to have a physical disorder ($N = 109$), nonpsychiatric consecutive admissions to the service ($N = 158$), and a group of referrals to the psychiatric emergency service and then interviewed with the SCID ($N = 150$). The prevalence of panic disorder and GAD in the full, nonpsychiatric sample was 2.7%, in contrast to 6.7% among patients with somatic complaints without a physical disorder and to 4.8% of psychiatric referrals.

| Marazziti et al., 1995 (30) | Outpatients seen in a neurology headache clinic (*N* = 73) | SCID | Psychiatric disorders were common in these subjects including: panic disorder (27.4%), (GAD) (24.7%), subthreshold panic disorder (19.2%), OCD (9.6%), cyclothymia (6.9%), social phobia (5.5%), current major depression (5.5%), dysthymia (5.5%), and simple phobia (4.1%). Panic disorder was more common in patients with migraine headaches, particularly the subgroup of migraine with aura, in contrast to subjects with tension headaches. |
| Spitzer et al., 1995 (31) | Adult patients in a primary care clinic (*N* = 1000) | PRIME-MD, SF-20 | Compared to patients without mental illness, patients with panic disorder demonstrated impairment on all scales. Anxiety disorders in general were associated with impaired social functioning and mental health, as well as significant number of excess disability days. When compared to physical disorders, mental disorders (including anxiety disorders) accounted for greater variance in all scales, including role functioning, general health, and social functioning, as well as mental health. |

Table 2 Continued

Author	Population	Diagnostic instrument(s)	Findings
Walker et al., 1995 (32)	Outpatients in a GI clinic	DIS, MOS	Compared to patients with IBD ($N = 40$), patients with IBS ($N = 71$) demonstrated significantly higher prevalence rates of current panic disorder, as well as lifetime rates of depression, GAD, somatization disorder, agoraphobia, and childhood rape and molestation. IBS patients also had a significantly higher mean number of psychiatric symptoms and diagnoses. Levels of disability in physical, emotional, family, social, and occupational functioning were comparable in both IBS and IBD groups, despite the absence of serious organic disease in the former group.
Brown et al., 1996 (33)	Primary care patients with major depression ($N = 157$)	DIS, SF-36	Compared to patients with depression and GAD or depression alone, patients with lifetime panic disorder (38%) demonstrated poor recovery in response to pharmacotherapy or psychotherapy. Patients with comorbid depression and a lifetime history of an anxiety disorder exhibited significantly more psychopathology and worse mental and physical health-related functioning at baseline when compared with medical patients with major depression alone.

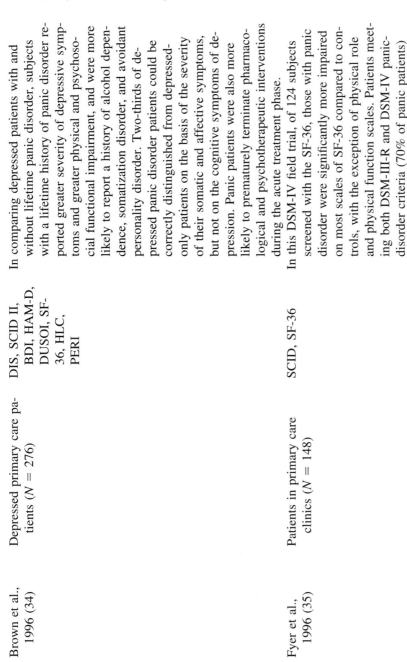

| Brown et al., 1996 (34) | Depressed primary care patients ($N = 276$) | DIS, SCID II, BDI, HAM-D, DUSOI, SF-36, HLC, PERI | In comparing depressed patients with and without lifetime panic disorder, subjects with a lifetime history of panic disorder reported greater severity of depressive symptoms and greater physical and psychosocial functional impairment, and were more likely to report a history of alcohol dependence, somatization disorder, and avoidant personality disorder. Two-thirds of depressed panic disorder patients could be correctly distinguished from depressed-only patients on the basis of the severity of their somatic and affective symptoms, but not on the cognitive symptoms of depression. Panic patients were also more likely to prematurely terminate pharmacological and psychotherapeutic interventions during the acute treatment phase. |
| Fyer et al., 1996 (35) | Patients in primary care clinics ($N = 148$) | SCID, SF-36 | In this DSM-IV field trial, of 124 subjects screened with the SF-36, those with panic disorder were significantly more impaired on most scales of SF-36 compared to controls, with the exception of physical role and physical function scales. Patients meeting both DSM-III-R and DSM-IV panic-disorder criteria (70% of panic patients) were significantly impaired on both self-perceived QOL and clinician-rated scales and 75% of this group were rated as moderately or more impaired by their attacks. |

Table 2 Continued

Author	Population	Diagnostic instrument(s)	Findings
Hahn et al., 1996 (36)	Adults in primary care clinics (N = 767)	DDPRQ, SF-20, PRIME-MD, self-report	Patients classified by their physicians as being difficult to treat (15%) were more likely to have a psychiatric diagnosis (67% vs. 25%), to be associated with greater functional impairment and health care utilization, and to have less satisfaction with their medical care. Psychiatric conditions strongly associated with difficulty were: multisomatoform disorder (OR 12.3), panic disorder (OR 6.9), dysthymia (OR 4.2), GAD (OR 3.4), major depression (OR 3.0), and probable alcohol abuse or dependence (OR 2.6).
Kaplan et al., 1996 (37)	Outpatients seeking treatment for general medical illnesses (N = 40) or for panic disorder (N = 40)	Semistructured clinical interview	IBS was diagnosed in 46.3% of panic patients in contrast to 2.5% of general medical controls.

| Olfson et al., 1996 (38) | Adult outpatients in an HMO ($N = 1001$) | SCID, SDS | Subthreshold psychiatric symptoms and associated disability were examined in primary care patients. After controlling for confounding effects of other variables, panic symptoms were significantly correlated with impairment through loss of work and greater use of mental health services, compared to depressive symptoms and major depression, which were correlated with impairment in all areas assessed. |
| Sherborne et al., 1996 (39) | Primary care patients with chronic medical illness, current depression, or subthreshold depression ($N = 2494$) | Modified DIS | Concurrent anxiety disorders were common (14–66%) in these patients. Patients with chronic medical illness (HTN, DM, MI, or CHF) or subthreshold depression had lower rates of panic disorder (lifetime 1.5–3.5%, current 1–1.7%) compared to patients with current major depression (lifetime 10.9%, current 9.4%). In general, primary care patients perceived that their need for care of personal or emotional problems was not satisfied (54.6–72.9%). |

CES-D = Center for Epidemiological Studies, depression scale; CIDI = Composite International Diagnostic Interview; DIS = Diagnostic Interview Schedule; GHQ = General Health Questionnaire; HADS = Hospital Anxiety and Depression Scale; HAM-A = Hamilton Anxiety Rating Scale; HAM-D = Hamilton Depression Rating Scale; HSC = Hopkins Symptom Checklist; MOS = Medical Outcomes Survey; PDRS = Panic Disorder Rating Scale; PRIME-MD = Primary Care Evaluation of Mental Disorders; SADS-LA = Schedule for Affective Disorders and Schizophrenia, Lifetime Version Modified for the Study of Anxiety Disorders; SCID-UP = Structured Clinical Interview for DSM-III, Upjohn Version; SF-20 = Short-form (20-item) General Health Survey; SF-36 = Short-form (36-item) General Health Survey.

anginal agents become ineffective over time, a diagnosis of crescendo angina may be made without consideration of a diagnosis of panic disorder as the cause of the symptoms. Alternatively, questions have been raised regarding the influence of the mechanisms of panic attacks on spasms of the cardiac microvasculature which, over time, may lead to ischemic damage, myocarditis, and progressive cardiomyopathy (19). In both cases, undiagnosed and untreated panic disorder can lead to worsening of chronic cardiac morbidity and mortality and progressive functional impairment.

Studies in Samples Under Evaluation for Gastrointestinal Symptoms

Gastrointestinal symptoms are commonly reported by individuals with panic disorder as demonstrated in the ECA study (27), and these symptoms have been associated with substantial physical impairment and disability. In a prospective study of patients seen in a gastrointestinal clinic, Walker and colleagues (32) examined the frequency of psychiatric diagnoses, sexual and physical victimization, and disability. Patients with either irritable bowel syndrome (IBS) ($N = 71$) or inflammatory bowel disease (IBD) ($N = 41$) underwent structured interviews to document psychiatric, GI, and victimization histories and completed self-report measures of personality, functional disability, and dissociation. The investigators found that 95% of IBS patients had a lifetime prevalence of at least one DSM III-R disorder, in contrast to 65% of IBD patients. In particular, IBS patients had significantly greater lifetime prevalence rates of current panic disorder, as well as major depression, somatization disorder, and childhood sexual abuse. In addition, despite the absence of objective findings of gastrointestinal pathology, the IBS patients demonstrated disability in personal, emotional, family, social, and occupational functioning that was equal to or greater than that reported by IBD patients. IBS patients also had significantly higher rates of physical symptoms without a medical basis.

In another study (37), investigators examined the prevalence of IBS in 41 patients seeking treatment for panic disorder compared to 40 patients seeking treatment for other medical illnesses in a general practitioner's office. After completing a semistructured clinical interview to assess gastrointestinal complaints, 19 subjects with panic disorder (46%) met criteria for IBS, compared to one (2.5%) of the nonpanic controls. The patients with panic disorder and IBS were also more likely to have heartburn and GI symptoms related to stress. In that the treatment of panic disorder can result in resolution of GI symptoms (42), individuals with similar presentations may experience an improvement in their physical impairment and disability with the appropriate diagnosis and treatment of their panic disorder.

Studies in Samples Under Evaluation for Neurological Symptoms

Neurological symptoms commonly reported by patients with panic disorder include dizziness and headache. In a study of patients with complaints of dizziness and referred for further otological evaluation, 75 patients were assessed using a structured psychiatric interview, self-report questionnaires of psychological distress, and a complete otological evaluation, including electronystagmogram (23). Patients with evidence of a peripheral vestibular disorder were compared to patients with otherwise normal vestibular function. Patients without evidence of vestibular dysfunction had a greater likelihood of a lifetime history of a psychiatric illness, particularly panic disorder, major depression, or somatization disorder. In addition, these patients reported more current and lifetime unexplained medical symptoms and more severe current anxiety, depressive, and somatic symptoms.

In another study (30), investigators examined 73 outpatients assessed in a neurology headache clinic. Patients were divided into groups based on headache subtype, including migraine without aura, migraine with aura, and tension headache, excluding individuals with other types of headache. All patients underwent a semistructured clinical interview to assess the prevalence of psychiatric disorders, including a spectrum of panic illness that included infrequent panic attacks or subthreshold panic disorder, as well as DSM-III-R criteria panic disorder. The most frequently observed psychiatric conditions were in the anxiety spectrum, particularly panic disorder (27.4%), generalized anxiety disorder (GAD) (24.7%), and subthreshold panic disorder (19.2%). Among the headache subgroups, panic disorder was more common in subjects with migraine headaches, particularly in those with migraine with aura.

There are many organic causes for these common neurological symptoms, which may range in severity from mildly irritating to disabling or incapacitating. In the majority of cases, medical evaluations are unable to provide a treatable etiology. This failure leads to further frustration for the patient and the clinician, with continued patient discomfort and suffering that could be minimized or alleviated by consideration of a diagnosis of panic disorder and institution of the appropriate therapy.

Studies in Primary Care Samples

Panic disorder is common in primary care patient populations, with worldwide prevalence estimates ranging from 1.1% to 13% for current panic disorder and from 1.5% to 30.2% for lifetime panic disorder. These patients report substantially elevated rates of somatic complaints and physical symptoms, as well as minor medical illnesses (26,28,43). Compared to nonpanic patients, they are more frequently referred for consultation and further medical evaluation and prescribed both non-psychiatric and psychiatric medications, contributing to overall greater utilization of health care resources (28,38,44).

Considerable disability and impairment have been demonstrated in these samples. Panic disorder has been associated with significant dysfunction in most domains of life quality, including physical function, bodily pain, role (including occupational) and social function, and mental health (11,28,36,38). These individuals are at a greater risk of being identified by care providers as "difficult patients" (36), making their treatment more challenging, and further frustrating—and potentially stigmatizing—them and/or their health care providers.

The disability associated with mental health concerns is demonstrated through both patient self-reports and elevated rates of comorbid psychopathology, particularly major depression, multiple phobias, and avoidant behavior (43). Of these conditions, major depression is the most common in primary care and has been studied in relation to panic disorder. One investigation examined panic disorder in patients with chronic medical illness (hypertension, diabetes, myocardial infarction, or congestive heart failure), current major depression, or subthreshold depression. The prevalence of current and lifetime panic disorder in subjects with current major depression was significantly greater than in the medical and subthreshold depression groups (current 9.4% vs. 1–1.7% and lifetime 10.9% vs. 1.5–3.5%, respectively), and these subjects reported less satisfaction with the care they were receiving (39). In another study, depressed patients with and without a lifetime history of panic disorder were compared. Individuals with comorbid panic disorder and depression demonstrated more severe depressive symptomatology, physical and psychosocial impairment, and comorbid alcohol dependence, somatization disorder, and avoidant personality disorder. Two-thirds of the depressed panic disorder patients were distinguishable from depressed-only patients on the basis of the severity of their somatic and affective symptoms, but not the cognitive symptoms of depression (34).

QUALITY OF LIFE IN PANIC DISORDER: STUDIES OF TREATMENT-SEEKING POPULATIONS

Studies of individuals seeking treatment for panic disorder or for infrequent panic attacks consistently demonstrate substantial functional impairment in these samples. Whether presenting for treatment to primary care providers or to mental health specialists, these patients report significant social, psychiatric, and medical morbidity associated with panic symptomatology (Table 3).

The adverse impact of panic disorder on personal happiness and role functioning have been well documented. Elevated rates of unemployment or partial employment have been reported, with patient perceptions that their inability to maintain a job is directly related to panic symptoms (56). Lower levels of social, family, and emotional functioning have also been noted in both patients with panic disorder or with infrequent panic attacks, particularly in contrast to levels noted in non-panic controls (39,49,52,54,55).

Similarly, the comorbid physical and mental disability in these individuals is impressive. The presentation of an array of somatic symptoms and related sequelae can be seen in patients as described

Table 3 The Prevalence and Social Morbidity of Panic Disorder: Studies of Patients with Panic Disorder or Infrequent Panic Attacks

Author	Population	Diagnostic instrument	Findings
Coryell et al., 1982 (45)	Inpatients with panic disorder (N = 113/125) and matched unipolar depressed controls (N = 112/125)	Chart review	A review of charts 35 years after the index admission showed that patients with panic disorder had significant excess mortality due to death by unnatural causes. Men with panic disorder also showed excess mortality due to circulatory system disease, while men and women in the unipolar depression group showed excess mortality. Suicide accounted for 20% and 16% of deaths in the panic and depressed groups, respectively.
Coryell et al., 1986 (46)	Outpatients in a university clinic (N = 155)	Structured interview (Feighner criteria)	At a 12-year follow-up contact and in comparison to matched surgical controls, men in the anxiety neurosis group (88% with a history of panic attacks) were twice as likely to die as controls, and this excess mortality was attributable to cardiovascular disease and suicide.

| Fawcett, 1988 (47) | Patients with major affective disorders (*N* = 955) | | 25 suicides were documented in the first 4 years of follow-up. While 8 suicides (32%) occurred in the first 6 months, a total of 13 (52%) occurred by the end of the first year of follow-up. Predictors of early suicide within the first year included panic attacks, as well as anhedonia, psychic anxiety associated with glucocorticoid changes, depressive turmoil, and moderate alcohol abuse. |
| Noyes et al., 1990 (48) | Outpatients recruited through news media for a clinical drug study (*N* = 30 panic patients, *N* = 30 controls) | SCID, SADS | Compared to controls, panic patients reported more frequent treatment for hemorrhoids, peptic ulcer, and irritable bowel syndrome, with a greater proportion of panic patients reporting irritable bowel syndrome compared to controls. Panic disorder patients also reported 5.7 symptoms per week compared to 1.5 symptoms in controls. Effective treatment for panic disorder resulted in a reduction in GI symptoms in all subjects. |

Table 3 Continued

Author	Population	Diagnostic instrument(s)	Findings
Massion et al., 1993 (49)	Naturalistic, longitudinal, multicenter study of a clinical population with anxiety disorders ($N = 357$)	SCID-P, SADS-L, LIFE, SF-36	Of patients with panic disorder ($N = 234$) or generalized anxiety disorder ($N = 63$), significant impairment was noted in emotional health, and functioning in role, marital, and social domains. In addition, in comorbid anxiety disorders with major depression, 9% had ever attempted suicide and 31% had been hospitalized. High rates of alcohol abuse or dependence histories were reported in 30% of panic patients, but 44% of those with panic without agoraphobia.
Noyes et al., 1993 (50)	7-year follow-up in outpatients diagnosed with panic disorder in a university-based anxiety clinic ($N = 69$)	Clinical interview, SRAS, PGI, SAS, FQ	Patients were interviewed to investigate environmental factors related to outcome. Those who were more severely ill on initial assessment had a worse outcome. Other variables associated with a poor outcome included specific developmental variables (e.g., separation from parent by death or divorce), high interpersonal sensitivity, low social class, and unmarried status.

Manassis et al., 1994 (51)	Mothers with anxiety disorders and their preschool children (N = 18)	SCID, AAI, SSP	14 mothers had panic disorder, 3 had generalized anxiety, 1 had OCD. High rates of insecurity were observed among the offspring.
Katon et al., 1995 (52)	Outpatients in primary care clinics with panic disorder (N = 62), intermittent panic (N = 19), and nonpanic controls (N = 61)	SCID, SF-36, SDS	Patients with infrequent panic attacks reported similar levels of disability in social, family, and vocational functioning compared to patients with panic disorder, and both panic groups had significantly more disability than nonpanic controls. While medical comorbidity was similar, panic patients has more psychiatric comorbidity than controls. Higher levels of neuroticism were observed in the panic groups than in controls.
Sherbourne et al., 1996 (53)	Outpatients with current panic disorder (N = 423) and nonpanic controls (N = 9839)	SF-20, SF-36	Patients with panic disorder had substantially lower levels of role functioning and mental health compared to controls, except for depressed patients who demonstrated comparable or higher levels of medical control of impairment compared to panic patients. Physical functioning and perception of current health were similar to those experienced by patients with hypertension and general population norms.

Table 3 Continued

Author	Population	Diagnostic instrument(s)	Findings
Hollifield et al., 1997 (54)	Patients with panic disorder (N = 62) and primary care clinic controls (N = 61)	SCID, SF-36	Patients with panic disorder were more impaired than controls on each SF-36 measure. In addition to panic phenomena, factors that contribute to severe impairment include major depression, increasing age and neuroticism, less education, and an interaction with age and panic.
Katerndahl and Realini, 1997 (55)	Community survey (PACT), including SCID, patients with panic disorder (N = 42), QOL panic attacks (N = 55), and nonpanic controls (N = 97)	SCID, QOL	QOL was significantly poorer in panic subjects than in nonpanic controls. Subjects with panic disorder demonstrated poorer QOL and panic-related disability than those with infrequent panic attacks. Predictors of QOL included comorbid depression, extent of social support, worry, and severity of chest pain. Predictors of work disability included panic frequency, illness attitudes, family dissatisfaction, and gender.

AAI = Adult Attachment Interview; FQ = Fear Questionnaire; LIFE = Longitudinal Interval Followup Evaluation; PGI = Patient Global Improvement scale; QOL = Quality of Life questionnaire developed for PACT; SADS-L = Schedule for Affective Disorders, Lifetime SAS: Social Adjustment Scale; SCID = Structured Clinical Interview for DSM; SCID-P = Structured Clinical Interview for DSM, Patient Version; SDS = Sheehan Disability Scale, SF-20 = Short-form (20 item) Health Survey; SF-36 = Short-form (36-item) Health Survey; SRAS = Self-Rated Anxiety Scale; SSP = Strange Situation Procedure.

above, as well as in treatment-seeking samples. For instance, in a study of GI symptoms in subjects seeking treatment for panic disorder compared to nonpanic controls, not only did individuals with panic disorder report more frequent occurrence and number of somatic GI symptoms as well as treatment for GI complaints, but all subjects also noted relief of GI distress after proper treatment of panic disorder (48). Comorbid psychiatric illnesses are also more common than in control groups, particularly depression and alcohol abuse or dependence (49,52,54).

Together, these influences may contribute to the excess mortality reported in samples with panic disorder. In a 35-year follow-up study of panic patients compared to unipolar depressed control subjects, those with panic disorder demonstrated significant excess mortality due to death by unnatural causes, while the subgroup of panic males showed excess mortality due to circulatory disease (45). In another 12-year follow-up study comparing mortality rates in subjects with anxiety neurosis (88% with a history of panic attacks) to nonpanic surgical controls, men in the anxiety neurosis group were twice as likely to die as controls, due to elevated rates of cardiovascular disease and suicide (46). Increased rates of suicide in patients with panic symptomatology have been reported in other studies as well (47,49), further underscoring the intrapsychic distress and desperation often experienced by these individuals.

Particular attention has been focused on one group of patients with panic disorder, namely, pregnant and postpartum women. While many believe that women are "protected" from psychiatric disorders during pregnancy (57,58) and at greater risk of exacerbation during the peurperium (59,60), meager data have been published in support of this opinion. The data available for panic disorder suggest a highly variable course of the panic disorder during, after, and between subsequent pregnancies. In a retrospective study of 46 women with pregravid panic disorder reporting a history of a total of 67 pregnancies, 66% of pregnancies were associated with stable or improved panic symptoms, while 33% were associated with antepartum exacerbation; subsequent pregnancies, however, were unlikely to be associated with the same outcome. The peurperium, by contrast, was associated with worsening in 63% of pregnancies (61). Similar results were observed by Cohen et al. (24) in a case series of pregnant women with pregravid panic disorder. The authors noted further that more severely ill patients were more likely to require antipanic medication at some point during their pregnancy. In a subsequent study focused on the postpartum period, Cohen et al. (25) reported peurperal exacerbation in only 35% of patients and found a significantly reduced risk of worsening in patients who received pharmacotherapy during the third trimester. Recognizing the potential risks and benefits of medication during pregnancy, these findings suggest that more severely ill women may benefit from antepartum and/or postpartum treatment of panic disorder to improve QOL during and after pregnancy.

In summary. while several factors are believed to contribute to the impairment observed in panic disorder, other features have been identified as predictive of poor QOL and occupational disability. Depression, older age, neuroticism, and a lower educational level have been reported to contribute to the dysfunction observed in panic disorder (54). Factors identified as predictive of poor QOL include depression, lack of social support, worrying, and increased severity of chest pain, while greater panic frequency, attitudes toward illness, family dissatisfaction, and male gender were predictive of work disability (55).

COST-EFFECTIVENESS: UNTREATED VS. TREATED PANIC DISORDER

In examining the costs associated with panic disorder, it is important to consider the impact of both direst and indirect costs. Direct costs include expenses related to health care utilization, such as doctor visits for general medical or mental health care, emergency-room visits, hospitalization, invasive diagnostic tests, and prescription medications. Indirect costs include expenses related to lost or reduced productivity in patients, such as greater number of sick days, unemployment, disability and financial assistance, lost leisure time, and social and family/home dysfunction. The lost productivity of family members who make adjustments and compromises in their lives to compensate for the deficits of the affected family member are also included in these estimates, further adding to the burden of indirect costs.

The expenditures associated with anxiety disorders in general and panic disorder in particular are substantial. It has been estimated that the economic cost of anxiety disorders in the United States in 1990 was $46.6 billion, 31.5% of all U.S. expenditures on mental illness. Less than 25% of this sum was related to the cost of direct medical treatment, with the remaining 75% attributable to reduced or lost productivity (62). Recognizing the wide prevalence of panic disorder, a large proportion of these expenses are likely to be accounted for by patients with panic disorder (see Table 4).

In the past, attention has been focused on the direct costs associated with panic disorder. In a study of service usage and expenditures in panic patients recruited for a clinical drug trial, health care utilization was quite varied (65). Of the 391 patients assessed, 70% accessed primary care physicians for mental health services for the current episode, in contrast to 47% who used specialty mental health services. Nearly half of the sample (47%) reported evaluation and/or treatment by a nonpsychiatric specialist. Overall, the authors estimated that the direct cost associated with the current episode of panic disorder in this sample was $1.3 million, noting that 10% of the sample were heavy utilizers of the health care system and accounted for 45% of the total expenditures.

Other data relating to the direct costs of panic disorder have focused on medical costs associated with a missed diagnosis of panic disorder. For example, it has been estimated that 10–30% of cardiac catheterizations in the United States result in a negative work-up. Other data indicate that over one-third of patients with chest pain and normal angiograms meet criteria for panic disorder. If approximately 10% of the 500,00 angiograms performed annually in the United States are negative (at a cost of approximately $2000 per test), and one-third of this group suffers from panic disorder, over $30 million is expended annually in the assessment of patients with chest pain associated with panic disorder (43,66). Despite negative medical evaluations, these patients will often continue to have somatic complaints, receive further work-ups and treatment, and experience continued disability due to their chest pain (67,68), further increasing the direct and indirect costs.

Although it is widely recognized that the indirect costs associated with anxiety disorders far exceed the direct costs, similar data concerning the indirect costs of panic disorder are limited. The social and economic cost of panic disorder was studied in a sample of 30 outpatients

Table 4 Quality of Life in Panic Disorder: Studies of Cost and Treatment Effectiveness

Author	Population	Diagnostic instrument	Findings
Sheehan et al., 1980 (79)	Patients with severely debilitating, longstanding endogenous anxiety (N = 57)	Clinical interview, SSABS, SWDS, WLFSS, RFSS, Zung, SCL-90	Patients were randomly assigned treatment with imipramine, phenelzine, or placebo, in conjunction with supportive group therapy. Patients receiving active medication showed significant improvement over baseline on all measures and when compared to placebo. Phenelzine was significantly superior to imipramine on the SWDS and SSPAS, with trends toward improvement on the other measures.
Edlund and Swann, 1987 (56)	Outpatients under examination for a biological study of panic disorder (N = 30)	SCID	63% of patients had previously received treatment for panic disorder, although few had received treatments generally recognized as effective. High rates of unemployment or parttime work were reported, and many subjects noted that this condition had impacted adversely on the quality of their work and/or on their ability to maintain a job. The loss due to total work disability was estimated at $33,674.

| Siegel et al., 1990 (63) | Attendees at a forum for individuals with panic disorder (*N* = 500) | DSM-III-R criteria | Of 65 subjects (13%) found to have panic disorder, 85% reported current mental health counseling and/or medication. 205 medical visits were reported in the previous month, 47% of which were mental health visits. Workdays missed averaged 1 per month for subjects employed full-time, with an average annual economic loss of $1093; when compared to the cost of workdays lost in the general U.S. population in full-time employment, the estimated excess cost of lost wages is $619 in subjects with panic disorder. Panic disorder subjects reported fewer "good days" in the past week compared to subjects with end-stage renal disease (3.2 vs. 4.8) and less overall life satisfaction (4.25 vs. 5.0). |

Table 4 Continued

Author	Population	Diagnostic instrument(s)	Findings
Salvador-Carulla et al., 1995 (64)	Outpatients in a psychiatric clinic with panic disorder ($N = 61$)	SCID-UP, VAS, PAAS, HAM-A, HAM-D	Significant improvement was demonstrated on ratings of general functioning, improvement, severity of symptoms, and level of disability in the 12 months between initial diagnosis and follow-up assessment. During this period, while direct costs increased by 59%, from $29,158 to $46,256, indirect costs attributable to lost productivity fell by 79%, from $65,643 to $13,883. (Costs in $U.S.)
Telch et al., 1995 (80)	Patients evaluated for a treatment outcome study of panic disorder ($N = 156$)	Clinical interview, SAS, SDS TPARF, SPRAS, FQ-Ago	While all patients displayed significant QOL impairment at baseline, CBT-treated subjects showed significant reductions in impairment that were maintained at follow-up, when compared to delayed-treatment controls. Anxiety and phobic avoidance were significantly associated with QOL, while frequency of panic attacks was not.

Brown et al., 1996 (33)	Primary care patients with major depression ($N = 157$)	DIS, SF-36	Compared to depressed patients with and without GAD, depressed patients with a lifetime history of panic disorder showed poor recovery in response to pharmacotherapy or psychotherapy.
Katschnig et al., 1996 (81)	Patients who had participated in a multinational drug trial ($N = 423$)	SCID-UP, PAAS	367 patients were interviewed 4 years after completion of the drug trial, 61% of whom suffered at least occasional panic attacks. Improvement was noted on work, family life/home, and social/leisure domains, with only 20% of patients continuing to report disability in these domains.
Jacobs et al., 1997 (82)	Outpatients in a clinical drug study of panic disorder ($N = 144$)	SCID, SF-36, WPIQ	Compared to the placebo group, patients receiving clonazepam exhibited twice as much improvement, demonstrating improvement on all measures of mental health–related QOL, 3 of 5 measures of health-related QOL, and both measures of work productivity. The placebo group showed improvement on only 3 mental health–related QOL measures. Patients with marked improvement on clinical measures of PD severity (especially avoidance and fear of the main phobia) showed greatest gains on the mental health–related component scale.

Table 4 Continued

Author	Population	Diagnostic instrument(s)	Findings
Leon et al., 1997 (65)	Outpatients with panic disorder ($N = 391$)	DSM-III criteria, Cross-National Survey	In a U.S. sample of patients in the Cross-National Collaborative Panic Study, over 70 used primary care for mental health services and 47% specialty mental health services for the current episode. The mean cost per panic episode was $3339, roughly half of which was for specialty mental health services. Among users, median expenses for primary care physicians was $518 and for specialty mental health services $2122.
Newman et al., 1997 (83)	Patients responding to advertisement for a clinical study of panic disorder ($N = 18$)	SCID, ACQ, FQTPRA, MIA, BSQ	Treatment with 12-session CBT (CBT12) was compared to 4-session computer-assisted CBT (CBT4-CA). Subjects showed significant improvement with both treatments at posttest, and these gains were maintained at 6-month follow-up.

| Sharp et al., 1997 (84) | Patients referred by general practitioners for panic disorder ($N = 193$) | Clinical interview, HAM-A, MADRS, CGI, GHQ, SDS | Subjects were randomly assigned to 1 of 5 treatment groups: fluvoxamine (FLU), placebo, CBT and FLU, CBT and placebo, or CBT alone. All active treatment groups showed significant improvement over placebo, with the CBT groups demonstrating the most robust and consistent changes. |

ACQ = Agoraphobic Cognitions Questionnaire; BSQ = Body Sensations Questionnaire; CBT = cognitive-behavioral therapy; CGI = Clinical Global Improvement scale; DIS = Diagnostic Interview Schedule; FQ-Ago = Agoraphobia scale of the Marks and Mathews Fear Questionnaire; FQTPRA = Fear Questionnaire Total Phobia Rating and Agoraphobia subscale; GHQ = General Health Questionnaire; HAM-A = Hamilton Anxiety Rating Scale; HAM-D = Hamilton Depression Rating Scale; MADRS = Montgomery Asberg Depression Rating Scale; MIA = Mobility Inventory for Agoraphobia; PAAS = Panic-Associated Symptom Scale; RFSS = Rubin Fear Survey Schedule; SAS = Social Adjustment Scale; SCID = Structured Clinical Interview for DSM; SCID-UP = Structured Clinical Interview for DSM-III-R, Upjohn Version; SCL-90 = Symptom Check List-90; SDS = Sheehan Disability Scale; SF-36 = Short-form (36 item) Health Survey; SPRAS = Sheehan Patient-Rated Anxiety Scale; SSABS = Symptom Severity and Avoidance Behavior Scale; SWDS = Social and Work Disability Scale; TPARF = Texas Panic Attack Record Form; VAS = Visual Analogue Scale; WLFSS = Wolpe Lang Fear Survey Schedule; WPIQ = Work Productivity and Impairment Questionnaire; Zung = Zung Self-Rating Depression Scale.

with panic disorder (56). Occupational dysfunction was common, with 53% of the sample unemployed, 23% partially employed, and 78% wanting to work more than at their current level. The quality of work performed had declined as a result of panic attacks or phobic avoidance in 83% of the sample, and 37% reported quitting or losing a job at some time as a result of their condition. Overall, the duration of occupational disability computed for this sample was 79.5 years. Other factors included in assessment of the indirect costs included increases in alcohol use (30%), limitations on activity lasting a year or more due to phobic avoidance (50%), and excess burden created for other family members. The authors estimated that the total loss of income due to work disability alone in this sample was between $532,650 and $1,332,382, or between $17,755 and $44,413 per patient.

There is great potential for these costs to be substantially reduced through the proper diagnosis and treatment of panic disorder. In a study of 61 outpatients with panic disorder, costs incurred in the 6-month period prior to the diagnosis of panic disorder were compared with the costs accumulated during the 6-month period following the year after the diagnosis and treatment of panic disorder (64). Estimates of total direct and indirect costs in the period prior to diagnosis were $29,158 and $65,643, respectively, or $478 and $1076 per patient. In the follow-up period after diagnosis and treatment, direct costs increased to $46,256 or $758 per patient, while indirect costs fell to $13,883 or $228 per patient, representing a net savings of $568 per patient. This change represents an impressive offset effect (a phenomenon whereby the provision of psychiatric care for the mentally ill reduces the use of nonpsychiatric services) of 94%, a figure significantly greater than that demonstrated in other psychiatric conditions (69,70).

TREATMENT CHOICES

A variety of pharmacological and psychotherapeutic treatments have been proven to be effective in the treatment of both the symptoms of panic disorder and the frequency and severity of panic attacks, including benzodiazepines, tricyclic antidepressants, monoamine oxidase inhibitors, selective serotonin-reuptake inhibitors, busprione, and cognitive-behavioral therapy (CBT) (71–78). Few data, however, are available pertaining to the response of QOL variables to these interventions (Table 4).

Medication Studies

In reviewing recent studies examining effects of pharmacotherapy alone on the QOL in panic disorder, improvement is noted consistently in a range of QOL domains. Medications studied have included imipramine, phenelzine, alprazolam, and clonazepam in comparison with placebo (79,81,82).

In a study of imipramine or phenelzine vs. placebo and in conjunction with supportive psychotherapy, improvement observed with either active medication was significantly better than with placebo on all outcome measures. While an overall trend was observed for further improvement with phenelzine over imipramine, a significant improvement was reported in work and social disability and in phobic avoidance in subjects treated with phenelzine (79).

In a more recent, placebo-controlled study of clonazepam, subjects treated with clonazepam demonstrated a significant twofold improvement on the Mental Health Component Scale (MCS) of the SF-36 in comparison to subjects receiving placebo. In addition, the clonazepam group showed significant improvement on all measures of mental health-related QOL (e.g., social functioning, role limits—emotional, vitality, general mental health, and MCS summary score), on measures of the Physical Component Scale (PCS) of the SF-36 (e.g., physical functioning, freedom from bodily pain, and general health perceptions), and in measures of work productivity. By comparison, the placebo group showed improvement on MCS measures of social functioning and vitality and in the summary MCS score only (82).

A third study has examined the effects of medication or placebo on panic disorder, assessing change after the initial treatment period and in follow-up several years later. In this study, subjects were treated with either alprazolam or imipramine vs. placebo and examined after 8 weeks of treatment and in follow-up 4 years later. After the initial treatment period, both medications were equally efficacious in contrast to placebo in the overall treatment of panic disorder. At 4-year follow-up, comparing baseline (BL) and follow-up (FU) assessments, sustained gains were noted on all measures of the Sheehan Disability Scale (SDS). The proportion of subjects reporting no or mild disability increased substantially between the BL and FU assessments on all life domains, including work (BL 22%, FU 88%), family and home life (BL 19%, FU 77%), and social life and leisure (BL 7%, FU 70%). Despite these changes, 60% of subjects continued to report occasional panic attacks and 40% reported persistence of phobic avoidance, although improved from 85% of subjects at baseline (81,85). Although these authors did not compare FU response between the treatment groups, these data suggest that patients can have improvement in QOL, even with persistence of symptoms after treatment with medication or placebo, but the results are more robust with the active medication.

Psychotherapy Studies

Several studies have examined the effect of psychotherapy on the QOL impairment in panic disorder. In a study of CBT, investigators compared the effects of 12-session group CBT over 8 weeks with treatment-delayed controls who received CBT at the end of the initial 8-week period. All subjects were assessed at baseline and at week 9; subjects in the initial CBT group were also assessed at 6-month follow-up. Substantial impairment was noted in both groups at baseline, with subjects reporting moderate to severe impact of symptoms on work (69%), social (80%), and family/home (62%) functioning. After the initial 8-week treatment period, individuals in the CBT treatment group showed significant improvement compared to controls on all measures of the SDS and the majority of measures of the Social Adjustment Scale (SAS) (e.g., work outside/inside of home, social/leisure, extended family, marital, and overall), and these gains were maintained at 6-month follow-up (80).

Another study has examined the effects of CBT administered under two different treatment conditions. One group of panic patients received 12-session individual CBT (CBT12) over 12 weeks; a second group received four-session individual CBT in conjunction with the use of a palmtop computer over 4 weeks (CBT4-CA). The computer was used both for daily symptom recording and as a treatment adjunct during these 4 weeks, followed by continued diary and treatment use in the 8 weeks following formal CBT training. While the CBT12 group showed significant improvement at week 13 compared to the CBT4-CA group, reductions in behavioral avoidance, panic-related cognitions, and fear and panic symptoms and overall satisfaction with treatment were demonstrated and maintained in both groups at 6-month follow-up (83).

Combined Medication and Psychotherapy Studies

Two other studies have investigated the impact of medication and/or psychotherapy, either individually or in combination, on QOL measures in panic disorder. Brown et al. (33) compared the effects of interpersonal therapy (IPT) to those of pharmacological treatment with nortriptyline in depressed subjects with lifetime GAD, lifetime panic disorder, or depression alone. Among their findings, the authors reported that while both standardized treatments were effective for depressed subjects with or without GAD, depressed subjects with panic disorder demonstrated poor recovery to either medication or psychotherapy, with longer time to recovery or a lack of response altogether. The authors concluded that these findings should be considered by primary care physicians in assessing depressed patients for lifetime anxiety disorders so that proper therapeutic interventions may be made.

More recently, Sharp et al. (84) examined the effects of individual and combined treatments of fluvoxamine, CBT, and placebo on global measures of treatment outcome. Subjects were randomized to treatment in one of the following groups: fluvoxamine (FL), placebo (PL), CBT and FL (CBT-FL), CBT and PL (CBT-PL), or CBT. Subjects who received active treatment with FL and/or CBT showed significant improvement over subjects in the PL-alone group on a range of measures; however, the CBT groups demonstrated the most robust and consistent changes. On the General Health Questionnaire, treatment with CBT with FL was better than FL alone, while treatment with FL was superior to PL with or without CBT. Using the SDS, subjects receiving active treatment reported significant improvement in work and social/life disability compared to placebo, while all treatment groups showed improvement in home/family life scores. Changes in the Clinical Global

Impressions improvement score (CGI-I) were also impressive. Based on ratings of much improved or very much improved, both patient and clinician reports showed significant change after treatment (patient ratings: FL and/or CBT 75–89% vs. PL 35%, clinician CGI ratings: FL and/or CBT 78–90% vs. PL 48%).

These findings demonstrate a range of improvement in life quality in patients with panic disorder who receive treatment. Whether given an active medication or placebo and/or psychotherapy, benefits were noted in all groups, with the gains frequently maintained for several years after the intervention.

ROLE OF MANAGED CARE

Managed health care is an evolving concept in the United States. Although affected by decisions of government and the judicial system, managed health care is influenced predominantly by the forces of individual managed care organizations. These organizations share common guiding principles but otherwise maintain independent and unique identities. One author (86) has described managed care plans as sharing the same common language but with individual, idiosyncratic dialects. Two features common to all managed care plans, however, are cost containment and, to achieve this, the sentinel role of the primary care physician. Recognizing prevalence of panic disorder in primary care practice, these issues have particular relevance to the treatment of patients with panic disorder.

Unquestionably, recent changes in the health care environment have introduced additional work and responsibilities for primary care physicians. At the same time, these developments may be viewed as a source of opportunity for managed care plans to become more actively involved in the development of programs to improve both diagnostic knowledge and patient care in panic disorder, while also containing health care expenditures. For instance, providing additional education to primary care physicians has been shown to promote more accurate identification of patients with specific mental illnesses and to alter treatment practices. In a study comparing diagnostic and treatment patterns for six mental illnesses in the primary care setting, physicians receiving an intervention (e.g., a 2-hour evening seminar) were compared with other colleagues in practice (87). Physicians in the intervention group overall demonstrated greater diagnostic accuracy, particularly for major depression, dysthymia, and agoraphobia with panic disorder. In addition, a strong influence was observed on treatment recommendations, especially for panic disorder and major depression. In a study of emergency-room patients with panic attacks, Swinson et al. (88) found improvements in patients who received a brief counselling intervention. Compared to subjects who received reassurance alone, patients who received exposure instruction demonstrated a significant reduction in panic attack frequency at 6 month follow-up, as well as a reduction in depressive symptoms at both 3- and 6-month follow-up.

Managed care organizations could provide a variety of other services to facilitate more cost-effective care for patients with panic disorder. Recognizing the time constraints placed on care providers, managed care plans could assist in the development of screening instruments for anxiety disorders in general and panic disorder in particular. Ratings scales currently in use include the Primary Care Evaluation of Mental Disorders (PRIME-MD) (89), the Symptoms Driven Diagnostic System for Primary Care (SDDS-PC) (90,91), the General Health Questionnaire (92), the Duke Anxiety Depression Scale (91), and the Brief Panic Disorder Screen (94). These and similar tools can aid physicians in more rapid recognition and accurate diagnosis of psychiatric conditions seen in routine practice.

There is also a role for managed care to provide support for patient and family education. The development of psychoeducational materials and the provision of access to health care workers with specialized training in education and supportive care for individuals with anxiety disorders would initially increase direct costs. However, over time, this cost would be reversed by the savings associated with direct-cost reductions due to diminished utilization of medical resources and with indirect savings related to improvement in functional status.

Identification of patients with panic disorder early in the course of their illness would result in a more efficient allocation of resources. By reducing the time to diagnosis and intervention, patient suffering could be minimized and quality of life enhanced. Unnecessary and costly specialty referrals and expensive diagnostic tests could also be eliminated.

SUMMARY

The importance of QOL as a measure of health status and of medical outcome is gaining wider recognition. Clearly, both medical and emotional conditions have significant impact on an individual's personal happiness, role fulfillment, and health status. As more standardized measures of QOL are developed, these characteristics can be systematically studied to provide an understanding of how features of QOL change over time and with the course of treatment. By enhancing QOL, both the patient and society benefit with improved patient health, compliance, and satisfaction, and a reduction in direct and indirect health care expenditures. The role of managed health care organizations in this process is evolving, as they strive to provide quality patient care while containing health care costs.

In the case of panic disorder, substantial functional impairment has been documented in both nonpsychiatric and psychiatric samples. Markedly elevated rates of health resource utilization are frequently observed, usage that is often unnecessary, inappropriate, and very costly. Furthermore, additional costs associated with lost productivity in patients and family members contribute enormously to the indirect cost of panic disorder. These costs, however, can be significantly reduced and QOL parameters dramatically improved with appropriate diagnosis and treatment. In this era of managed health care, managed care organizations will have an increasing role in and responsibility for facilitating these changes.

REFERENCES

1. Ware JE, Sherbourne CD. The MOS 36-item Short-form Health Survey (SF-36). I. Conceptual framework and item selection. Med Care 1992; 30:473–483.
2. Brazier JE, Harper R, Jones NM. Validating the SF-36 health survey

questionnaire: new outcome measure for primary care. Br Med J 1992; 305:160–164.

3. McHorney CA, Ware JE, Raczek AE. The MOS 36-item Short-form Health Survey (SF-36). II. Psychometric and clinical tests of validity in measuring physical and mental health constructs. Med Care 1993; 31: 247–263.

4. Reilly MC, Zborzek AS, Dukes EM. The validity and reproducibility of a work productivity and impairment instrument. Pharmacoeconomics 1993; 4:353–365.

5. Robins LN, Helzer JE, Croughland JL, Williams JBW, Spitzer RL. NIMH Diagnostic Interview Schedule. Version III. Public Health Service (PHS), publication ADM-T-42-3 (5-8-81). Rockville, MD: NIMH, 1981.

6. What quality of life? The WHOQOL Group: World Health Organization Quality of Life Assessment. World Health Forum 1996; 17:354–356.

7. Klerman GL, Weissman MM, Ouellette R, Johnson J, Greenwald S. Panic attacks in the community: social morbidity and health care utilization. JAMA 1991; 265:742–746.

8. Edlund MJ. The economics of anxiety. Psychiatr Med 1990; 8:15–26.

9. Brown G, Harris TO. Aetiology of anxiety and depressive disorders in an inner-city population. 1. Early adversity. Psycholog Med 1993; 23: 143–154.

10. Angst J. Comorbidity of panic disorder in a community sample. Clin Neuropharmacol 1992; 14(suppl 1A):176A–177A.

11. Ormel J, Von Korff M, Ustan B, Pini S, Korten A, Oldehinkel T. Common mental disorders and disability across cultures: results from the WHO Collaborative Study on Psychological Problems in General Health Care. JAMA 1994; 272:1741–1748.

12. Goldberg R, Morris P, Christian F, Badger J, Chabot S, Edlund M. Panic disorder in cardiac outpatients. Psychosomatics 1990; 31:168–173.

13. Beitman BD, Mukerji V, Flaker G, Basha IM. Panic disorder, cardiology patients, and atypical chest pain. Psychiatr Clin North Am 1988; 11: 387–397.

14. Cormier LE, Katon W, Russo J, Hollifield M, Hall ML, Vitaliano PP. Chest pain with negative cardiac diagnostic studies: relationship to psychiatric illness. J Nerv Ment Dis 1988; 176:351–358.

15. Katon W, Von Korff M, Lin E, et al. Distressed high-utilizers of medical care: DSM-III-R diagnoses and treatment needs. Gen Hosp Psychiatry 1990; 12:355–362.

16. Markowitz JS, Weissman MM, Ouellette R, Lish JD, Klerman GL. Quality of life in panic disorder. Arch Gen Psychiatry 1989; 46:984–992.
17. Leon AC, Portera L, Weissman MM. The social costs of anxiety disorders. Br J Psychiatry 1995; 166(suppl 27):19–22.
18. Katon W, Vitaliano PP, Russo J, Cormier L, Anderson K, Jones M. Panic disorder: epidemiology in primary care. J Fam Practice 1986; 23:233–239.
19. Kahn JP, Drusin RE, Klein DF. Idiopathic cardiomyopathy and panic disorder: clinical association in cardiac transplant candidates. Am J Psychiatry 1987; 144:1327–1330.
20. Wuslin LR, Hillard JR, Geier P, Hissa D, Rouan GW. Screening emergency room patients with atypical chest pain for depression and panic disorder. Int J Psychiatr Med 1988; 18:315–323.
21. Brown FW, Golding JM, Smith GR. Psychiatric comorbidity in primary care somatization disorder. Psychosom Med 1990; 52:445–451.
22. Chignon JM, Lepine JP, Ades J. Panic disorder in cardiac outpatients. Am J Psychiatry 1993; 150:780–785.
23. Sullivan M, Clark MR, Katon WJ, Fischl M, Russo J, Dobie RA, Voorhees R. Psychiatric and otologic diagnoses in patients complaining of dizziness. Arch Intern Med 1993; 153:1479–1484.
24. Cohen LS, Sichel DA, Dimmock JA, Rosenbaum JF. Postpartum course in women with preexisting panic disorder. J Clin Psychiatry 1994; 55:289–292.
25. Cohen LS, Sichel DA, Dimmock JA, Rosenbeum JF. Impact of pregnancy on panic disorder: a case series. J Clin Psychiatry 1994; 55:284–288.
26. Hollifield M, Katon W, Morojele N. Anxiety and depression in an outpatient clinic in Lesotho, Africa. Int J Psychiatry Med 1994; 24:179–188.
27. Lydiard RB, Greenwald S, Weissman MM, Johnson J, Drossman DA, Ballenger JC. Panic disorder and gastrointestinal symptoms: findings from the NIMH Epidemiologic Catchment Area Project. Am J Psychiatry 1994; 151:64–70.
28. Simpson RJ, Kazmierczak T, Power KG, Sharp DM. Controlled comparison of characteristics of patients with panic disorder. Br J Gen Practice 1994; 44:352–356.
29. Klein E, Lin S, Colin V, Lang R, Lenox RH. Anxiety disorders among patients in a general emergency service in Israel. Psychiatr Services 1995; 46:488–492.
30. Marazziti D, Toni C, Pedri S, Bonuccelli U, Pavese A, Muratorio A, Battista Cassano G, Akiskal HS. Headache, panic disorder, and depres-

sion: comorbidity or a spectrum? Neuropsychobiology 1995; 31:125–129.

31. Spitzer RL, Kroenke K, Linzer M, Hahn SR, Williams JBW, deGruy FV, Brody D, Davies M. Health-related quality of life in primary care patients with mental disorders: results from the PRIME-MD 1000 study. JAMA 1995; 274:1511–1517.

32. Walker EA, Gelfand AN, Gelfand MD, Katon WJ. Psychiatric diagnoses, sexual and physical victimization, and disability in patients with irritable bowel syndrome or inflammatory bowel disease. Psycholog Med 1995; 25:1259–1267.

33. Brown C, Schulberg HC, Madonia MJ, Shear MK, Houck PR. Treatment outcomes for primary care patients with major depression and lifetime anxiety disorders. Am J Psychiatry 1996; 153:1293–1300.

34. Brown C, Schulberg HC, Shear MK. Phenomenology and severity of major depression and comorbid lifetime anxiety disorders in primary medical care practice. Anxiety 1996; 2:210–218.

35. Fyer A, Katon W, Hollifield M, Rassnick H, Mannuzza S, Chapman T, Ballenger JC. The DSM-IV Panic Disorder Field Trial: panic attack frequency and functional disability. Anxiety 1996; 2:157–166.

36. Hahn SR, Kroenke K, Spitzer RL, Brody D, Williams JBW, Linzer M, deGruy FV. The difficult patient: prevalence, psychopathology, and functional impairment. J Gen Intern Med 1996; 11:1–8.

37. Kaplan DS, Masand PS, Gupta S. The relationship of irritable bowel syndrome (IBS) and panic disorder. Ann Clin Psychiatry 1996; 8:81–88.

38. Olfson M, Broadhead E, Weissman MM, Leon AC, Farber L, Hoven C, Kathol R. Subthreshold psychiatric symptoms in a primary care group practice. Arch Gen Psychiatry 1996; 53:880–886.

39. Sherbourne CD, Jackson CA, Meredith LS, Camp P, Wells KB. Prevalence of comorbid anxiety disorders in primary care outpatients. Arch Fam Med 1996; 5:27–34.

40. Katon W, Hall ML, Russo J, Cormier L, Hollifield M, Vitaliano PP, Beitman BD. Chest pain: the relationship of psychiatric illness to coronary angiographic results. Am J Med 1988; 84:1–9.

41. Svensson TH. Peripheral autonomic regulation of the locus ceruleus neurons in the brain: putative implications for psychiatric and psychopharmacology. Psychopharmacology 1987; 92:1–7.

42. Lydiard RB, Laraia MT, Howell EF, Ballenger JC. Can panic disorder present as irritable bowel syndrome? J Clin Psychiatry 1986; 47:470–473.

43. Katon W. Panic disorder: epidemiology, diagnosis, and treatment in primary care. J Clin Psychiatry 1986; 47(suppl 10):21–27.
44. Katon WJ. Chest pain, cardiac disease, and panic disorder. J Clin Psychiatry 1990; 51(suppl 5):27–30.
45. Coryell W, Noyes R, Clancy J. Excess mortality in panic disorder: a comparison with primary unipolar depression. Arch Gen Psychiatry 1982; 39:701–703.
46. Coryell W, Noyes R, House JD. Mortality among outpatients with anxiety disorders. Am J Psychiatry 1986; 143:508–510.
47. Fawcett J. Predictors of early suicide: identification and appropriate intervention. J Clin Psychiatry 1988; 49(suppl):7–8.
48. Noyes R, Cook B, Garvey M, Summers R. Reduction of gastrointestinal symptoms following treatment for panic disorder. Psychosomatics 1990; 31:75–79.
49. Massion AO, Warshaw MG, Keller MB. Quality of life and psychiatric morbidity in panic disorder and generalized anxiety disorder. Am J Psychiatry 1993; 150:600–607.
50. Noyes R, Clancy J, Woodman C, Holt CS, Suelzer M, Christiansen J, Anderson DJ. Environmental factors related to the outcome of panic disorder: a seven year followup study. J Nerv Ment Dis 1993; 181:529–538.
51. Manassis K, Bradley S, Goldberg S, Hood J, Swinson RP. Attachment in mothers with anxiety disorder and their children. J Am Acad Child Adolesc Psych 1994; 33:1106–1113.
52. Katon W, Hollifield M, Chapman T, Mannuzza S, Ballanger J, Fyer A. Infrequent panic attacks: psychiatric characteristics and functional disability. J Psychiatr Res 1995; 29:121–131.
53. Sherbourne CD, Wells KB, Judd LL. Functioning and well-being of patients with panic disorder. Am J Psychiatry 1996; 153:213–218.
54. Hollifield M, Katon W, Skipper B, Chapman T, Ballenger JC, Mannuzza S, Fyer AJ. Panic disorder and quality of life: variables predictive of functional impairment. Am J Psychiatry 1997; 154:766–772.
55. Katerndahl DA, Realini JP. Quality of life and panic-related work disability in subjects with infrequent panic and panic disorder. J Clin Psychiatry 1997; 58:153–158.
56. Edlund MJ, Swann AC. The economic and social costs of panic disorder. Hosp Commun Psychiatry 1987; 38:1277–1280.
57. Kendell RE, Wainwright S, Hailey A, Shannon B. The influence of childbirth on psychiatric morbidity. Psycholog Med 1976; 6:297–304.
58. Zajicek E. Psychiatric problems during pregnancy. In: Wolkind S, Zaji-

cek E, eds. Pregnancy: A Psychological and Social Study. London: Academic Press, 1981:57–73.

59. Kendell RE, McGuire RJ, Connor Y. Mood changes in the first weeks after childbirth. J Affect Disord 1981; 3:317–326.

60. Paffenbarger RA. Epidemiological aspects of mental illness associated with childbearing. In: Brockington IF, Kumar R, eds. Motherhood and Mental Illness. New York: Grune & Stratton, 1982.

61. Northcott CJ, Stein MB. Panic disorder in pregnancy. J Clin Psychiatry 1994; 55:539–542.

62. Dupont RL, Rice DP, Miller LS, Shiraki SS, Rowland CR, Harwood HJ. Economic costs of anxiety disorders. Anxiety 1996; 2:167–172.

63. Siegel L, Jones WC, Wilson JO. Economic and life consequences experienced by a group of individuals with panic disorder. J Anxiety Disord 1990; 4:201–211.

64. Salvador-Carulla L, Segui J, Fernancez-Cano P, Canet J. Costs and offset effect in panic disorder. Br J Psychiatry 1995; 166(suppl 27):23–28.

65. Leon AC, Olfson M, Portera L. Service utilization and expenditures for the treatment of panic disorder. Gen Hosp Psychiatry 1997; 19:82–88.

66. Beitman BD, Lamberti JW, Mukerji V, DeRosear L, Basha I, Schmid L. Panic disorder in patients with angiographically normal coronary arteries. Psychosomatics 1987; 28:480–484.

67. Ockene IS, Shay MJ, Alpert JS, et al. Unexplained chest pain in patients with normal coronary arteriograms. N Engl J Med 1980; 303:1249–1252.

68. Lavey EB, Winkle RA. Continuing disability of patients with chest pain and normal coronary arteriograms. J Chronic Dis 1979; 32:191–196.

69. Borus JF, Olendzki MC, Kessler L, Burns BJ, Brandt UC, Broverman CA, Henderson PR. The "offset effect" of mental health treatment on ambulatory medical care: utilization and charges. Arch Gen Psychiatry 1985; 42:573–580.

70. Hankin JR, Kessler LG, Goldberg ID, Steinwachs DM, Starfield BH. A longitudinal study of offset in the use of nonpsychiatric services following specialized mental health care. Medical Care 1983; 21:1099–1110.

71. Rickels K, Case G, Downing RW, et al. Long-term diazepam therapy and clinical outcome. JAMA 1983; 250:767–771.

72. Cohn JB, Wilcox CS. Long-term comparison of alprazolam, lorazepam, and placebo in patients with anxiety disorder. Pharmacotherapy 1984; 4:93–98.

73. Zitrin CM, Klein DR, Woerner MG. Treatment of agoraphobia with

group exposure in vivo and imipramine. Arch Gen Psychiatry 1980; 37: 63–72.

74. Tyrer P, Candy J, Kelly D. A study of the clinical effects of phenelzine and placebo in the treatment of phobic anxiety. Psychopharmacologia 1973; 32:237–254.

75. Goa KL, Ward A. Buspirone: a preliminary review of its pharmacological properties and therapeutic efficacy as an anxiolytic. Drugs 1986; 32: 114–129.

76. Rickels K, Weisman K, Norstad N, et al. Buspirone and diazepam in anxiety: a controlled study. J Clin Psychiatry 1982; 43:81–86.

77. Mavissalalian M. Antidepressant medications for panic disorder. In: Mavissakalian M, Prien R, eds. Long-term Treatments of Anxiety Disorders. Washington, DC: American Psychiatric Association Press, 1996: 265–284.

78. Barlow DH, Lehman CL. Advance in the psychosocial treatment of anxiety disorders: implications for national health care. Arch Gen Psychiatry 1996; 53:727–735.

79. Sheehan DV, Ballenger J, Jacobson G. Treatment of endogenous anxiety with phobic, hysterical and hypochondriacal symptoms. Arch Gen Psychiatry 1980; 37:51–59.

80. Telch MJ, Schmidt NB, Jaimez TL, Jacquin KM, Harrington PJ. Impact of cognitive-behavioral treatment on quality of life in panic disorder patients. J Consult Clin Psychol 1995; 5:823–830.

81. Katschnig H, Amering M, Stolk JM, Ballenger JC. Predictors of quality of life in a longterm followup study in panic disorder patients after a clinical drug trial. Psychopharmacol Bull 1996; 32:149–155.

82. Jacobs RJ, Davidson JRT, Gupta S, Meyerhoff AS. The effects of clonazepam on quality of life and work productivity in panic disorder. Am J Managed Care 1997; 3:733–736.

83. Newman MG, Kenardy J, Herman S, Taylor CB. Comparison of palmtop-computer-assisted brief cognitive-behavioral treatment to cognitive-behavioral treatment for panic disorder. J Consult Clin Psychol 1997; 65:178–183.

84. Sharp DM, Power KG, Simpson RJ, Swanson V, Anstee JA. Global measures of outcome in a controlled comparison of pharmacological and psychobiological treatment of panic disorder and agoraphobia in primary care. Br J Gen Practice 1997; 47:150–155.

85. Cross-National Collaborative Panic Study, Second Phase Investigators. Drug treatment of panic disorder: comparison of efficacy of alprazolam, imipramine, and placebo. Br J Psychiatry 1992; 160:191–202.

86. Rapaport MH, Cantor JJ. Panic disorder in a managed care environment. J Clin Psychiatry 1997; 58(suppl 2):51–55.

87. Andersen SM, Harthorn BH. Changing the psychiatric knowledge of primary care physicians: the effects of a brief intervention on clinical diagnosis and treatment. Gen Hosp Psychiatry 1990; 12:177–190.

88. Swinson RP, Soulios C, Cox BJ, Kuch K. Brief treatment of emergency room patients with panic attacks. Am J Psychiatry 1992; 149:944–946.

89. Spitzer RL, Williams JBW, Kroenke K, Linzer M, Hahn SR, Williams JB, deGruy FV III, Brody D, Davies M. Utility of a new procedure for diagnosing mental disorders in primary care: the PRIME-MD 1000 Study. JAMA 1994; 272:1749–1756.

90. Broadhead WE, Leon AC, Weissman MM, Barrett JE, Blacklow RS, Gilbert TT, Keller MB, Olfson M, Higgins ES. Development and validation of the SDDS-PC screen for multiple mental disorders in primary care. Arch Fam Med 1995; 4:211–219.

91. Olfson M, Leon AS, Broadhead WE, Weissman MM, Barrett JE, Blacklow RS, Gilbert TT, Higgins ES. The SDDS-PC: a diagnostic aid for multiple mental disorders in primary care. Psychopharmacol Bull 1995; 31:415–420.

92. Goldberg D, Williams P. A User's Guide to the General Health Questionnaire. Windsor, England: NFER/Nelson, 1988.

93. Parkerson GR, Broadhead WE. Screening for anxiety and depression in primary care with the Duke Anxiety-Depression Scale. Fam Med 1997; 29:177–181.

94. Apfeldorf WA, Shear MK, Leon AC, Portera L. A brief screen for panic disorder. J Anxiety Disord 1994; 4:71–78.

Appendix

Diagnostic and Symptom Assessment of Panic Disorder

Michael W. Otto, Susan J. Penava, and Mark H. Pollack

Massachusetts General Hospital
and Harvard Medical School
Boston, Massachusetts

The study of panic disorder has benefited from the diversity of theoretical, methodological, and treatment perspectives that have been brought to bear by clinical and applied researchers. Nonetheless, the synthesis of this information into a meaningful whole requires consistency in the manner in which diagnostic and symptom severity indices are applied. This issue received direct attention in the National Institute of Health's Consensus Development Conference on the Treatment of Panic Disorder. Subsequently, a 2-day conference was organized with the goal of recommending standards for assessment. In their report on this conference, Shear and Maser (1) summarize recommendations and issues for both diagnostic and symptom assessment, including assessment of panic frequency, anticipatory anxiety, phobic fear and avoidance, and global impairment. The following sections provide brief reviews of several assessment measures for each of these domains.

DIAGNOSTIC ASSESSMENT

The goal of diagnostic assessment is to confirm the presence of panic disorder, and investigate comorbid conditions that may alter its presentation or course. Shear and Maser (1) identified five structured interviews that were found to be acceptable for this purpose: the Anxiety Disorders Interview Schedule–Revised (ADIS-R) (2), the Composite International Diagnostic Interview (CIDI) (3), the Diagnostic Interview Schedule (DIS) (4), the Schedule for Affective Disorders–Lifetime, Anxiety (SADS-LA) (5), and the Structured Clinical Interview for DSM-III-R (SCID) (6). Revised versions appropriate for the DSM-IV are available for the SCID (SCID-IV) (7) and the ADIS (ADIS-IV) (8). The SCID, because of its early development, has enjoyed the most popularity of use in controlled treatment trials, but it is followed closely by the ADIS-R. In a recent meta-analysis of 43 controlled studies between 1974 and 1994 (9), 19 studies reported use of a structured diagnostic interview. The SCID was used in 10 (53%) studies, followed by the ADIS/R in eight studies (42%), and the SADS-L in one study (5%). None of these panic disorder treatment studies reported use of the CIDI or the DIS.

In addition to diagnostic assessment, the ADIS-R includes a number of clinician-rated severity indices. For panic disorder, these indices include ratings of distress and disability, as well as fear and avoidance ratings across a range of typical agoraphobic situations. Hamilton anxiety and depression rating scales (see below) are also included in the ADIS-R assessment inteview.

SCREENING FOR PANIC DISORDER IN PRIMARY CARE

Psychiatric disorders are common in primary care practices, and the majority of patients with psychiatric illness present and are treated in the general medical setting. The recognition that undetected psychiatric disorders are associated with increased medical utilization and other costs, as well as marked distress and disability for patients, has spurred efforts to screen for psychiatric disorders in primary care settings. There is at present no "gold standard" for screening of panic disorder in the primary care setting, but a number of potentially useful instruments currently exist, and others are in development.

Primary Care Evaluation of Mental Disorders (Prime-MD): a two-part screening instrument consisting of a 26-item patient self-report questionnaire and follow-up interview modules. Five major groups of psychiatric illness are targeted—mood, anxiety, somatoform, alcohol, and eating disorders—and panic disorder is one of 18 specific disorders assessed. The Prime-MD has the advantage of being time-efficient, requiring an average of 5 to 10 minutes to follow-up patients' self-report of symptoms; it also offers an acceptable level of agreement with diagnoses derived by psychiatric interview (10). The specificity of this instrument is strong for mood, alcohol, and eating disorders, but is more moderate for anxiety disorders, including panic and somatoform disorders. This instrument is copyrighted by Pfizer Pharmaceuticals, Inc., and an interactive voice response (IVR) format is in development.

Symptom Driven Diagnostic Screen-Primary Care (SDDS-PC): a two-part instrument that screens for six psychiatric disorders—major depression, panic disorder, generalized anxiety disorder, obsessive-compulsive disorder, and alcohol and drug dependence—as well as suicidal ideation (11). A 26-item patient screen is used to trigger follow-up questions. An automated computer version (which incorporates toll-free telephone access by patients for initial screening, with information faxed to the clinician for follow-up) is also being evaluated. The sensitivity and specificity appear to be relatively adequate for this instrument for mood and anxiety disorders, and somewhat less so for alcohol and drug abuse disorders. The SDDS-PC system is available through the Pharmacia Upjohn Company.

Autonomic Nervous System Questionnaire (ANS): recently, McQuaid and Stein (12) utilized the seven-item ANS to assess whether patients had experienced recent panic attacks. They reported good sensitivity and specificity on this measure for detecting panic disorder.

ASSESSMENT OF PANIC FREQUENCY

Daily assessment of panic attacks, in the form of self-report diaries, has been recommended as essential to studies of panic disorder (1). Panic diaries frequently detail the duration and severity of panic episodes, as well as information on whether attacks were situationally cued or "unexpected," and whether full or limited symptom attacks were experienced.

When panic diaries are assigned, care needs to be taken to ensure that patients share the same definitions of symptoms as the research staff. This is particularly important for the differentiation of episodes of anticipatory anxiety from limited or full panic attacks. Patients should be provided with clear examples of each; diagrams of symptom profiles are helpful for this purpose. Occasional reconfirmation of the definition of specific symptom domains can help reduce patient ''drift'' from these definitions during the course of a study.

Because frequency of panic episodes may be highly variable across days or weeks, prolonged baseline monitoring of panic frequency is desirable before initiation of treatment. Shear and Maser (1) discuss the compromise between an optimal 1-month monitoring period and the practical demands for a brief baseline period in treatment outcome studies, noting that a 2-week monitoring period is desirable.

ASSESSMENT OF PANIC-RELATED FEARS

Anxiety Sensitivity Index (ASI) (13): anxiety sensitivity refers to fears of anxiety-related sensations based on beliefs that these sensations have harmful or dangerous consequences (14,15). This fear can be assessed by the 16-item, self-report ASI (16). According to normative data (17), patients with panic disorder and/or agoraphobia score at a mean of 35.9 on the ASI. Patients with posttraumatic stress disorder score at a mean of 31.6, and patients with other anxiety disorders tend to score in the mid-20s. Healthy control subjects score much lower (mean = 19.0; SD = 9.1) (17). Moderate elevations on the ASI (mean scores in the mid-20s) have also been found for patients with major depressive disorder without comorbid panic disorder (18,19).

Inclusion of a measure of fears of anxiety symptoms such as the ASI has been recommended to be part of standardized assessment for panic disorder (1), and results to date suggest that the ASI is sensitive to clinical improvement (20). The ASI predicts the prospective emergence of panic attacks among infrequent panickers, the emergence of panic among individuals free of a history of panic, and the maintenance of panic disorder among untreated patients (16,21). In addition, the ASI is a predictor of the biological provocation of anxiety and panic (22–

24), and the prospective emergence of panic in adults undergoing psychosocial stress (25).

Body Sensations Questionnaire (BSQ) (26): a 17-item self-report measure that, like the ASI, assesses the fear of bodily sensations. Patients respond to each item on a five-point scale, with responses ranging from ''not frightened or worried by this sensation'' to ''extremely frightened by this sensation.'' Higher scores indicate a higher degree of fear. Chambless and colleagues (26) found the BSQ to have high internal consistency and a moderate test–retest reliability. This scale has been shown to distinguish between agoraphobic patients and normal controls, and to be sensitive to change during treatment (26).

Agoraphobia Cognitions Questionnaire (ACQ) (26): this 14-item, self-report questionnaire assesses the frequency of thoughts about possible negative consequences of symptoms of anxiety. Subjects respond to each item on a five-point scale, indicating the frequency with which they have each thought when feeling anxious. The total score is the average of individual item ratings. The ACQ has been found to have high internal consistency and adequate test–retest reliability (26). The ACQ, like the BSQ, has also been found to discriminate patients with panic disorder from healthy control subjects and to be sensitive to change during the course of treatment (26).

Panic Beliefs Questionnaire (PBQ) (27): a 42-item self-report questionnaire used to assess catastropic beliefs about panic attacks. Each item is rated on a six-point scale, ranging from ''totally disagree'' to ''totally agree,'' with higher scores indicating greater beliefs that panic attacks are harmful and dangerous. The PBQ has been found to have high internal reliability (alpha = 0.94) and adequate concurrent validity with other cognitive measures of panic and anxiety (28).

ASSESSMENT OF AGORAPHOBIC AVOIDANCE

Fear Questionnaire (FQ) (29): one of the most widely used self-report measures of treatment outcome in studies of agoraphobia (30). The NIMH-SUNY Albany conference on anxiety disorders recommended it as a standard measure for all research studies on phobias (31). In fact, it was utilized in 15 of the 43 (35%) studies reviewed in the meta-analysis by Gould et al. (9) of treatment-outcome studies. This 15-item, self-report questionnaire asks subjects to rate the degree to which they would avoid various situations, with higher scores indicating greater avoidance. In addition to the total score, three five-item subscale scores can also be calculated: agoraphobia (FQ-Ag), social phobia (FQ-Soc), and avoidance of situations related to blood/injury phobia (FQ-BI). Michelson and Mavissakalian (32) reported adequate test–retest correlations over a 4-month interval, Mizes and Crawford (33) provide normative data, and Oei et al. (34) reported that the FQ-Ag and FQ-Soc subscales discriminate between agoraphobics and social phobics.

Mobility Inventory (MI) (35): a seven-item self-report scale that measures avoidance of a variety of situations. Higher scores reflect a greater degree of avoidance. The questionnaire also includes one item that assesses panic frequency. Chambless et al. (35) reported high internal consistency and good test–retest reliability for this scale. The MI has also been shown to discriminate between agoraphobic patients and social phobics, and was found to be sensitive to change during treatment (35).

Behavioral Avoidance Tests (BATs): as opposed to the reliance on patients' self-report, BATs provide a behavioral measure of agoraphobic avoidance. BATs typically require patients to walk a specified course that includes exposure to standard agoraphobic situations (e.g., a crowded urban shopping center and a crowded bus stop). Patients are asked to walk the course alone, continuing until they experience intolerable anxiety or complete the course. The level of anxiety and the degree of completion of the course provide measures of avoidance. Both standardized and idiosyncratic courses have been used (36). Standardized courses have at times been criticized for offering too limited a range of agoraphobic stimuli. Idiosyncratically constructed courses avoid this criticism (each course is designed relative to a patient's hierarchy of avoided situations), although the individualized hierarchies may make meaningful comparisons between patients difficult.

ASSESSMENT OF GENERALIZED ANXIETY

Beck Anxiety Inventory (BAI) (37): a 21-item self-report measure that assesses the severity of anxiety. Items are common symptoms of anxiety, and subjects indicate on a four-point scale the degree to which they have been bothered by each symptom over the past week. Scores range from 0 to 63, with higher scores indicating greater severity of anxiety symptoms. The scale has been found to have high internal consistency and high test–retest reliability over a 1-week interval ($r = 0.75$).

Hamilton Rating Scale for Anxiety (HRSA or HAM-A) (39): a 14-item, clinician-administered instrument that assesses the severity of anxious symptomatology. All responses are rated on a 0-to-4 scale, with higher scores indicating a greater severity of symptoms. The HAM-A is commonly applied in treatment-outcome studies as a measure of general anxiety, although it tends to be weighted toward somatic symptoms. For many patients with panic disorder, these somatic symptoms may occur exclusively in the context of a panic attack; hence, researchers must decide for any given study whether to consider or ignore these symptoms in completing the HAM-A. If the goal of the HAM-A rating is to capture general or anticipatory anxiety symptoms, symptoms occurring only in the context of a panic attack should not be rated. Although the original HAM-A provides raters with no guidance for assigning item-severity ratings, structured interview guides that provide clear anchor points have been developed and are now undergoing empirical testing. Scoring methods for the HAM-A have also been developed that reduce the overlap between the Hamilton anxiety and Hamilton depression (see below) rating scales (40).

GLOBAL MEASURES

Clinician Global Impression of Severity (CGI-S) (41): clinician global ratings have been especially popular in pharmacological research studies. The measure, which is designed to provide an overview of symptom severity, is assessed by clinicians using a seven-point scale ranging from 1 (''normal, not at all ill'') to 7 (''extremely ill, among the most ill patients seen''). The potential benefit of such a global measure of overall disability is offset by the prominent absence of anchor points for assigning ratings. Clinicians must judge severity according to their own experiences with patients, and construct their own algorithm for collapsing the varied symptoms of panic disorder—panic frequency and severity, anticipatory anxiety, avoidance, and role dysfunction—into a single rating. Although internal standards may easily be developed at any one site, the potential for between-site variation is huge, especially given the possibility that the general severity of patients may vary significantly from site to site.

To counter these problems, anchor points for a panic-specific CGI-severity score have been developed (MGH Panic CGI-S; see chart). Individual anchor points are provided for each of four domains of functioning: panic frequency, anticipatory anxiety, avoidance, and role disability. Clinicians consider the level of functioning in each domain, then select a single global score that provides the best clinical summary of these domains.

The well-anchored CGI-S score also provides an excellent score for judging relapse and remission of panic disorder. A CGI-S score of 1 or 2 defines patients who are essentially free of panic attacks (i.e., no panic episodes or no more than one mild panic episode in the last month), are free of significant anticipatory anxiety or avoidance, and who report no effects of the disorder on role functioning. In longitudinal studies, these scores have been used to define remission in a manner similar to "high endstate functioning" (see below) measures used in other studies. For example, to identify consistent treatment gains, Otto et al. (42) used a CGI score of 1 or 2 for 2 consecutive months to define remission, and scores above 2 for 2 consecutive months to define relapse.

Clinician Global Impression of Improvement (CGI-I) (41): CGI-I scores provide global judgments of improvement in relevant clinical symptoms over time, and range from 1 ("markedly improved") to 7 ("markedly worse"), with a rating of 4 indicating no change in symptoms. Although this measure provides an intuitively pleasing method to sum up improvement across treatment, it is replete with methodological difficulties. Assigning an improvement rating requires the clinician to keep in mind the degree of severity experienced by a patient at the beginning of a trial. This daunting task is made more difficult by the natural demand characteristics inherent in a trial, and the fact that clinical raters may fill in for one another across the course of a trial. It is tempting to suggest that CGI-I raters keep track of both

Massachusetts General Hospital Anchor Points for the Panic CGI

Please indicate the level of severity in each column by circling the symptom levels best reflecting the patient's current status.

CGI rating	Panic symptoms	Level of anxiety	Level of avoidance	Level of functioning
Normal	Normal	Normal	Normal	No difficulties
Borderline mentally ill	Mild panic ≤1× mo	Infrequent anticipatory anxiety; no other fear	None to rare avoidance	No effect on functioning; no distress about symptoms
Mildly ill	Mild panic <1× wk and >1× mo	Mild, infrequent anticipatory anxiety; mild fear	Only infrequent activities with no consequences	No significant effect; mild concern and distress about symptoms
Moderately ill	Panic episodes >1× wk, moderate to severe intensity	Mild to moderate fear, anticipatory anxiety more days than not	>1× wk, nonrequired social activities avoided	No significant decrease in role functioning; exerts some effort to maintain normal functioning
Markedly ill	Panic episodes almost daily (e.g., >5× wk) of significant severity	Severe fear; anticipatory anxiety almost daily	Some required and desired activities avoided	Impairment of required role functioning; may require assistance
Severely ill	Daily with little change in intensity	Daily severe fear and anticipatory anxiety	Daily; cannot do many/most required or desired activities	Severe impairment of required role functioning (e.g., quit or was demoted or fired)
Extremely severe illness	Incapacitating	Incapacitating	Homebound or hospitalized due to incapacitating panic or avoidance	Total impairment of role functioning

Overall Panic Disorder Severity Rating (CGI-S) (please check)

1. _____ Normal
2. _____ Borderline mentally ill
3. _____ Mildly ill
4. _____ Moderately ill
5. _____ Markedly ill
6. _____ Severely ill
7. _____ Among the most severely ill

initial and current severity with CGI-S ratings, but with such data at hand there is no need for the CGI-I rating.

Patient Global Impression (PGI) scores: PGI ratings have some of the same benefits and limitations as the CGI ratings presented above. It is likely that patients may better remember their baseline functioning, and may thus be able to provide a more valid rating of improvement.

However, because patients may not have the same standards for judging improvement, large variations in these scores are likely. PGI-severity scores offer the potential of more consistent ratings, as long as anchor points are used.

COMPOSITE MEASURES

To provide overall estimates of improvement during the study period, as well as descriptions of subjects' overall level of posttreatment functioning, several investigators have utilized composite scores constructed from the particular outcome measures included in the studies. Guidelines to establish clinically significant change during the course of treatment were outlined by Himadi et al. (43), and outcome measures based on these guidelines have been utilized in a number of treatment-outcome studies of panic disorder. Two examples of the use of composite measures to provide categorical outcome measures are: 1) responder status, which assesses the degree of change in symptomatology across the course of treatment (e.g., Refs. 44–46), and 2) endstate functioning, which assesses a subject's level of functioning after treatment (46–48). For example, high or low endstate functioning has been determined by establishing cutoff scores for a group of measures such as clinician-rated severity, patient-rated severity, a rating of phobic anxiety and phobic avoidance, and results of a behavioral avoidance test (e.g., Ref. 46). Composite scores have the general advantage of combining ratings by both clinicians and patients, as well as ratings of both anxiety and avoidance.

Panic Disorder Severity Scale (PDSS) (49): modeled after the Yale-Brown Obsessive-Compulsive Scale (Y-BOCS) (50). The PDSS is a seven-item scale that assesses seven dimensions of panic disorder: panic frequency, distress during panic attacks, anticipatory anxiety, situational fear and avoidance, fear and avoidance of sensations, and interference in or impairment of work and/or social functioning. Responses to each item on this clinician-rated instrument are rated on a 0-to-4 scale (0 = none; 4 = extreme). The composite score is the average of scores on the seven items. The PDSS has been found to have good interrater reliability (intraclass correlation coefficient = 0.87 to

0.88), with interrater reliability of the individual items ranging from 0.74 to 0.87. As may be expected of a composite measure, the internal consistency of the total score is modest (Cronbach's alpha = 0.65). Although the PDSS was developed as a clinician-rated instrument, it has been applied as a patient-rated instrument in studies (51).

ASSESSMENT OF QUALITY OF LIFE AND FUNCTIONAL IMPAIRMENT

Assessment of quality of life in psychiatric patients is a rapidly evolving area of interest, with a number of instruments available or being developed to help in documenting the distress and disability associated with mental illness and the impact of treatment. Three instruments that have been used in assessing quality of life in association with panic disorder are 1) the Sheehan Disability Scale, 2) the Medical Outcome Study Short Form-36 (SF-36), and 3) the Quality of Life Enjoyment and Satisfaction Questionnaire (Q-LES-Q).

The **Sheehan Disability Scale,** designed to assess functional impairment in panic patients, is a three-item, self-rated scale of impairment that addresses the impact of symptomatology on work, social, and family functioning. It has the advantage of being brief and easily administered, but offers clinicians little guidance for making ratings. The instrument has demonstrated moderate reliability and validity in patients with panic disorder, is sensitive to change in impairment over time, and discriminates symptomatic from asymptomatic patients (52).

The **Medical Outcome Study Short Form-36 (SF-36)** is a widely used, relatively brief, self-report instrument that assesses health-related quality of life. It is scored from 0 to 100, with higher scores indicating better health. The SF-36 is composed of eight subscales that assess limitations in physical activities because of health problems; limitations in social activities because of physical and emotional problems; limitations in usual-role activities because of physical health problems; bodily pain; general mental health; limitations in usual-role activities because of emotional problems; vitality; and general health perceptions (53). Validity and reliability of the SF-36 have been established in large general population samples as well as in groups with heart disease, chronic lung problems, diabetes, hypertension, osteoarthritis, and major depression. The SF-36 has also been used to document impairment in populations of patients with panic disorder (54,55).

The **Quality of Life Enjoyment and Satisfaction Questionnaire (Q-LES-Q)** is a self-report measure used to assess well-being and function in psychiatric patients (56). It comprises 83 items divided into eight domains assessing a number of areas of function. It has been used to document impairment in panic disorder patients and is sensitive to change with treatment. One analysis suggests that it may aid in the discrimination of pharmacological versus placebo response (57).

ASSESSMENT OF DEPRESSION AND ASSOCIATED SYMPTOMS

Depression frequently co-occurs with panic disorder, and depressive symptoms frequently improve with panic treatment.

Beck Depression Inventory (BDI) (58,59): a 21-item self-report measure of symptoms of depression that is widely used in both research and clinical practice. Each item assesses a particular symptom of depression; total scores range from 0 to 63, with higher scores indicating greater severity. It is easy to administer and has good face validity, as well as adequate internal consistency and test–retest reliability. The BDI has also been found to correlate highly with other measures of depression and to discriminate between psychiatric patients and normal controls (38).

Hamilton Rating Scale for Depression (HRSD or HAM-D) (60,61): a 17-item clinician-administered instrument that assesses the severity of depressive symptomatology. Whereas the BDI tends to emphasize cognitive symptoms, the HAM-D emphasizes somatic symptoms. Internal consistency of the HAM-D has been reported to be adequate (62), and this scale also has been found to discriminate between depressed patients and control subjects (62). The HAM-D has been found to be sensitive to clinical change (e.g., Ref. 63). Like the HAM-A, little guidance is given in the original version for assigning specific severity ratings, but a structured interview guide is now available that provides such guidance as well as a uniform structure for inquiring about symptoms (64).

Hopkins Symptom Checklist (SCL-90) (65,66): a general, self-report measure of psychiatric symptoms that consists of 90 items, each being rated on a five-point scale. Subjects are asked to rate how problematic the particular symptom has been to them over the past week (responses range from ''not at all'' to ''extremely''). The scale provides a total score as well as nine subscales: somatization, obsessive-compulsive, interpersonal sensitivity, depression, anxiety, hostility, phobic anxiety, paranoid ideation, and psychoticism. The total scale score has been used as a measure of general psychiatric symptomatology, and the phobic anxiety subscale has been used as a measure of the severity of phobic fears in a number of treatment-outcome studies (e.g., Ref. 67).

REFERENCES

1. Shear MK, Maser JD. Standardized assessment for panic disorder research. Arch Gen Psychiatry 1994; 51:346–354.
2. DiNardo PA, Barlow DH. Anxiety Disorders Interview Schedule, Revised (ADIS-R). New York: Graywind Publications, 1988.
3. Robins LN, Wing J, Wittchen HU, Helzer JE, Babor TF, Burke J, Farmer A, Jablensky A, Pickens R, Regier DA, Sartorius N, Towle LH. The composite international diagnostic interview: an epidemiologic instrument suitable for use in conjunction with different diagnostic systems and in different cultures. Arch Gen Psychiatry 1989; 45:1069–1077.
4. Robins LN, Helzer JE, Croughan J, Ratliffe KS. National Institute of Mental Health Diagnostic Interview Schedule: its history, characteristics, and validity. Arch Gen Psychiatry 1981; 38:381–389.
5. Manuzza S, Fyer A, Klein D, Endicott J. Schedule for Affective Disorders-Lifetime, Anxiety (SADS-LA): rationale and conceptual development. J Psychiatr Res 1986; 20:317–325.
6. Spitzer RL, Williams JBW, Gibbon M, First MB. Structured Clinical Interview for DSM-III-R: Patient Version (SCID-P 6/1/88). New York: Biometrics Research Department, New York State Psychiatric Institute, 1988.
7. First MB, Spitzer RL, Gibbon M, Williams JBW. Structured Clinical Interview for DSM-IV Axis I Disorders: Patient Edition (SCID-I/P, Version 2.0). New York: Biometrics Research Department, New York State Psychiatric Institute, 1996.

8. DiNardo PA, Brown TA, Barlow DH. Anxiety Disorders Interview Schedule for DSM-IV: Lifetime Version (ADIS-IV). San Antonio, TX: Psychological Corporation, 1994.

9. Gould RA, Otto MW, Pollack MH. A meta-analysis of treatment outcome for panic disorder. Clin Psychol Rev 1995; 15:819–844.

10. Spitzer RL, Williams JBW, Kroenke K, et al. Utility of a new procedure for diagnosing mental disorders in primary care: the PRIME-MD 1000 study. JAMA 1994; 272:1749–1756.

11. Weissman MM, Olfson M, Leon AC, Broadhead WE, Gilbert TT, Higgin ES, Barrett JE, Blacklow RS, Keller MB, Hoven C. Brief diagnostic interviews (SDDS-PC) for multiple mental disorders in primary care. Arch Fam Med 1995; 4:220–227.

12. McQuaid JR, et al. Use of brief psychiatric screening measures in a primary care sample. Presented at 31st Annual Convention of the Association for the Advancement of Behavior Therapy, Miami Beach, FL, 1997.

13. Reiss S, Peterson RA, Gursky DM, McNally RJ. Anxiety sensitivity, anxiety frequency and the prediction of fearfulness. Behav Res Ther 1986; 24:1–8.

14. Reiss S. The expectancy model of fear, anxiety and panic. Clin Psychol Rev 1991; 11:141–153.

15. Reiss S, McNally RJ. The expectancy model of fear. In: Reiss S, Bootzin RR, eds. Theoretical Issues in Behavior Therapy. New York: Academic Press, 1985:107–121.

16. Taylor S, ed. Anxiety Sensitivity: Theory, Research and Treatment of the Fear of Anxiety. Hillsdale, NJ: Lawrence Erlbaum Associates. In press.

17. Peterson RA, Reiss S. Anxiety Sensitivity Index Revised Test Manual. Worthington, OH: International Diagnostic Services, 1992.

18. Otto MW, Pollack MH, Fava M, Uccello R, Rosenbaum JF. Elevated Anxiety Sensitivity Index scores in patients with major depression: correlates and changes with antidepressant treatment. J Anxiety Disord 1995; 9:117–124.

19. Taylor S, Koch WJ, Woody S, McLean P. Anxiety sensitivity and depression: how are they related? J Abnorm Psychol 1996; 105:474–479.

20. Otto MW, Reilly-Harrington N. The impact of treatment on anxiety sensitivity. In Taylor S, ed. Anxiety Sensitivity: Theory, Research and Treatment of the Fear of Anxiety. Hillsdale, NJ: Lawrence Erlbaum. In press.

21. Ehlers A. A 1-year prospective study of panic attacks: clinical course

and factors associated with maintenance. J Abnorm Psychol 1995; 104: 164–172.

22. Eke M, McNally RJ. Anxiety sensitivity, suffocation fear, trait anxiety, and breath-holding duration as predictors of response to carbon dioxide challenge. Behav Res Ther 1996; 34:603–607.

23. Rapee RM. Psychological factors influencing the affective response to biological challenge procedures in panic disorder. J Anxiety Disord 1995; 9:59–74.

24. Telch MJ, Harrington PJ. Anxiety sensitivity and expectedness of arousal in mediating affective response to 35% carbon dioxide inhalation. Pesented at the 26th annual AABT Convention, Boston, 1992.

25. Schmidt NB, Lerew DR, Jackson RJ. The role of anxiety sensitivity in the pathogenesis of panic: prospective evaluation of spontaneous panic attacks during acute stress. J Abnorm Psychol 1997; 106:355–364.

26. Chambless DL, Caputo GC, Bright PN, Gallagher R. Assessment of fear of fear in agoraphobics: the Body Sensations Questionnaire and the Agoraphobic Cognitions Questionnaire. J Consulting Clin Psychol 1984; 52:1090–1097.

27. Greenberg RL. Panic disorder and agoraphobia. In: Williams JMG, Beck AT, eds. Cognitive Therapy in Clinical Practice: An Illustrative Casebook. London: Routledge and Kegan Paul, 1989.

28. Brown GK, Beck AT, Greenberg RL, Newman CF, Beck J, Tran G, Clark D, Reilly N, Betz F. The role of beliefs in the cognitive treatment of panic disorder. Presented at the World Congress of Cognitive Therapy, Toronto, Ontario, June 1992.

29. Marks IM, Mathews AM. Brief standard self-rating for phobic patients. Behav Res Ther 1979; 17:263–267.

30. Mavissakalian M. The Fear Questionnaire: a validity study. Behav Res Ther 1986; 24:83–85.

31. Barlow DH, Wolfe BE. Behavioral approaches to anxiety disorders: a report on the NIMH-SUNY Albany Research Conference. J Clin Consult Psychol 1981; 49:448–454.

32. Michelson L, Mavissakalian M. Temporal stability of self-report measures in agoraphobia research. Behav Res Ther 1983; 21:695–698.

33. Mizes JS, Crawford J. Normative values on the Marks and Mathews fear questionnaire: a comparison as a function of age and sex. J Psychopathol Behav Assessment 1986; 8:253–262.

34. Oei TPS, Moylan A, Evans L. Validity and clinical utility of the Fear Questionnaire for anxiety disorder patients. Psycholog Assessment 1991; 3:391–397.

35. Chambless DL, Caputo GC, Jasin SE, Gracely EJ, Williams C. The Mobility Inventory for agoraphobia. Behav Res Ther 1985; 23:35–44.

36. deBeurs E, Lange A, Van Dyck R, Blonk RWB, Koele P. Behavioral assessment of avoidance in agoraphobia. J Psychopathol Behav Assessment 1991; 13:285–300.

37. Beck AT, Epstein N, Brown G, Steer RA. An inventory for measuring clinical anxiety: psychometric properties. J Consulting Clin Psychol 1988; 56:893–897.

38. Beck AT, Steer RA, Garbin MG. Psychometric properties of the Beck Depression Inventory: twenty-five years of evaluation. Clin Psychol Rev 1988; 8:77–100.

39. Hamilton M. The assessment of anxiety states by rating. Br J Med Psychol 1959; 32:50–55.

40. Riskind JH, Beck AT, Brown GB, Steer RA. Taking the measure of anxiety and depression: validity of reconstructed Hamilton scales. J Nerv Ment Dis 1987; 175:474–479.

41. Guy W, ed. ECDEU Assessment Manual for Psychopharmacology. Publication ADM 76–336. Rockville, MD: US Department of Health, Education and Welfare, 1976.

42. Otto MW, Pollack MH, Sabatino SA. Maintenance of remission following cognitive-behavior therapy for panic disorder: possible deleterious effects of concurrent medication treatment. Behav Ther 1996; 27:473–482.

43. Himadi WG, Boice R, Barlow DH. Assessment of agoraphobia. II. Measurement of clinical change. Behav Res Ther 1986; 24:321–332.

44. Barlow DH, O'Brien GT, Last CG. Couples treatment of agoraphobia. Behav Ther 1984; 15:41–58.

45. Barlow DH, Craske MG, Cerny JA, Klosko JS. Behavioral treatment of panic disorder. Behav Ther 1989; 20:261–282.

46. Michelson L, Mavissakalian M, Marchione K. Cognitive, behavioral, and psychophysiological treatments of agoraphobia: a comparative outcome investigation. Behav Ther 1988; 19:97–120.

47. Marchione KE, Michelson L, Greenwald M, Dancu C. Cognitive behavioral treatment of agoraphobia. Behav Res Ther 1987; 5:319–328.

48. Mavissakalian M, Michelson L. Self-directed in-vivo exposure practice in behavioral and pharmacological treatments of agoraphobia. Behav Ther 1983; 14:506–519.

49. Shear MK, Brown TA, Barlow DH, Money R, Sholomskas DE, Woods

SW, Gorman JM, Papp LA. Multicenter Collaborative Panic Disorder Severity Scale. Am J Psychiatry 1997; 154:1571–1575.

50. Goodman WK, Price LH, Rasmussen SA, Mazure C, Fleischmann RL, Hill CL, Heninger GR, Charney DS. The Yale-Brown Obsessive-Compulsive Scale. I. Development, use, and reliability. Arch Gen Psychiatry 1989; 46:1006–1011.

51. Penava SJ, Otto MW, Maki KM, Pollack MH. Rate of improvement during cognitive-behavioral group treatment for panic disorder. Behav Res Ther. In press.

52. Leon A, Shear MK, Portera L, Klerman GL. Assessing impairment in patients with panic disorder: the Sheehan Disability Scale. Soc Psychiatry Psychiatr Epidemiol 1992; 27:78–82.

53. Ware JE, Sherbourne CD. The MOS 36-Item Short-Form Health Survey (SF-36). I. Conceptual Framework and Item Selection. Med Care 1992; 30:473–483.

54. Candilis PJ, McLean RYS, Otto MW, Manfro GG, Worthington JJ, Penava SJ, Pollack MH. Quality of life in patients with panic disorder. Submitted.

55. Sherbourne CD, Wells KB, Judd LL. Functioning and well-being of patients with panic disorder. Am J Psychiatry 1996; 153:213–218.

56. Endicott J, Nee J, Harrison W, Blumenthal R. Quality of life enjoyment and satisfaction questionnaire: a new measure. Psychopharmacol Bull 1993; 29:321–326.

57. Wolkow R, Judd L, Rapaport M, Clary CM. Quality of life differences in sertraline and placebo responsive panic disorder patients. Presented at the 36th Annual Meeting of the American College of Neuropsychopharmacology (ACNP), Kamuela, Hawaii, 1997.

58. Beck AT, Ward CH, Mendelson M, Mock J, Erbaugh J. An inventory for measuring depression. Arch Gen Psychiatry 1961; 4:561–571.

59. Beck AT, Rush AJ, Shaw BF, Emery G. Cognitive Therapy of Depression. New York: Guilford Press, 1979.

60. Hamilton M. A rating scale for depression. J Neurol Neurosurg Psychiatry 1960; 23:56–62.

61. Hamilton M. Development of a rating scale for primary depressive illness. Br J Soc Clin Psychol 1967; 6:278–296.

62. Rehm LP, O Hara MW. Item characteristics of the Hamilton Rating Scale for Depression. J Psychiatr Res 1985; 19:31–41.

63. Knesevich JW, Biggs JT, Clayton PJ, Ziegler VE. Validity of the Hamilton Rating Scale for Depression. Br J Psychiatry 1977; 131:49–52.

64. Williams JBW. A structured interview guide for the Hamilton Depression Rating Scale. Arch Gen Psychiatry 1988; 45:742–747.

65. Derogatis LR, Lipman RS, Covi L. SCL-90: An outpatient psychiatric rating scale: preliminary report. Psychopharmacol Bull1973; 9:13–18.

66. Derogatis LR. SCL-90 administration, scoring, and procedures manual. I. Baltimore: Johns Hopkins University Press, 1977.

67. Uhde TW, Stein MB, Vittone BJ, Siever LJ, Boulenger JP, Klein E, Mellman TA. Behavioral and physiologic effects of short-term and long-term administration of clonidine in panic disorder. Arch Gen Psychiatry 1989; 46:170–177.

Index

ACQ, fears assessment, 327
Adjunctive cognitive-behavioral
    therapy (CBT), in preg-
    nancy, 237
Adjunctive lithium, 166
Affectionate constraint, 124
Affectionless control, 124
Agoraphobia, 11, 13, 41, 94, 95,
    118
  cognitive-behavioral therapy
    (CBT) and pharmacother-
    apy, 171
  onset, 105
Agoraphobia Cognitions Question-
    naire (ACQ), 327
Agoraphobic avoidance assess-
    ment, 327–328
Agoraphobic situations, avoidance
    of, 182
Alcohol abuse, 15

Alcohol-causes-panic hypothesis,
    substance use disorders and
    PD, 258
Alcohol dependence vs. PD, 255–
    256
Alcoholics, 252–254
  benzodiazepines (BZDs) and,
    263
Alcoholism, depression and, 103
Alprazolam, 14, 21, 162–165, 210
  behavior therapy, 40
  Cross National Collaborative
    Panic Study, 39
  neurochemical abnormalities,
    62, 63
  PD and comorbid depression, 44
  prenatal exposure, 235
  quality-of-life studies, 309–310
American Psychiatric Association
    treatment module, 20

Amitriptyline, pregnancy and, 238
Antecedents, 93–135
Anticipatory anxiety, 45
Antidepressants, 39, 45, 155–161,
    166
  benzodiazepines (BZDs), 171
  discontinuation studies, 42
  pregnancy, 230
  relapse, 44
  selective serotonin-reuptake in-
    hibitors (SSRIs), 155–159
Antipanic medications
  recommended doses, 167t
  reproductive safety, 233–236
Antipanic treatment, medical condi-
    tions, 168
Anxiety assessment, 328–329
Anxiety difficulties, 46
Anxiety disorders
  behavioral inhibition, 112t–113t
  women, 229–230
Anxiety-management skills, 188–
    189
Anxiety neurosis, 38
Anxiety patients
  follow-up, 38
  follow-up studies, 38
Anxiety proneness, 105–106
Anxiety sensitivity, 117–119, 185
Anxiety Sensitivity Index (ASI)
  factors, 117–118
  fears assessment, 326–327
Anxiety state, 38
Anxiogenic effect, benzodiaze-
    pines (BZDs), 218
Anxiogenic health habits, 212
Arrhythmias, 9–10
ASI
  factors, 117–118
  fears assessment, 326–327

Assessments, diagnostic and symp-
    tom, 323–335
Asthma, 13
Atenolol, 165
Autonomic Nervous System Ques-
    tionnaire (ANS), 325
Avoidant coping strategies, 128

Beck Anxiety Inventory (BAI),
    328–329
Beck Depression Inventory (BDI),
    334
Behavioral Avoidance Tests
    (BATs), 328
Behavioral experiments, 187–188
Behavioral inhibitions, 48
  anxiety disorders, 112t–113t
  genetic contributions, 108
Behavioral inhibitor experience,
    122–123
Behavioral patterns, 120–121
Behavioral tendencies, 120
Behavior therapy, 40
Benzodiazepines (BZDs), 21, 62,
    72, 154, 157t, 162–166
  abuse-prone individuals, 262–
    263
  alcoholics, 263
  antidepressants, 171
  anxiogenic effect, 218
  discontinuation, 169
  neonatal toxicity, 234–235
  pregnancy, 230, 237
  prenatal exposure, 234, 235
  receptors, 64, 65, 66
  treatment resistance, 219, 220, 221
Beta-blockers, 165, 209
Bodily sensations
  interoceptive exposure, 187
  misinterpretation, 185, 187

Bodily symptoms and panic provocation, 186
Body Sensations Questionnaire (BSQ), for fears assessment, 327
Brain-electrical activity mapping (BEAM), for substance abuse/dependence and PD, 260
Brain regions implicated in PD, 74
Breastfeeding, psychotropic medications and, 238–239
Bupropion, 209
Buspirone, 165, 209
BZD/GABA dysfunction, clinical relevance, implications, and treatment, 64–66

Caffeine, 60
  anxiety production, 168
Calcium channel blocker, treatment resistance, 220
Candidate genes, 101
Carbamazepine, 209
Cardiology patients, 7
Cardiovascular physiology, clinical relevance and implications, 73–74
Cardiovascular risk factors, 10
Cardiovascular symptoms, 6–10
  quality-of-life studies, 277, 290
CASI, 118–119
Catecholamines, 116
CCK, clinical relevance, implications, and treatment, 66–68
Cerebrospinal fluid, alcoholics and PD, 259
Cerebrovascular disease, 11
CGIS scores, 163–164
Chest pains, 6

Childhood anxiety disorders, 104–107
  clinical implications, 134–135
  and parental behavior, 124–129
  physiological differences, 116–117
  precursors, 104–107
  temperament, 107–116
  temperamental behavioral inhibition, 111
Childrens Anxiety Sensitivity Index (CASI), 118–119
Choking symptoms, 13
Cholecystokinin (CCK), clinical relevance, implications, and treatment, 66–68
Chronic obstructive pulmonary disease (COPD), 14
Clinical Global Impression Improvement and Severity Scales, 158
Clinical Global Impression-Severity (CGI-S)
  global ratings, 329–330
  scores, 163–164, 166
Clinical neurophysiology, relevance and implications, 70–74
Clinician Global Impression of Improvement (CGI-I), global ratings, 330–331
Clomipramine, 160
  vs. paroxetine, 155, 158
Clonazepam, 21, 39, 162–165
  prenatal exposure, 235
  quality-of-life studies, 309–310
  valproate, 221
Clonidine, 166
  growth hormone (GH), 59, 60
Cocaine and anxiety production, 168

Cognitive-behavioral interventions, 37, 39, 41–42 (*see also* Cognitive-behavioral therapy)
Cognitive-behavioral model, 183–186, 184f
Cognitive-behavioral therapy (CBT), 14, 154, 181–196
  agoraphobia, 171
  applications, 193–194
  components, 186–189
  discontinuation process, 169
  follow-up, 41–43
  medications, 192
    imipramine, 189
    selective serotonin-reuptake inhibitors (SSRIs), 189
    tolerance, 214
  neurochemical abnormalities, 60, 63
  treatment considerations, 186–189
  treatment-outcome findings, 189–192
  pharmacological alternatives, 189
  pregnancy, 237
  psychopharmacologists, 194–196
  quality-of-life studies, 310–311
Cognitive distortions, 119–120
Cognitive factors, aggravated, 212
Cognitive interventions, exposure, 187
Cognitive restructuring, 187
Cognitive vulnerability factors, 117–121
Combination treatments, 169–171, 191–192, 219t, 221

CO_2 metabolism, clinical relevance, implications, and treatment, 62–64
Community studies of PD prevalence, 274t–275t
Comorbid depression, 44
Comorbidity contributions, 216
Complex partial seizure disorder, 208
Composite measures, 332–333
Conduct-disordered, 128
Congenital malformations, 235, 236
COPD, 14
Corticotropin-releasing factor (CRF), 68
Cortisol, salivary, 109
Cost-effectiveness of untreated *vs.* treated, 300–308
Cost issues, 3
CRF, 68
Cross National Collaborative Panic Study, 162–163
  alprazolam and imipramine, 39

Depakote, treatment resistance, 220
Depression
  alcoholism and, 103
  assessment, 334–335
Desipramine, 160
Developmental model, 45–47
Diagnosis, 4–17
  assessment, 323–335
  goal, 323–324
  tools, 324
Diagnostic Interview Survey (DIS), quality-of-life, 271
Diathesis model, 45

Diazepam, 39, 162, 164
  prenatal exposure, 235
Differential diagnosis, 16–17
DIS, quality-of-life, 271
Discontinuation process
  benzodiazepines (BZDs), 169
  cognitive-behavioral therapy
    (CBT), 169
Discontinuation studies, pharmaco-
    therapy, 42–43
Dizziness, 11
Drug treatment, 156t–157t
DSM drift, 248
Dyspnea, 13

Early antecedents, 93–135
ECA study, 6
  panic/anxiety/substance use dis-
    orders, 249–250
  quality of life, 273
EEGs
  abnormalities, 71
  clinical relevance and implica-
    tions, 71–73
EKG monitoring study, 73
Electrical stimulation, LC, 58
Emergency rooms, 5–6
Emotional overinvolvement, 126
Environmental factors, 46, 121–
    133
Environmental stressors, 109
Epidemiological studies, 153,
    294t–298t
Epidemiologic Catchment Area
    (ECA) study, 6
  panic/anxiety/substance use dis-
    orders, 249–250
  quality of life, 273
Escape behaviors, 183

Etiology, 207–208
  model, 133–134, 183–184
Etiopathological interest in sub-
    stance use disorders and
    PD, 259
Exogenous factors, 215–216
Exposure interventions, cognitive,
    187
Expressed emotion, 126

Family studies, 46, 48, 95–100
Fear and alarm mechanisms, 66–
    68, 70–71, 154
Fear behaviors, 68
Fear Questionnaire (FQ), agorapho-
    bic avoidance assessment,
    327–328
Fears, role of, 183
Fears assessment
  Agoraphobia Cognitions Ques-
    tionnaire (ACQ), 327
  Anxiety Sensitivity Index (ASI),
    326–327
  Panic Beliefs Questionnaire
    (PBQ), 327
Fight-or-flight alarm reaction, ini-
    tial panic, 183
Fluoxetine, 159
  exposed children, 235
  in pregnancy, 237, 238
Fluvoxamine, 159
  prenatal exposure, 236
Follow-up
  of anxiety patients, 38
  of cognitive-behavioral therapy
    patients, 41–42
  studies, 38–41
Functional impairment assessment,
    333–334

GABA-BZD complex, treatment resistance, 220
GABA neuronal system, 64, 65, 66
Gabapentin, 166
Gamma-aminobutyric acid (GABA)
    neuronal system, 64, 65, 66
    panic/anxiety/alcohol intermix, 259
Gastrointestinal (GI) symptoms, 13
    quality-of-life studies, 290–291
Generalized anxiety assessment, 328–329
General medicine, 1–21
Genetic epidemiology, 104t
Genetics, 94–104
    behavioral inhibitions, 108
    substance use disorders and PD, 259–260
Genome scans, 101
GH
    clonidine, 59, 60
    responses, 69
GI symptoms, 13
    quality-of-life studies, 290–291
Global measures, 329–332
Gradual taper, 42
Growth hormone (GH)
    clonidine, 59, 60
    responses, 69

Half-life agents, 42
HAM-A for anxiety assessment, 329
HAM-D for depression assessment, 334
Hamilton Rating Scale for Anxiety (HRSA or HAM-A), 329
Hamilton Rating Scale for Depression (HRSD or HAM-D), 334
HARP study, 43
Harvard Anxiety Research Program (HARP) study, 43
Harvard-Brown Anxiety Disorders Project, substance abuse/dependence and PD, 261
Headache, 10–11
Hepatic 2D6 microsomal enzyme system, 220
Hidden psychiatric morbidity, 2
Holter monitoring, 8
Hopkins Symptom Checklist (SCL-90) for depression assessment, 335
HPA-axis dysregulation, clinical relevance, implications, and treatment, 68–70
HRSA for anxiety assessment, 329
HRSD for depression assessment, 334
5-HT dysfunction, clinical relevance, implications, and treatment, 61–62
5-HT1A receptor agonists flesinoxan, 165
Hypercortisolemia, in developing brain, 236
Hypertension, 9
Hyperthyroidism, 208
Hyperventilation syndrome, 12
Hypothalamic-pituitary-adrenal (HPA) axis, clinical relevance, implications, and treatment, 68–70

Iatrogenic anxiety, 217–218
IBS, 13

Imipramine, 39–43, 63, 160, 161, 164, 210
  cognitive-behavioral therapy (CBT), 189
  Cross National Collaborative Panic Study, 39
  discontinuation, 42
  pregnancy, 238
  quality-of-life-studies, 309–310
  substance abuse/dependence and PD, 262
Inheritance, of neurochemistry, 109
Initial panic, fight-or-flight alarm reaction, 183
International Classification of Diseases (ICD-10), and quality of life, 272
Interoceptive exposure, 188
  bodily sensations, 187
Ipsapirone, 165
Irritable bowel syndrome (IBS), 13

Lactate and panic, clinical relevance, implications, and treatment, 62–64
Late luteal phase dysphoric disorder (LLPDD), 15–16
LC, 58, 59, 60
Life stressors, 129–133
Lithium, 166
  augmentation, 221
LLPDD, 15–16
Locus ceruleus (LC), 58, 59, 60
Longitudinal course, 37–50
Lorazepam, 162

Magnetic resonance spectroscopy (MRS) techniques, 66
Maintenance model, 183–184

Maintenance treatment, 45, 169
Managed care, role of in PD, 312–314
Management, primary care steps in, 19
MAO, 116
MAOIs, 21, 38, 154–156, 161
  neurochemical abnormalities, 60
  pregnancy, 238
  prenatal exposure, 236
  substance abuse/dependence and PD, 263
  treatment adequacy, 209
  treatment resistance, 219, 219t, 220, 221
Maprotiline, 160
Marijuana, and anxiety production, 168
Massachusetts General Hospital Longitudinal Study of Panic Disorder, 43, 49
MCPAS, 158
MCS, quality-of-life, 271
Medical conditions
  antipanic treatment and, 168
  PD resemblance to, 17t
Medical history, 17
Medical model, 154
Medical Outcome Study Short Form-36 (SF-36) for functional impairment assessment, 333–334
Medical work-up, 17–18
Medication
  anxiety production and, 168
  cognitive-behavioral therapy (CBT) and, 192
  intolerance, 213
  and psychotherapy, quality-of-life-studies, 311–312

[Medication]
quality-of-life-studies, 309–310
resistance to, 219–221
tolerance, cognitive-behavioral
therapy (CBT) and, 214
trial, 213
Mendelian inheritance patterns,
101
Meniere's syndrome, 12
Mental Component Scale (MCS),
quality-of-life, 271
Metabolite 3-methoxy-4-hydrox-
phenethyleneglycol
(MHPG), 59, 60, 109
MI, agoraphobic avoidance assessment, 328
Mitral valve prolapse (MVP), 8–9,
116
Mobility Inventory (MI) for agoraphobic avoidance assess-
ment, 328
Molecular-genetic analyses, 100–
104
Molecular genetics, 57
Monoamine oxidase inhibitors
(MAOIs), 21, 38, 154–156,
161
neurochemical abnormalities, 60
pregnancy, 238
prenatal exposure, 236
resistance to, 219, 219t, 220,
221
substance abuse/dependence and
PD, 263
treatment adequacy, 209
MRI abnormalities, 71
MRS techniques, 66
Multicenter Panic Anxiety Scale
(MCPAS), 158

Multiple medical causes, 207
MVP, 8–9, 116

Nadolol, 165
National Comorbidity Survey
(NCS) for panic/anxiety/
substance use disorders,
250–252
NCS for panic/anxiety/substance
use disorders, 250–252
Nefazodone, 209
Neonatal toxicity
benzodiazepines (BZDs), 234–
235
data, 236
NE system, 58–61
Neurobehavioral consequences of
prenatal exposure, 235–236
Neurobiology of panic disorder,
57–78
Neurochemical abnormalities, 58–
70
Neurochemistry, inheritance of, 109
Neuroimaging, 57, 74, 76t–78t
Neurological symptoms, 10–12
quality-of-life-studies, 291–292
Neurotic disorders, 114
N-methyl-D-aspartate (NMDA), 70
Non-alcoholic substance use disor-
ders, 260–261
Noradrenergic dysfunction, clinical
relevance, implications, and
treatment, 58–61
Norepinephrine (NE), panic/
anxiety/alcohol intermix,
259
Norepinephrine (NE) system, 58–
61
Nortriptyline, 160

Obsessive-compulsive disorder
(OCD), 105
Onset factors, 46
Oral cleft risk, benzodiazepines
(BZDs) and, 237–238
Overanxious disorder, 105
Overprotectiveness, 126

Palpitations, 6, 8
Panic attacks
clinical and nonclinical pan-
ickers, 182–183
phobic responses, 183
vs. PD, 18
Panic Beliefs Questionnaire
(PBQ) for fears assessment,
327
Panic Disorder Severity Scale
(PDSS), composite assess-
ment, 332–333
Panic frequency assessment, 325–
326
Panic provocation, bodily symp-
toms of, 186
Panic-related fears assessment,
326–327
Parental behavior and child anxi-
ety, 124–129
Parental control, 127
Parental influences, 121–129
Parental overprotection, 124
Parental restrictiveness, 127
Parent–child experiences, 123
Parenting styles, 47
Paroxetine, 210
vs. clomipramine, 155, 158
prenatal exposure, 236
Paroxysmal supraventricular tachy-
cardia (PSVT), 9

Pathological anxiety
animal models, 47
treatment and development, 47–
50
Patient Global Evaluation rating, 158
Patient Global Impression (PGI)
scores, global ratings, 331–
332
PBQ for fears assessment, 327
PCS for quality-of-life, 271
PDSS for composite assessment,
332–333
PFTs, 14–15
PGI scores, global ratings, 331–332
Pharmacotherapy, 37, 153–171
CBT, 189
agoraphobia, 171
choices, 308–312
pregnancy, 237
puerperium, 234
Phenelzine, 63, 161
prenatal exposure, 236
quality-of-life-studies, 309–310
Pheochromocytoma, 9
Phobic anxiety syndrome, 262
Phobic avoidance, 44–45
Phobic responses in panic attacks,
183
Physical Component Scale (PCS)
for quality of life, 271
Physiological differences, child-
hood precursors, 116–117
Platelet monoamine oxidase
(MAO), 116
PMS, 15–16
Postpartum period
definition, 229
exacerbation of PD in, 232
studies, 232–233

Posttraumatic stress disorder
    (PTSD), 16, 69, 70, 71,
    118
Power-assertive, 126
Pregnancy (*see also* Prenatal expo-
    sure)
    amitriptyline, 238
    antidepressants, 230
    antidepressants and benzodiaze-
        pines (BZDs), 230
    anxiety about fetal outcome,
        237
    benzodiazepines (BZDs), 237
    cognitive-behavioral therapy
        (CBT), 237
    definition, 229
    fluoxetine, 237, 238
    imipramine, 238
    monoamine oxidase inhibitors
        (MAOIs), 238
    pharmacotherapy discontinua-
        tion, 237
    studies, 230–231
    tricyclic antidepressants (TCAs),
        235, 237, 238
Premenstrual syndrome (PMS),
    15–16
Prenatal exposure
    benzodiazepines (BZDs), 234,
        235
    monoamine oxidase inhibitors
        (MAOIs), 236
    psychotropic agents, 236–239
    psychotropic medications, 233,
        234
    selective serotonin-reuptake in-
        hibitors (SSRIs), 236
Prevalence, 153, 272–273
Prevalence and social morbidity
    studies, 294t–298t

Primary care, 1–21
    patients, symptoms list for, 4–5
    samples in quality-of-life-stud-
        ies, 292–293
    screening, 324–325
Primary Care Evaluation of Men-
    tal Disorders (Prime-MD)
    screening instrument, 324–
    325
Prime-MD screening instrument,
    324–325
Propranolol, 165
Proximate triggering events, 130
PSVT, 9
Psychiatric history, importance of,
    17
Psychogenic dizziness, 12
Psychopharmacologists and cogni-
    tive-behavioral therapy
    (CBT), 194–196
Psychotherapy
    choices, 308–312
    quality-of-life-studies, 310–311
    medication, 311–312
    trial, 210
Psychotropic medications
    breastfeeding, 238–239
    prenatal exposure, 233, 234
    risks, 236–239
PTSD, 16, 69, 70, 71, 118
Puerperium, pharmacological treat-
    ment in, 234
Pulmonary functioning tests
    (PFTs), 14–15

Quality of life
    assessment, 333–334
    characteristics, 271
    community, 273, 276
    measures, 270–272

[Quality of life]
  studies
    cardiac symptoms, 277, 290
    cost and treatment effective-
      ness, 302t–307t
    gastrointestinal symptoms,
      290–291
    medication, 309–310
    neurological symptoms, 291–
      292
    nonpsychiatric populations,
      276–293
    primary care samples, 292–293
    psychotherapy, 310–311
    psychotherapy and medica-
      tion, 311–312
    treatment-seeking popula-
      tions, 293–300
Quality of Life Enjoyment and Satisfaction Questionnaire
  (Q-LES-Q), 334

Recognition, steps for increasing,
  3–4
Relapse, 40, 41, 42, 45, 166, 168
Relapse predictors, 192–193
Relapse risk in pregnancy, 239–240
REM latency, 72
Reproductive physiology, 232
Reproductive safety of antipanic
  medications, 233–236
Respiratory symptoms, 13–15
Response predictors, 192–193
Risk factors, 133–134
Risk indicators, 132t–133t

Safety behaviors, 183
Salivary cortisol, 109
School-phobic youngsters, 126
Screening, primary care, 324–325

SDDS-PC, screening instrument, 325
Self-medication hypothesis
  substance abuse/dependence and
    PD, 261
  substance use disorders and PD,
    257–258
Selective serotonin-reuptake inhibitors (SSRIs), 21, 154–159
  cognitive-behavioral therapy
    (CBT), 189
  follow-up studies, 38, 40, 43
  intolerance, 214
  neurochemical abnormalities, 62
  prenatal exposure, 236
  relapse and, 44
  resistance to, 219, 220
  substance abuse/dependence and
    PD, 263
  treatment adequacy, 208–210
Sertraline, 158–159
  prenatal exposure, 236
SF-36
  functional impairment assess-
    ment, 333–334
  quality of life, 271
Sheehan Disability Scale for functional impairment assessment, 333
Short-form Health Survey (SF-36)
  for quality-of-life, 271
Single-photon emission computed
  tomography (SPECT) neu-
  roreceptor imagining techniques, 65–66
Sinus tachycardia, 9
Sleep panic, 72–73
Smothering symptoms, 13
Social morbidity and prevalence
  studies, 294t–298t
Social phobia, 105

Sodium valproate, 209
SPECT nueroreceptor imagining
    techniques, 65–66
SSRIs (see Selective Serotonin-
    Reuptake Inhibitors)
Startle Studies, clinical relevance
    and implications, 70–71
Statistics on primary care and PD,
    1–2
Stepwise exposure, 195
Stress response
  NE system, 58
Substance abuse, 15
Substance use disorders
  comorbidity with PD, 257–259
  panic and anxiety disorders,
    247–252
  and PD patients, 254–255
Substance use disorders and PD
  alcohol-causes-panic hypothesis,
    258
  coexistence, 256
  epidemiological studies, 264
  etiopathological interest, 259
  genetic link, 259–260
  self-medication hypothesis,
    257–258
  treatment, 261–264
Susceptibility genes, mapping dif-
    ficulty, 101
Sustaining treatment response,
    168–169
Symptom assessment, 323–335
Symptom Driven Diagnostic
    Screen-Primary Care
    (SDDS-PC) screening in-
    strument, 325
Symptoms, 4–17
Syncopal symptoms, 72
Syncope, 12

Tachycardia, 6, 9
TCAs (*see* Tricyclic antidepres-
    sants)
Temperament, childhood precur-
    sors, 107–116
Temperamental behavioral inhibi-
    tion and childhood anxiety
    disorders, 111
Tertiary amines in pregnancy,
    238
Tranylcypromine, 161
  prenatal exposure, 236
Traumatic events, 129–133
Trazodone, 209
Treatment, 19–21
  adequacy studies, 208–211
    trials, factors in, 209
  choices, 308–312
  cognitive-behavioral therapy
    (CBT), 186–189
  effectiveness, untreated vs.
    treated, 300–308
  failure, reasons for, 208
  focused, 154
  follow-up, 38–41
  intolerance, studies of, 211–215
  in pregnancy and planning,
    236–239
  psychopharmacological, 21
  refractoriness
    definition, 206
    determinants, 207–218
    prevalence, 206–207
  resistance
    factors, 215–218
    medication approaches, 219–
      221
    misnomer, 205
  substance use disorders and PD,
    261–264

Treatment-outcome findings in cognitive-behavioral therapy (CBT), 189–192
Treatment-resistant panic disorder, clinical approach, 205–221
Treatment-seeking populations, quality-of-life-studies in, 293–300
Triazolobenzodiazepine, 162
Tricyclic antidepressants (TCAs), 10, 21, 154–156, 160–161
  follow-up studies, 38, 39, 40, 44
  intolerance, 214
  neurochemical abnormalities, 60, 62
  pregnancy, 235, 237, 238
  resistance to, 219, 221
  substance abuse/dependence and PD, 263
  treatment adequacy, 209, 210
Triggering events, 130
Triple therapy, 221
Twin studies, 46, 95–100

Underrecognition, 2–3
Unimodal treatment, 216–217

Valproate, 166
  and clonazepam, 221
Valproic acid, 72
  resistance to, 220
Venlafaxine, 165, 209
Verapamil, treatment resistance to, 220
Vestibular abnormalities, 11–12
Vestibular dysfunction, 12
Vestibular neuritis, 12
Virginia Twin Registry, 99
Vulnerability factors, 117–121

Work Productivity Impairment (WPI) questionnaire for quality-of-life, 271
World Health Organization (WHO)
  primary care study, 18
  quality of life, 271–272

About the Editors

Jerrold F. Rosenbaum is the Director of Outpatient Psychiatry and the Chief of the Clinical Psychopharmacology Unit at Massachusetts General Hospital, as well as an Associate Professor of Psychiatry at Harvard Medical School, Boston, Massachusetts. The author or coauthor of more than 200 journal articles and the editor or coeditor of seven books, he is a Fellow of the American Psychiatric Association, a founding and board member of the American Society of Clinical Psychopharmacology, and a member of the Society of Biological Psychiatry, the American College of Psychiatrists, and the American College of Neuropsychopharmacology, among others. Dr. Rosenbaum received the B.A. degree (1969) from Yale College and the M.D. degree (1973) from the Yale University School of Medicine.

Mark H. Pollack is the Director of the Anxiety Disorders Program at the Massachusetts General Hospital and an Associate Professor of Psychiatry at Harvard Medical School, Boston, Massachusetts. He is the coeditor of the book *Challenges in Clinical Practice: Pharmacologic and Psychosocial Strategies* and ''Progress Notes'' of the American Society of Clinical Psychopharmacology, as well as the author or coauthor of more than 100 journal articles, reviews, book chapters, and abstracts. A recipient of a career development award from the National Institute of Mental Health to study the longitudinal course of panic disorder, Dr. Pollack serves on the scientific advisory board of the Anxiety Disorders Association and is a fellow of the American Psychiatric Association. Dr. Pollack received the B.A. degree (1978) from the University of Virginia and the M.D. degree (1982) from the New Jersey Medical School.